Before We Are Born

Essentials of Embryology and Birth Defects

Fourth Edition

Before We Are Born

Essentials of Embryology and Birth Defects

KEITH L. MOORE, B.A., M.Sc., Ph.D., F.I.A.C., F.R.S.M.

Professor of Anatomy and Cell Biology
Faculty of Medicine, University of Toronto
Toronto, Ontario, Canada

Visiting Professor of Clinical Anatomy
Department of Anatomy, Faculty of Medicine
University of Manitoba
Winnipeg, Manitoba, Canada

T.V.N. PERSAUD, M.D., Ph.D., D.Sc., F.R.C.Path. (Lond.)

Professor and Head, Department of Anatomy
Professor of Pediatrics and Child Health
Associate Professor of Obstetrics, Gynecology and
  Reproductive Sciences
University of Manitoba, Faculties of Medicine and Dentistry

Consultant in Pathology and Clinical Genetics
Health Sciences Centre
Winnipeg, Manitoba, Canada

W. B. SAUNDERS COMPANY *Philadelphia/London/Toronto/Montreal/Sydney/Tokyo*
A Division of Harcourt Brace & Company

W. B. SAUNDERS COMPANY
A Division of Harcourt Brace & Company

The Curtis Center
Independence Square West
Philadelphia, PA 19106

Library of Congress Cataloging-in-Publication Data

Moore, Keith L.
    Before we are born : essentials of embryology and birth defects / Keith L.
Moore, T.V.N. Persaud. — 4th ed.
      p. cm.
    Includes bibliographical references and index.
    ISBN 0-7216-4665-4
    1. Embryology, Human. I. Persaud, T. V. N. II. Title.
    [DNLM: 1. Anomalies. 2. Embryology. QS 604 M822b 1993]
    QM601.M757 1993
    612.6′4—dc20
    DNLM/DLC
                                             92-48476

Front cover: Photograph of a human embryo of about 56 days. Courtesy of Dr. Kazumasa Hoshino, former Professor of Anatomy and Director of Congenital Anomaly Center, Faculty of Medicine, Kyoto University, Kyoto, Japan.

Before We Are Born   ISBN 0–7216–4665–4

Printed in the United States of America.

Last digit is the print number: 9   8   7   6   5   4   3   2

*To our wives, children and
grandchildren*

PREFACE

This fourth edition welcomes *Dr. T.V.N. (Vid) Persaud,* Professor and Head of the Department of Anatomy at the University of Manitoba with whom I have worked for many years. He is also Professor of Pediatrics and Child Health and Associate Professor of Obstetrics, Gynecology and Reproductive Sciences. An award-winning teacher of embryology and gross anatomy, Dr. Persaud is conducting modern research in embryology and teratology. The current edition of this book will reflect his basic and clinical knowledge, and his vigour.

This synoptic volume of human embryology presents the basic facts and concepts of normal and abnormal development that are essential for students of medicine and the associated health sciences. This book is a digest of *The Developing Human. Clinically Oriented Embryology,* 5th edition. Persons wishing more information about any of the subjects therefore should refer to our more comprehensive text also published by W.B. Saunders.

An important part of this book are the *Commonly Asked Questions* which appear at the end of each chapter. Over the years we have been asked these and other questions by students, colleagues, physicians, and lay people. Because of misconceptions derived from newspaper articles and discussions on television and radio, we have done our best to give answers that are supported by current research and medical practice. In this edition there are many more references and suggestions for reading about current research on human development and treatment of congenital anomalies.

The chapters are organized so they present a systematic and logical approach that explains how an embryo and fetus develop. In addition to being updated, the material has been modified to include more material that is useful in clinical practice. This material will be helpful to those taking courses involving problem-solving. Several new illustrations and ultrasound images have been prepared for this edition. We have also included some scanning electron micrographs of the developing human embryo. The original illustrations were prepared mainly by Mr. Glen Reid in the Faculty of Medicine of the University of Manitoba. Others were prepared by Angela Cluer and David Mazierski in the Instructional Media Services at the University of Toronto. All new illustrations were prepared by Sari O'Sullivan of Toronto. We are indebted to all these artists for their skill in presenting difficult concepts in an understandable way. Illustrations prepared by other persons and from other books have also been used through the courtesy of the authors and publishers. We are very grateful to them for permitting us to use their work.

Many of our colleagues helped with the preparation of this edition; it is our pleasure to acknowledge their help. Professor Anne Agur, Associate Professor of Anatomy and Cell Biology, University of Toronto, Toronto, Ontario; Dr. Margaret W. Thompson, Professor

Emeritus, Department of Molecular and Medical Genetics, University of Toronto, Toronto, Ontario; Dr. Raymond Gasser, Department of Anatomy, Louisiana State University, School of Medicine, New Orleans; Dr. A.E. Chudley, Professor of Pediatrics and Child Health, Director of Clinical Genetics, Health Sciences Centre, University of Manitoba, Winnipeg, Manitoba; Dr. E.A. Lyons, Professor of Radiology and Obstetrics and Gynecology and Head of the Department of Radiology, Health Sciences Centre, University of Manitoba, Winnipeg, Manitoba. Those who have contributed photographs are individually acknowledged in the figure legends. Barbara Clune in Winnipeg, and Marion Moore in Toronto, did all the wordprocessing and helped with the review of the manuscript. Lawrence McGrew, Medical Editor, W.B. Saunders Company and his colleagues have been most helpful with our work. To all these people, we extend our sincere thanks. Last, but not least, we thank our wives, Marion and Gisela for their tolerance and support.

KEITH L. MOORE
T.V.N. PERSAUD

CONTENTS

1

INTRODUCTION TO EMBRYOLOGY. 1

Stages of Human Development 1
Importance of Embryology. 6
Historical Highlights 7
Descriptive Terms 10
Commonly Asked Questions 10

2

HUMAN REPRODUCTION 11

The Reproductive Organs. 11
Gametogenesis. 14
The Gametes. 15
Female Reproductive Cycles 19
Transportation of Gametes. 23
Viability of Gametes. 24
Summary 24
Commonly Asked Questions 24

3

THE FIRST WEEK OF HUMAN DEVELOPMENT. 26

The Beginning of Human Development. 26
Cleavage of the Zygote 31
Summary 32
Commonly Asked Questions 32

4

THE SECOND WEEK OF HUMAN DEVELOPMENT 35

Formation of the Bilaminar Embryonic Disc. 35
Completion of Implantation and Early Embryonic Development 35
Implantation Sites of the Blastocyst 39
Spontaneous Abortion of Early Embryos. 43
Summary 43
Commonly Asked Questions 44

5

THE THIRD WEEK OF HUMAN DEVELOPMENT 45

Formation of the Trilaminar Embryo 45
Gastrulation: Formation of the Germ Layers 45
Neurulation 49
The Allantois 51
Development of Somites 51
Development of the Intraembryonic Coelom 53
Development of the Primitive Cardiovascular System 54
Development of Chorionic Villi 55
Summary 57
Commonly Asked Questions 58

6

THE FOURTH TO EIGHTH WEEKS OF HUMAN DEVELOPMENT 59

Development of Tissues, Organs, and Body Form 59
Phases of Development 59
Folding of the Embryo 59
Germ Layer Derivatives 61
Control of Embryonic Development 61
Highlights of the Fourth to Eighth Weeks 63
Estimation of Embryonic Age 69
Summary 76
Commonly Asked Questions 76

7

THE NINTH TO THIRTY-EIGHTH WEEKS OF HUMAN DEVELOPMENT 78

The Fetal Period 78
Estimation of Fetal Age 78
Highlights of the Fetal Period 80
Factors Influencing Fetal Growth 85
Perinatology 88
Summary 92
Commonly Asked Questions 92

8

THE PLACENTA AND FETAL MEMBRANES 94

The Placenta 94
Uterine Growth During Pregnancy 103
Parturition (Childbirth) 104
The Placenta, Umbilical Cord, and Fetal Membranes After Birth 106
The Yolk Sac 110
The Allantois 111
Twin and Other Multiple Pregnancies 111
Summary 116
Commonly Asked Questions 116

9

HUMAN BIRTH DEFECTS AND THEIR CAUSES 118

Anomalies Caused by Genetic Factors. 119
Anomalies Caused by Environmental Factors 128
Anomalies Caused by Multifactorial Inheritance. 139
Summary 140
Commonly Asked Questions. 140

10

BODY CAVITIES, PRIMITIVE MESENTERIES, AND THE DIAPHRAGM. 142

The Embryonic Body Cavity 142
Development of the Diaphragm. 148
Summary 150
Commonly Asked Questions. 151

11

THE BRANCHIAL OR PHARYNGEAL APPARATUS. 152

The Branchial (Pharyngeal) Arches. 152
The Pharyngeal Pouches. 159
The Branchial (Pharyngeal) Grooves. 159
The Branchial (Pharyngeal) Membranes. 159
Branchial (Pharyngeal) Anomalies 161
Development of the Thyroid Gland 161
Development of the Tongue 165
Development of Salivary Glands 167
Development of the Face. 168
Development of Nasal Cavities 169
Development of the Palate 169
Summary 177
Commonly Asked Questions. 178

12

THE RESPIRATORY SYSTEM. 180

Development of the Larynx 181
Development of the Trachea 181
Development of Bronchi and Lungs. 182
Summary 185
Commonly Asked Questions. 186

13

THE DIGESTIVE SYSTEM. 188

The Foregut. 188
The Midgut 193
The Hindgut 198
Summary 201
Commonly Asked Questions. 202

14

THE UROGENITAL SYSTEM 204

The Urinary System 204
The Suprarenal Glands 212
The Genital System 213
Summary 224
Commonly Asked Questions 225

15

THE CARDIOVASCULAR SYSTEM 227

Early Heart Development 227
The Primitive Circulation 231
Completion of Heart Development 231
Congenital Anomalies of the Heart and Great Vessels 237
The Aortic Arches 242
The Fetal Circulation 246
The Postnatal Circulation 249
Summary 249
Commonly Asked Questions 250

16

THE MUSCULOSKELETAL SYSTEM 252

Development of Bone and Cartilage 252
Development of Joints 255
Development of the Vertebral Column 255
Development of Ribs 259
Development of the Skull 260
Limb Development 263
Limb Defects 267
The Muscular System 271
Summary 273
Commonly Asked Questions 273

17

THE NERVOUS SYSTEM 275

Development of the Spinal Cord 275
Development of the Brain 286
The Peripheral Nervous System 298
Summary 298
Commonly Asked Questions 299

18

THE EYE AND EAR 301

The Eye 301
The Ear 308
Summary 313
Commonly Asked Questions 313

19

THE SKIN, CUTANEOUS APPENDAGES, AND TEETH 315

Skin 315
Hair 316
Sebaceous Glands 317
Sweat Glands 317
Nails.. 318
Mammary Glands 318
Teeth... 320
Summary 324
Commonly Asked Questions.. 324

ANSWERS TO COMMONLY ASKED QUESTIONS 326

INDEX... 339

1

INTRODUCTION TO EMBRYOLOGY

Human development begins when an oocyte (ovum) from a female is fertilized by a sperm (spermatozoon) from a male. Development involves many changes that transform a single cell, the **zygote** (fertilized ovum), into a multicellular human being. Most developmental changes occur before birth, (i.e., during the embryonic and early fetal periods), but important changes also occur during later periods of development: the perinatal period, infancy, childhood, adolescence, and adulthood.

Human embryology is the science concerned with the origin and development of a human being from a zygote to the birth of an infant.

STAGES OF HUMAN DEVELOPMENT

Development can be divided into *prenatal* (before birth) and *postnatal* (after birth) periods, but it is important to understand that human development is a continuous process that begins at fertilization (conception). Birth is a dramatic event during development, and important developmental changes occur after birth (e.g., in the teeth and female breasts). Most developmental changes are completed by the age of 25.

The developmental stages that occur before birth are illustrated in the *Timetables of Human Prenatal Development* (Figs. 1–1 and 1–2). The following list explains the terms used in these timetables and in discussions of developing humans during the prenatal period.

ZYGOTE. This cell, formed by the union of an ovum and a sperm (Gr. *zygōtos*, yolked together), represents the *beginning of a human being*. The common expression "fertilized ovum" refers to the zygote.

CLEAVAGE. Division or cleavage of the zygote by mitosis[1] forms daughter cells called *blastomeres*. These cells become smaller at each succeeding cell division.

MORULA. When 12 or more blastomeres have formed, the ball of cells resulting from cleavage of the zygote is called a *morula* and resembles the berrylike fruit known as the mulberry (L. *morus*). The morula stage is reached about three days after fertilization, just as the developing human is about to enter the uterus from the uterine tube.

BLASTOCYST. After the morula passes from the uterine tube into the uterus, a cavity forms in it known as the *blastocyst cavity*. This converts the morula into a blastocyst.

EMBRYO. The cells of the blastocyst that give rise to the embryo appear as an *inner cell mass*, often referred to as the **embryoblast** (Gr. *blastos*, germ). The term embryo is not usually used until the beginning of the third week. The *embryonic period* extends from the third week to

Text continued on page 6

---

[1] A method of division of a cell by means of which two daughter cells receive identical complements of chromosomes. For details of this process, see Thompson et al. (1991).

1

TIMETABLE OF HUMAN PRENATAL DEVELOPMENT
1 to 6 weeks

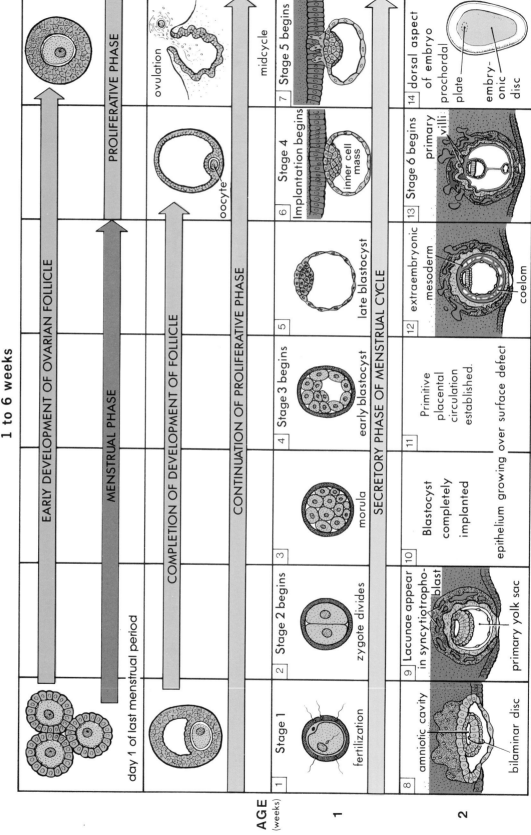

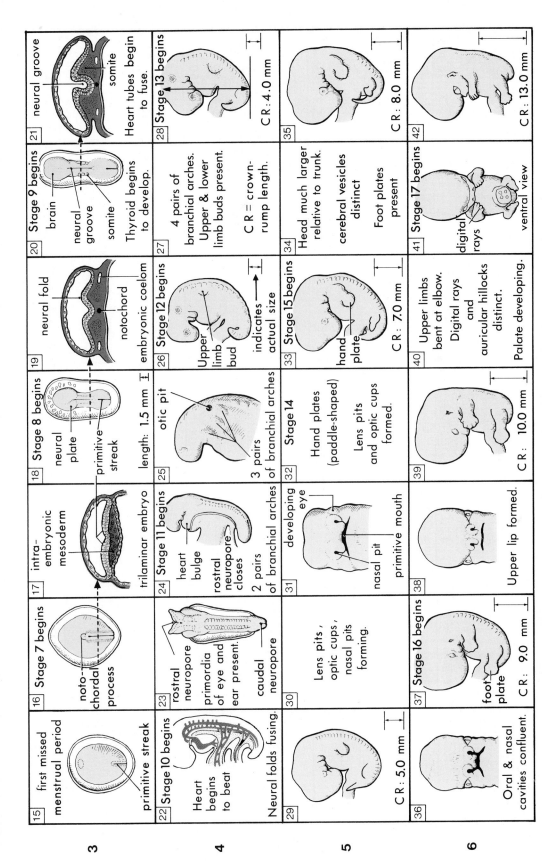

Figure 1–1. Development of an ovarian follicle containing an oocyte, ovulation, and the phases of the menstrual cycle are illustrated first. *Human development begins at fertilization,* about 14 days after the onset of the last normal menstruation. Cleavage of the zygote in the uterine tube, implantation of the blastocyst, and early development of the embryo are also shown. The main features of developmental stages in human embryos are illustrated. For a full discussion of embryonic development, see Chapter 6. Students should make no attempt to memorize these tables or details of the stages.

TIMETABLE OF HUMAN PRENATAL DEVELOPMENT
7 to 38 weeks

AGE (weeks)

Week 7

43 CR: 16.0 mm

44 Stage 18 begins

45 Tip of nose distinct.

Digital rays appear in foot plates.

CR: 17.0 mm

46 Loss of villi

Smooth chorion forms.

47 genital tubercle

urogenital membrane

anal membrane

♀ or ♂

48 Stage 19 begins

Trunk elongating and straightening.

49 CR: 18 mm

Week 8

50 Upper limbs longer & bent at elbows.

Fingers distinct.

51 Eyelids beginning

Anal membrane perforated

Urogenital membrane degenerating.

Testes and ovaries distinguishable.

52 Stage 21 begins

53 Stage 21

External genitalia still in sexless state but have begun to differentiate.

54 Stage 22 begins

genital tubercle

urethral groove

anus

♀ or ♂

55 Beginnings of all essential external & and internal structures are present.

56 Stage 23

CR: 30 mm

Week 9

57 Beginning of fetal period.

58

59 Genitalia show some ♀ characteristics but still easily confused with ♂.

60 phallus

urogenital fold

labioscrotal fold

perineum

♀

61 Genitalia show fusion of urethral folds.

Urethral groove extends into phallus.

62 phallus

urogenital fold

labioscrotal fold

perineum

♂

63 CR: 50 mm

Week 10

64 Face has human profile.

Note growth of chin compared to day 44.

65

66 Face has human appearance.

67 clitoris

labium minus

urogenital groove

labium majus

♀

68 Genitalia have ♀ or ♂ characteristics but still not fully formed.

69 glans penis

urethral groove

scrotum

♂

70 CR: 61 mm

The Fetal Period

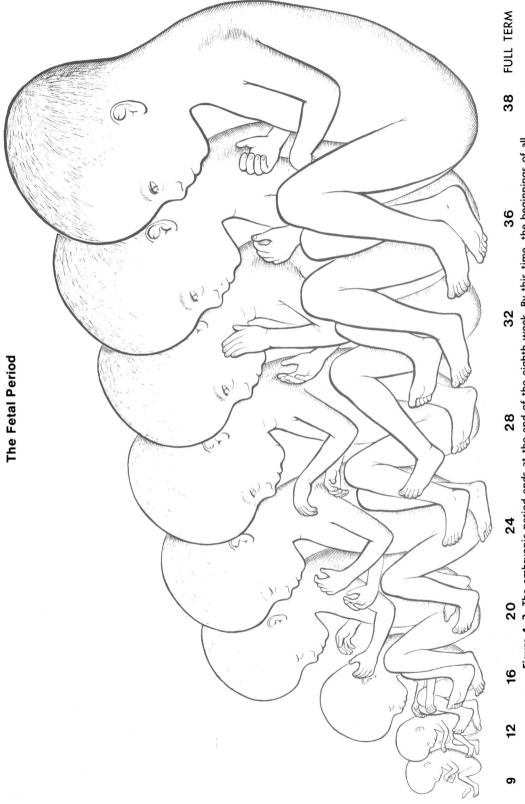

9   12   16   20   24   28   32   36   38   FULL TERM

Figure 1–2. The embryonic period ends at the end of the eighth week. By this time, the beginnings of all essential structures are present and the embryo has a human appearance. The fetal period, extending from the ninth week until birth, is characterized by growth and elaboration of structures. Sex is clearly distinguishable by 12 weeks. The above 9- to 38-week fetuses are about half actual size. For more information about fetal development, see Chapter 7.

5

the end of the eighth week, at which time the primordia of all major structures are present, and characteristics appear that give the embryo a distinctly human appearance.

CONCEPTUS. This term refers to the embryo and its membranes, i.e., the *products of conception or fertilization.* The term refers to all structures that develop from the zygote, both embryonic and extraembryonic; hence, it includes the embryo as well as its associated membranes, e.g., the amnion and chorionic sac (see Chapter 8).

FETUS (L. offspring). After the embryonic period (eighth week), the developing human is called a fetus. During the *fetal period* (ninth week to birth), differentiation and growth of the tissues and organs formed during the embryonic period occur. Although developmental changes are not so dramatic as those occurring during the embryonic period, they are very important because they enable the tissues and organs to function. The rate of body growth is remarkable, especially during the third and fourth months, and weight gain is phenomenal during the terminal months.

PRIMORDIUM (L. *primus,* first + *ordior,* to begin). This term refers to the first indication of an organ or structure, i.e., its earliest stage of development. The term *anlage* has a similar meaning, e.g., the primordium or anlage of the upper limb appears as a bud on about day 26 (Fig. 1–1).

TRIMESTER. This is a period of *three calendar months.* Obstetricians commonly divide the nine-month period of gestation (stages of intrauterine development) into three trimesters. The most critical stages of development occur during the first trimester.

ABORTION (L. *abortio,* to miscarry). This term refers to the birth of an embryo or a fetus before it is *viable* (mature enough to survive outside the uterus). *Threatened abortion* is a common complication in about 25 per cent of pregnancies. Despite every effort to prevent abortion, about one half of these pregnancies ultimately abort. All terminations of pregnancy that occur naturally or are induced before 20 weeks are abortions.

About 15 per cent of all recognized pregnancies end in *spontaneous abortions* (i.e., they occur naturally), usually during the first 12 weeks. Legally induced abortions, often called *elective abortions,* are usually produced by suction curettage (evacuation of the embryo and its membranes by suction from the uterus). Some abortions are induced because of the mother's poor health or to prevent the birth of a severely malformed child (e.g., one without most of its brain). A *missed abortion* is the retention of a conceptus in the uterus after death of the embryo or fetus.

ABORTUS. This term refers to the aborted products of a conception, i.e., the embryo/fetus and its associated membranes, such as the amnion and chorionic sac. An embryo or nonviable fetus and its membranes weighing less than 500 gm is called an abortus, but often they are referred to as aborted embryos or fetuses.

MISCARRIAGE. This term refers to an interruption of pregnancy during the later stages of pregnancy, i.e., spontaneous expulsion of the products of conception after the twentieth week. In medical descriptions, it is common to use the term *premature birth* for the expulsion of a mature fetus.

IMPORTANCE OF EMBRYOLOGY

The study of prenatal stages of development, especially those occurring during the embryonic period, helps us to understand the normal relationships of adult body structures and the causes of congenital anomalies. In other words, *embryology illuminates anatomy* and explains how abnormalities develop.

The embryo is vulnerable to large amounts of radiation, viruses, and certain drugs during the third to eighth weeks (see Chapter 9). The knowledge physicians have regarding normal development and the causes of congenital anomalies aids in giving the embryo the best possible chance of developing normally. Much of the modern practice of obstetrics involves what could be called applied or *clinical embryology.*

Because some of their patients may have disorders resulting from maldevelopment (e.g., spina bifida and congenital heart disease), the significance of embryology is readily apparent to pediatricians. Progress in surgery, especially in the prenatal and pediatric age groups, has made knowledge of human development more clinically significant. Understanding and correction of most congenital anomalies (e.g., cleft palate and cardiac defects) depend on an understanding of normal development and the deviations that have occurred.

HISTORICAL HIGHLIGHTS

If I have seen further, it is by standing on the shoulders of giants.

SIR ISSAC NEWTON, ENGLISH MATHEMATICIAN, 1643–1727

This statement, made over 300 years ago, emphasizes that each new study of a problem rests on a base of knowledge established by earlier investigators. Every age gives explanations according to the knowledge and experience of its people; therefore, we should be grateful for their ideas and neither sneer at them nor consider our ideas final.

A brief *Sanskrit treatise* on ancient Indian embryology is thought to have been written in 1416 B.C. This scripture of the Hindus, called *Garbha Upanishad*, describes ancient ideas concerning the embryo. It states, "From the conjugation of blood and semen the embryo comes into existence. During the period favorable for conception, after sexual intercourse, (it) becomes a *kalada* (one-day-old embryo). After remaining seven nights, it becomes a vesicle. After a fortnight, it becomes a spherical mass. After a month, it becomes a firm mass. After two months, the head is formed. After three months, the limb regions appear." Although the dates of appearance of the structures are inaccurate, the sequence is correct.

The **Greeks** made many important contributions to the science of *embryology* (Persaud, 1984; Dunston, 1990). The first recorded embryological studies are in the books of **Hippocrates,** the famous Greek physician of the 5th century B.C. In the 4th century B.C., **Aristotle** wrote the first known account of embryology, in which he described development of chick and other embryos. **Galen** (2nd century A.D.) wrote a book entitled *On the Formation of the Foetus* in which he described the development and nutrition of fetuses.

Growth of science was slow during the **middle ages,** and no embryological investigations are known to us. It is cited, however, in the *Koran* or *Qur'an* (7th century A.D.), The Holy Book of the Muslims, that human beings are produced from a *mixture of secretions* from the male and female. Several references are made to the creation of a human being from a *nufta* (small drop). It is also stated that the resulting organism settles in the woman like a seed six days after its beginning. (The human blastocyst begins to implant in the lining or endometrium of the uterus about six days after fertilization.) Reference is also made to the leechlike appearance of the early embryo. (The embryo of 22 to 24 days resembles a leech or bloodsucker.) The embryo is also said to resemble a "chewed substance," like gum or wood. (The somites of the early embryos shown in Chapter 6 somewhat resemble teethmarks in a chewed substance.)

The composition and sequential development of the embryo in relation to the planets and each month of pregnancy were described by *Constantinus Africanus* during the 11th century. In the 15th century, **Leonardo da Vinci** made accurate drawings of dissections of the pregnant uterus and associated fetal membranes (Fig. 1–3).

In 1651 **Harvey** studied chick embryos with simple lenses and made observations on the circulation of blood. He believed that after entering the womb, the sperm changed into an egg-like substance, which then developed into an embryo. *Early microscopes were simple* (Fig. 1–4), but they opened a new field of observation. In 1672 **de Graaf** observed little chambers (undoubtedly what we now call blastocysts) in the rabbit's uterus and concluded that they came from organs he called *ovaries.*

Malpighi, in 1675, studying what he believed to be unfertilized hen's eggs, observed early embryos. As a result, he thought the egg

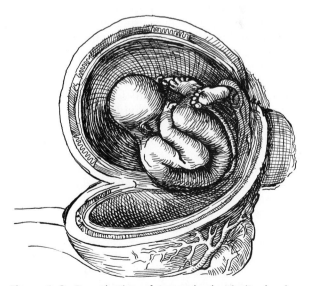

Figure 1–3. Reproduction of Leonardo da Vinci's drawing (15th century A.D.) showing a fetus in a uterus that has been incised and opened.

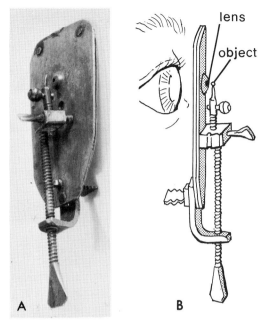

Figure 1–4. *A*, Photograph of a 1673 Leeuwenhoek microscope. *B*, Drawing of a lateral view illustrating its use. The object was held in front of the lens on the point of the short rod, and the screw arrangement was used to adjust the object under the lens. After the development of this crude instrument, embryologists were able to observe the early stages of development.

contained a miniature chick. Despite this, his observations on the developing chick were good.

In 1677, **Hamm and Leeuwenhoek** first observed the human sperm using an improved microscope, but they did not understand the sperm's role in fertilization. They thought it contained a miniature, preformed human being (Fig. 1–5). In 1775, **Spallanzani** showed that both the ovum and sperm were necessary for the initiation of a new individual. From his experiments, Spallanzani concluded that the sperm was the fertilizing agent that initiated development.

Great advances were made in embryology when the *cell theory* was established in 1839 by **Schleiden and Schwann.** The concept that the body was composed of cells and cell products soon led to the realization that the embryo developed from a single cell called the *zygote.* They discovered and demonstrated the cellular nature of tissues. Great progress was made in our understanding of prenatal development through the improved techniques developed by **Wilhelm His** (1831–1904) for the fixing, sectioning, and staining of tissues, and reconstruc-

tion of human embryos. **Hans Spemann** received the Nobel Prize in 1935 for discovering the phenomenon of primary induction, i.e., how one tissue determines the fate of another.

Edwards and Steptoe pioneered the technique of human *in vitro fertilization* which led to the birth of the first "test tube baby" in 1978.

The *principles of heredity* were developed in 1865 by an Austrian monk named **Mendel,** but biologists did not understand the significance of these principles in the study of mammalian development for many years.

Fleming observed chromosomes in 1878 and suggested their probable role in fertilization. The first significant observations on human chromosomes were made by **von Winiwarter** in 1912. In 1923, **Painter** concluded that there were 48 chromosomes. This number was accepted until 1956 when **Tjio and Levan** reported finding only 46 chromosomes. This number is now universally accepted.

Recent advances in the field of **molecular biology** have led to the application of sophisticated techniques (e.g., *recombinant DNA technology,* chimeric models, transgenic mice and so

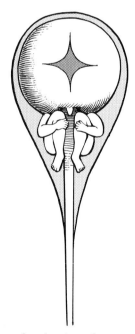

Figure 1–5. Copy of a drawing of a sperm by Hartsoeker. The miniature human being within it was thought to enlarge after it entered an ovum. Other embryologists in the 17th century thought the oocyte contained a miniature, preformed human being that enlarged when it was stimulated by a sperm.

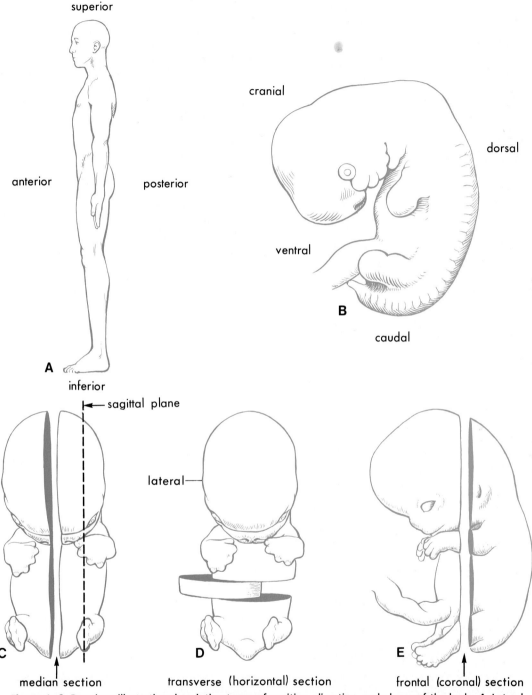

Figure 1–6. Drawings illustrating descriptive terms of position, direction, and planes of the body. *A*, Lateral view of a human adult in the anatomical position. *B*, Lateral view of a five-week embryo. *C* and *D*, Ventral views of six-week embryos. *E*, Lateral view of a seven-week embryo.

forth) for studying embryonic development (see Moore and Persaud [1993] for more information and references).

DESCRIPTIVE TERMS

In anatomy and embryology several terms of position and direction are used, and various planes of the body are referred to in sections. All descriptions of the adult are based on the assumption that the body is erect, with the upper limbs by the sides and the palms directed anteriorly (Fig. 1–6A). This is called the **anatomical position.**

The terms anterior or *ventral* and posterior or *dorsal* are used to describe the front or back of the body or limbs and the relations of structures within the body to one another. When describing embryos, dorsal and ventral are always used (Fig. 1–6B).

Superior or *cranial* (cephalic) and inferior or *caudal* are used to indicate the relative levels of different structures. In embryos, cranial and caudal are used to denote relationships to the head and tail ends, respectively. Distances from the source of attachment of a structure are designated as *proximal* or *distal,* e.g., in the lower limb the knee is proximal to the ankle and the ankle is distal to the knee.

The *median plane* is a vertical plane passing through the center of the body, dividing it into right and left halves (Fig. 1–6C). The terms *lateral* and *medial* refer to structures that are respectively farther from or nearer to the median plane of the body. A *sagittal plane* is any vertical plane passing through the body parallel to the median plane (Fig. 1–6C).

A *transverse* or *horizontal plane* refers to any plane that is at right angles to both the median and frontal planes (Fig. 1–6D). A *frontal* or *coronal plane* is any vertical plane that intersects the median plane at a right angle; it divides the body into front (anterior or ventral) and back (posterior or dorsal) parts (Fig. 1–6E).

Commonly Asked Questions

1. Should I learn to reproduce the timetables of human development and know the criteria for the various stages?
2. What is the difference between the terms *conceptus* and *embryo?* What are the products of conception?
3. Why are we asked to study human embryology? Does it have any practical value?
4. I have heard that animal and human embryos look alike. Is this true?
5. Doctors date a pregnancy from the first day of the last normal menstrual period (LNMP), but the embryo does not start to develop until about two weeks later. Why do they do this?
6. Is the zygote a human being? When does human development begin?

The answers to these questions are given on page 326.

REFERENCES

Biggers JD: Arbitrary partitions of prenatal life. *Human Reprod* 5:1, 1990.

De Pomerai D: *From Gene to Animal.* 2nd ed. New York, New York, Cambridge University Press, 1991.

Dunstan GR (ed): *The Human Embryo. Aristotle and the Arabic and European Traditions.* Exeter, University of Exeter Press, 1990.

Horder TJ, Witkowski JA, Wylie CC (eds): *A History of Embryology.* Cambridge, Cambridge University Press, 1986.

Meyer AW: *The Rise of Embryology.* Stanford, Stanford University Press, 1939.

Moore KL: A scientist's interpretation of references to embryology in the Qur'an. *JIMA* 18:15, 1986.

Moore KL, Persaud TVN: *The Developing Human. Clinically Oriented Embryology.* 5th ed. Philadelphia, WB Saunders, 1993.

Needham J: *A History of Embryology.* 2nd ed. Cambridge, Cambridge University Press, 1959.

Oppenheimer JM: Problems, concepts and their history. *In* Willier BH, Weiss PA, Hamburger V (eds): *Analysis of Development.* New York, Hafner Publishing Co, 1971.

O'Rahilly R: One hundred years of human embryology. *In* Kalter H (ed): *Issues and Reviews in Teratology,* vol. 4. New York, Plenum Press, 1988, pp 81–128.

O'Rahilly R, Müller F: *Developmental Stages in Human Embryos.* Washington, DC, Carnegie Institution of Washington, 1987.

Persaud TVN: *Problems of Birth Defects: From Hippocrates to Thalidomide and After.* Baltimore, University Park Press, 1977.

Persaud TVN: *Early History of Human Anatomy.* Springfield, Charles C Thomas, 1984.

Rossant J, Joyner AL: Towards a molecular-genetic analysis of mammalian development. *Trends in Genet* 5:277, 1989.

Slack JMW: *From Egg to Embryo.* 2nd ed. New York, Cambridge University Press, 1991.

Thompson MW, McInnes RR, Willard HF: *Thompson & Thompson's Genetics In Medicine.* 5th ed. Philadelphia, WB Saunders, 1991.

2

HUMAN REPRODUCTION

Human beings have a limited life span; consequently, for humankind to survive, there must be a mechanism for the production of new individuals. Human reproduction, like that of most animals, involves the fusion of germ cells or **gametes**—an oocyte (ovum) from the female and a sperm (spermatozoon) from the male. Each cell brings a half share of genetic information to the union so that the united cell or **zygote** receives the genetic information required for directing the development of a new human being. The reproductive system in both sexes is designed to ensure the successful union of the sperm and ovum, a process known as *fertilization* (conception).

Before **puberty**, male and female children are not strikingly different except for their genitalia. The sexual maturation that normally occurs during puberty results in considerable differences in appearance, so that the sexually mature male is distinctly masculine and the female is unmistakably feminine. Puberty encompasses the period during which the child, who is incapable of reproduction, is transformed into a person who is capable of reproduction. These changes involve the gross appearance, as well as alterations in the reproductive organs and psyche. The time period of puberty varies between the sexes, as does the age of onset.

Puberty in females is usually between the ages of 12 and 15 years, but **menarche** (first menstruation) often occurs in 11-year-old girls. *Puberty in males* usually begins later (13 to 16 years), but signs of sexual maturity may appear in 12-year-old boys.

Puberty begins when secondary sex characteristics first appear (e.g., the development of breasts in females and the increase in the size of the penis and testes in males) and ends when the person is fully capable of reproduction. Puberty is not a single event but a process of growth and development spanning several years. Although the most obvious changes are in the reproductive system, puberty affects the whole body (e.g., an increase in the growth rate—the *pubertal growth spurt*). Girls are often taller and heavier than boys of the same age during early puberty.

THE REPRODUCTIVE ORGANS

Each sex has reproductive or *sex organs*, which produce and transmit the *germ cells* or gametes from the *sex glands* or gonads to the site of fertilization (Fig. 2–1). The penis, the sex organ in the male, deposits the sperms (spermatozoa) produced by the *testes* in the female genital tract (Fig. 2–10). In the female, the *vagina* is a temporary receptacle for the penis and sperms.

The Female Reproductive Organs

The oocytes or *ova* (female germ cells or gametes) are produced by two oval-shaped **ovaries**

11

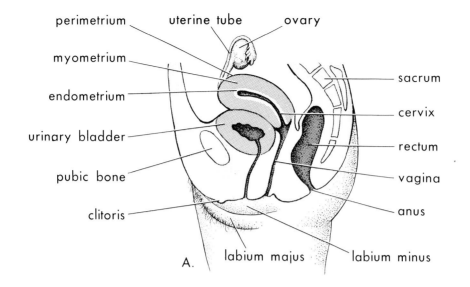

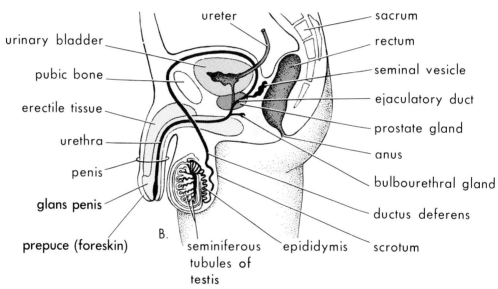

Figure 2-1. Schematic sagittal sections of the pelvic region showing the reproductive organs. *A*, Female. *B*, Male. The ovaries are the sex glands of the female, and the testes (testicles) are the sex glands of the male. There are two ovaries in the normal female, both located in the pelvis. There are two testes in the normal male, both located in the scrotum. The vagina, the female copulatory organ, is an elastic tube (7 to 9 cm long) that leads from the uterus to the outside of the body. It stretches during sexual intercourse and childbirth. The penis is the male copulatory organ and the organ for urination. Sperms leave the urethra during sexual intercourse and are deposited in the vagina (see Fig. 2-10).

located in the superior part of the pelvic cavity, one on each side of the uterus (Fig. 2–1A). When released from the ovary at *ovulation* (Fig. 2–8), the secondary oocyte, often called an ovum, passes into one of two trumpet-shaped *uterine tubes* (Figs. 2–1A and 2–2A). These tubes open into the pear-shaped *uterus* (womb),

which protects and nourishes the embryo and fetus until birth.

STRUCTURE OF THE UTERUS (Fig. 2–2). The uterus is a thick-walled, pear-shaped organ. It varies considerably in size but is usually 7 to 8 cm in length, 5 to 7 cm in width at its superior part, and 2 to 3 cm in thickness. *The uterus* *consists of two main parts*, the **body** and **cervix**. The *fundus* is the rounded superior part of the uterine body. The wall of the body of the uterus consists of three layers: (1) a thin external layer of peritoneum called the *perimetrium*, (2) a thick, smooth muscle layer or *myometrium*, and (3) a thin internal lining layer or *endometrium*.

THE VAGINA (Figs. 2–1*A* and 2–2*A*). The vagina is a muscular tube that passes to the exterior from the cervix, the inferior end of the uterus.

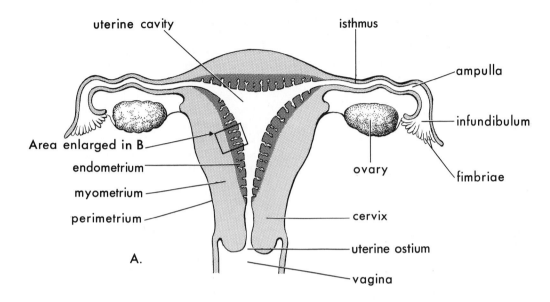

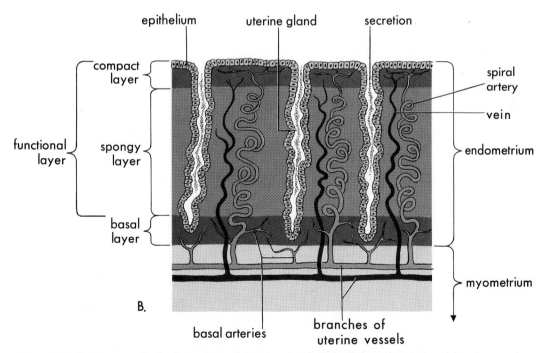

Figure 2–2. *A*, Diagrammatic frontal section of the uterus and uterine tubes. The ovaries and vagina are also illustrated. *B*, Detail of the area outlined in *A*. The endometrium (lining of the uterus) is composed of three layers (compact, spongy, and basal), which are subject to cyclic changes in response to ovarian secretory activity (see Fig. 2–7). The functional layer of the endometrium is sloughed off during menstruation, the monthly endometrial shedding and discharge of bloody fluid from the uterus.

The vagina is the female organ that receives the male organ or penis during *sexual intercourse* (see Fig. 2–10). It also serves as a temporary receptacle for sperms before they begin their passage through the uterus and uterine tubes.

THE EXTERNAL SEX ORGANS (Figs. 2–1 and 2–3). The external genitalia, or sex organs of the female, are known collectively as the *vulva* (pudendum). Two external folds of skin called the *labia majora* (large lips) conceal the opening of the vagina. Inside these labia are two smaller folds of mucous membrane called the *labia minora* (small lips). The *clitoris*, a small erectile organ, is at the superior junction of these folds. The clitoris, the morphological equivalent of the penis, is important in the sexual excitement of a female.

The vagina and urethra open into a cavity known as the *vestibule* (the cleft between the labia minora).

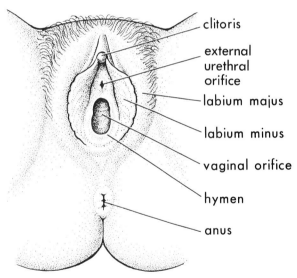

Figure 2–3. The female external genital organs are known collectively as the vulva. The opening at the inferior end of the alimentary canal, the anus, is also shown. In most women the labia majora are together and conceal the labia minora. The labia have been spread apart in this drawing to demonstrate the internal parts of the vulva. The hymen is a thin, incomplete fold of mucous membrane that surrounds the vaginal orifice. The labia majora are fatty folds of skin; whereas, the labia minora are thin folds of pink mucous membrane. The clitoris, 2 to 3 cm in length, is homologous with the penis in the male. Unlike the penis, the clitoris is not traversed by the urethra. The clitoris is composed of erectile tissue and, like the penis, is capable of enlargement upon tactile stimulation. It is highly sensitive and important in the sexual excitement of the female.

The Male Reproductive Organs

The parts of the male reproductive system (Fig. 2–1B) include the testis, epididymis, ductus (vas) deferens, prostate, seminal vesicles, bulbourethral glands, ejaculatory ducts, urethra, and scrotum. The *sperms* (male germ cells or gametes) are produced in the *testes*, two oval-shaped glands which are suspended in the scrotum, a loose pouch of skin (Fig. 2–1B).

Each **testis** consists of many highly coiled *seminiferous tubules* which produce the sperms. The sperms pass into a single, complexly coiled tube, the *epididymis*, where they are stored. The sperms are not mature (i.e., capable of fertilizing ova) when they leave the testes. It takes days for the sperms to mature in the epididymis, located alongside the testis (Fig. 2–1B).

From the inferior end of the epididymis, a long straight tube, the *ductus deferens* (vas deferens) carries the sperms from the epididymis to the ejaculatory duct. The ductus deferens passes from the scrotum through the inguinal canal into the abdominal cavity. It then descends into the pelvis where it fuses with the duct of the seminal vesicle to form the *ejaculatory duct,* which enters the urethra.

The *urethra* is a tube leading from the urinary bladder to the outside of the body; its spongy part runs through the *penis* (Fig. 2–1B). Within the penis the urethra is surrounded by three columns of spongy *erectile tissue.* During sexual excitement this tissue fills with blood under increased pressure. This causes the penis to become erect and thus able to enter the vagina during sexual intercourse. Ejaculation of *semen* (sperms mixed with seminal fluid produced by various glands: seminal vesicles, bulbourethral glands, and prostate) occurs when the penis is further stimulated. Consequently, the urethra transports both urine and semen but not at the same time.

GAMETOGENESIS

Gametogenesis (gamete or germ cell formation) is the process of formation and development of specialized generative cells called gametes or germ cells (see Fig. 2–5). This process, which involves the chromosomes and cytoplasm of the gametes, prepares these specialized sex cells for *fertilization* (union of male and female gametes, i.e., the sperm and ovum). During ga-

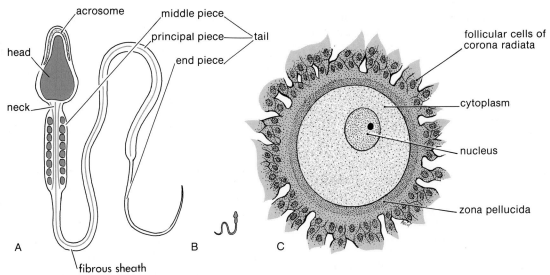

Figure 2–4. *A,* Drawing showing the main parts of a human sperm or spermatozoon (× 1250). The head, composed mostly of the nucleus, is partly covered by the acrosome, which contains enzymes that are released during fertilization. *B,* A sperm drawn to about the same scale as the ovum. *C,* Drawing of a human ovum (secondary oocyte) (× 200) surrounded by the zona pellucida, an elastic membrane, and the corona radiata, composed of follicular cells that accompanied it during ovulation (see Fig. 2–8).

metogenesis the chromosome number is reduced by half, and the shape of the cells is altered, especially the male sex cells.

THE GAMETES

The *sperm* (spermatozoon) and *oocyte* (ovum), the male and female gametes, are highly *specialized sex cells* (Figs. 2–4 and 2–5). They contain half the usual number of chromosomes (i.e., 23 instead of 46). The number of chromosomes is reduced during a special type of cell division called **meiosis.** This type of cell division occurs during the formation of gametes *(gametogenesis).* The gamete-forming process is known as *spermatogenesis* in males and *oogenesis* (ovogenesis) in females (Fig. 2–5).

Meiosis consists of two cell divisions during which the chromosome number is reduced to half (23, the *haploid* number) that which is present in other cells in the body (46, the *diploid* number). During the final stages of maturation, the chromosomes in each of the 23 pairs separate from each other and are distributed to different cells. Each mature germ cell (sperm or ovum), therefore, contains one member of each pair of the chromosomes present in the immature germ cell (primary spermatocyte or primary

oocyte). In summary, *meiosis halves the number of chromosomes* and resorts the genes received from the mother and father.

The significance of meiosis is that it provides for constancy of the chromosome number from generation to generation by producing *haploid germ cells.* It also allows the independent assortment of maternal and paternal chromosomes and genes among the gametes. *Crossing over,* by relocating segments of the maternal and paternal chromosomes, "shuffles" the genes and thereby produces a recombination of genetic material. Consequently, each gamete carries a mixture of maternal and paternal genes. Fertilization results in a new cell, the zygote, which has a mixture of genes from the parents.

Spermatogenesis

The term spermatogenesis refers to the entire sequence of events by which primitive germ cells known as *spermatogonia* are transformed into mature germ cells called spermatozoa (*sperms* for brevity). This maturation process begins at *puberty* (13 to 16 years) and continues into old age (Fig. 2–5).

The **mature sperm** (spermatozoon) is a free-swimming, actively motile cell consisting of a *head* and a *tail* (Fig. 2–4A). The head, forming

NORMAL GAMETOGENESIS

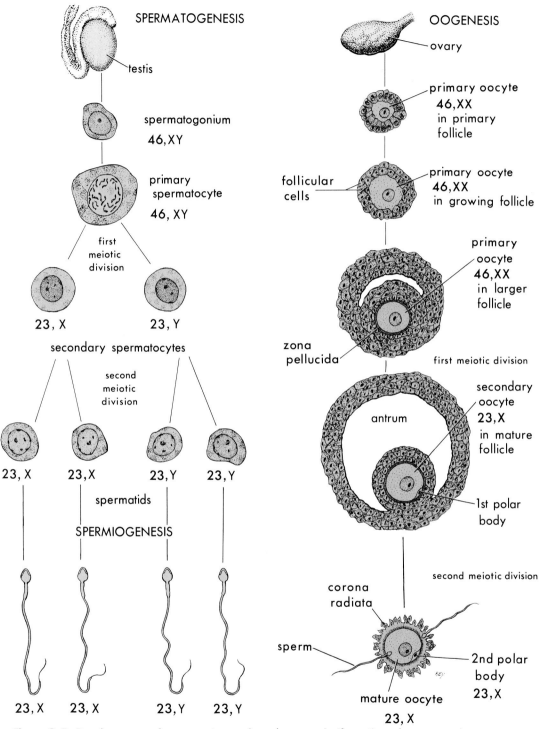

Figure 2–5. Drawings comparing spermatogenesis and oogenesis (formation of sperms and ova, respectively). Oogonia are not shown in this figure because all of them differentiate into primary oocytes before birth. The chromosome complement of the germ cells is shown at each stage. The number designates the total number of chromosomes, including the sex chromosome(s) shown after the comma. Note that: (1) following the two meiotic divisions, the diploid number of chromosomes, 46, is reduced to the haploid number, 23; (2) *four sperms* form from one primary spermatocyte, whereas only *one* mature ovum results from maturation of a primary oocyte; and (3) the cytoplasm is conserved during oogenesis to form one large cell, the mature oocyte or ovum. The polar bodies, nonfunctional cells that soon degenerate, also contain the haploid number of chromosomes.

Figure 2–6. Drawings illustrating the last phase of spermatogenesis known as *spermiogenesis.* During this process the rounded spermatids are transformed into elongated sperms (spermatozoa). Note the loss of cytoplasm, the development of the tail, and the formation of the acrosome. The acrosome, derived from the Golgi region of the spermatid, contains enzymes that are released at the beginning of the fertilization process and assist the sperm in penetrating the corona radiata and zona pellucida.

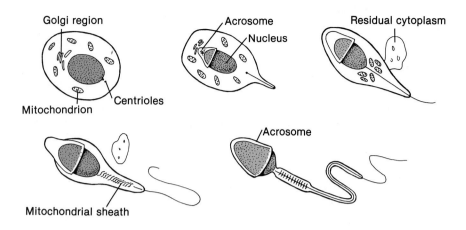

most of the bulk of the sperm, contains the nucleus of the cell which has 23 chromosomes. The anterior two-thirds of the head is covered by the *acrosome* (acrosomal cap), an organelle containing enzymes that facilitate sperm penetration during fertilization (see Chapter 3). The tail of the sperm consists of three segments: the *middle piece* (midpiece), *principal piece,* and *end piece.* The tail provides the motility of the sperm, assisting with its transport to the site of fertilization in the ampulla of the uterine tube (Fig. 2–2A). The middle piece of the tail contains the energy-producing cytoplasmic and mitochondrial apparatus. The junction between the head and tail is called the *neck* of the sperm (Fig. 2–4A).

The early germ cells called *spermatogonia,* which have been dormant in the seminiferous tubules of the testes since the fetal period, begin to increase in number at puberty. After several mitotic cell divisions, the spermatogonia grow and undergo gradual changes which transform them into *primary spermatocytes* (Fig. 2–5), the largest germ cells in the seminiferous tubules of the testes.

Each primary spermatocyte subsequently undergoes a reduction division[1] called the *first meiotic division* to form two haploid *secondary spermatocytes,*[2] which are about half the size of

---

[1] This process of chromosome reproduction by an atypical method of cell division is called *meiosis*; it consists of two specialized divisions called the first and second meiotic divisions (see Fig. 2–5).

[2] In humans, body cells and early sex cells have 46 chromosomes (the diploid number). Mature sex cells have 23 chromosomes (the haploid number).

primary spermatocytes. Subsequently, the secondary spermatocytes undergo a *second meiotic division* to form four haploid *spermatids.* They are about half the size of secondary spermatocytes. During this division, there is no further reduction in the number of chromosomes.

The spermatids are gradually transformed into *mature sperms* by a process known as **spermiogenesis.** During this metamorphosis (change in form), the nucleus condenses, the acrosome forms, and most of the cytoplasm is shed (Fig. 2–6). Spermatogenesis, including spermiogenesis, requires many days for completion and normally continues throughout the reproductive life of a male.

Oogenesis

The term *oogenesis* (ovogenesis) refers to the sequence of events by which oogonia are transformed into ova. This maturation process begins during the fetal period, but is not completed until after *puberty* (12 to 15 years). Oogenesis, a recurring process, is *part of the ovarian cycle* (Fig. 2–7). Except during pregnancy, these cycles occur monthly during the reproductive period of females.

During early fetal life, primitive ova called *oogonia* proliferate by mitotic division. These oogonia enlarge to form *primary oocytes* before birth (Fig. 2–5). By the time of birth all primary oocytes have completed the prophase of the first meiotic division. These oocytes remain in prophase until puberty. Shortly before ovulation a primary oocyte completes the *first meiotic division.* Unlike the corresponding stage of spermatogenesis, however, the division of cytoplasm

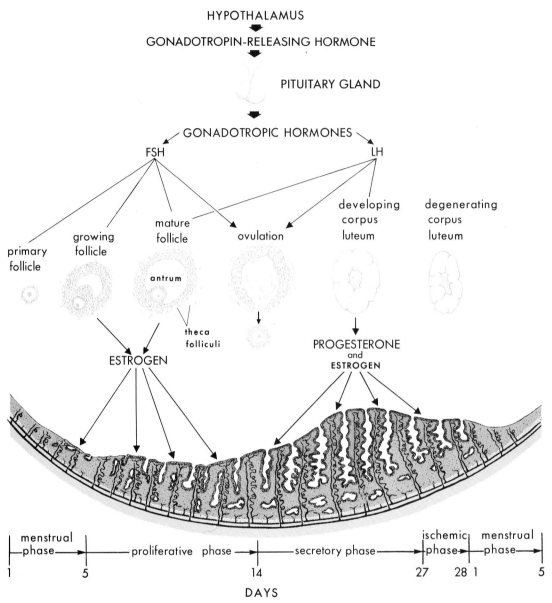

HYPOTHALAMUS

GONADOTROPIN-RELEASING HORMONE

PITUITARY GLAND

GONADOTROPIC HORMONES

FSH   LH

developing   degenerating
corpus   corpus
luteum   luteum

mature
follicle   ovulation

growing
follicle

primary
follicle

antrum

theca
folliculi

PROGESTERONE
and
ESTROGEN

ESTROGEN

| menstrual | proliferative phase | secretory phase | ischemic | menstrual |
| phase | | | phase | phase |

1   5   14   27   28 1   5

DAYS

Figure 2–7. Schematic drawing illustrating the interrelations of the hypothalamus of the brain, hypophysis cerebri (pituitary gland), ovaries, and endometrium. One complete menstrual cycle and the beginning of another are shown. Changes in the ovaries called the ovarian cycle are promoted by the gonadotrophic hormones (FSH and LH). Hormones from the ovaries (estrogens and progesterone) promote changes in the structure and function of the endometrium, called the endometrial or uterine cycle. Thus, the cyclical activity of the ovary is intimately linked with changes in the uterus. The ovarian cycles are under the rhythmic endocrine control of the adenohypophysis, the anterior part of the pituitary gland, and this, in turn, is dominated by the influence of neurosecretory cells in the hypothalamus of the brain.

is unequal. The *secondary oocyte* receives almost all the cytoplasm, and the *first polar body* receives hardly any (Fig. 2–5); this small nonfunctional cell soon degenerates.

At ovulation the nucleus of the secondary oocyte begins the *second meiotic division*, but pro-

gresses only to metaphase where division is arrested. If the secondary oocyte is fertilized by a sperm (Fig. 2–5; see also Fig. 3–1), the second meiotic division is completed. Again, most cytoplasm is again retained by one cell, the *mature ovum* (Fig. 2–5). The other nonfunctional cell called the *second polar body* is very small; it soon degenerates.

The ovum released at ovulation is surrounded by a covering of amorphous material known as the *zona pellucida* and a layer of follicular cells called the *corona radiata* (Fig. 2–4C). Compared with ordinary cells, the secondary oocyte is large and just visible to the unaided eye as a tiny speck. Up to two million primary oocytes are usually present in the ovaries of a newborn female infant. Most of these oocytes regress during childhood so that by puberty no more than 40,000 remain. Of these, only about 400 mature and are expelled at ovulation during the reproductive period (about 30 years).

It is important to realize that primary oocytes that develop toward the end of the reproductive period have been dormant in arrested first meiotic division for at least 30 years. As it is known that the incidence of children with anomalies resulting from chromosomal abnormalities (e.g., the Down syndrome) increases with maternal age, it appears that the extended first meiotic division makes the primary oocyte susceptible to damage by environmental agents (e.g., radiation).

Comparison of Male and Female Gametes

The sperm and secondary oocyte (ovum) are dissimilar in several ways because of their adaptation for specialized roles in reproduction. Compared with the sperm the ovum is massive (Fig. 2–4) and immotile; whereas, the microscopic sperm is highly motile. The ovum has an abundance of cytoplasm; the sperm has very little. The sperm bears little resemblance to an ovum or to any other cell because of its specialization for motility.

With respect to sex chromosome constitution, *there are two kinds of normal sperm* (Fig. 2–5): 22 autosomes plus an X chromosome (i.e., 23,X); and 22 autosomes plus a Y chromosome (i.e., 23,Y). *There is only one kind of normal ovum:* 22 autosomes plus an X chromosome (i.e., 23,X). This difference in sex chromosome complement forms the basis of primary sex determination (see Chapter 3).

Abnormal Gametes

The ideal maternal age for reproduction is considered to be from 18 to 35 years. The likelihood of chromosomal abnormalities in the ova

and the embryo increases significantly after the age of 35. It is also undesirable for the father to be old because the likelihood of gene mutation (alteration) increases with paternal age. The older the father at the time of conception, the more likely he is to have accumulated mutations that the embryo might inherit. This relationship does not hold for all dominant mutations and is not present, or at least has not been recognized, in older mothers.

Ionizing radiation is a strong *mutagen* (producer of mutations). It is therefore wise to reduce as much as possible the exposure of the gonads (ovaries or testes) to radiation during the reproductive period (e.g., from diagnostic and therapeutic x-rays).

NUMERICAL CHROMOSOMAL ABNORMALITIES IN GAMETES. During meiosis, homologous chromosomes sometimes fail to separate and go to opposite poles of the cell. As a result of this error of cell division known as *nondisjunction* (nonseparation), some germ cells have 24 chromosomes and others have only 22.

If a gamete with 24 chromosomes fuses with a normal one during fertilization, a zygote with 47 chromosomes forms (see Fig. 9–1). This condition is called *trisomy* because of the presence of three representatives of a particular chromosome, instead of the usual two; for example, people with the *Down syndrome* have 47 chromosomes (see Fig. 9–4) due to the presence of three number 21 chromosomes.

If a gamete with only 22 chromosomes fuses with a normal one, a zygote with 45 chromosomes forms. This condition is known as *monosomy* because only one representative of the particular chromosome pair is present; for example, people with the *Turner syndrome* have 45 chromosomes due to the absence of a sex chromosome (see Fig. 9–3).

MORPHOLOGICAL ABNORMALITIES OF SPERMS. Up to 10 per cent of sperms in a sample of semen may be grossly abnormal (e.g., two heads or tails), but it is generally believed that they do not fertilize oocytes due to their lack of normal motility. Most, if not all, morphologically abnormal sperms are unable to pass through the mucus in the cervical canal. X-rays, severe allergic reactions, and certain antispermatogenic agents are believed to increase the percentage of abnormally shaped sperms. Such sperms are not believed to affect fertility unless their number exceeds 20 per cent.

FEMALE REPRODUCTIVE CYCLES

Commencing at puberty and normally continuing throughout the reproductive years, human females undergo monthly reproductive or sexual cycles involving the hypothalamus, pituitary gland (hypophysis cerebri), ovaries, and uterus (Fig. 2–7). Cyclic changes in structure and function also occur in the uterine tubes, vagina, and mammary glands. The reproductive cycles prepare the female reproductive system for pregnancy.

Small blood vessels carry *gonadotropin-releasing hormones* (GnRH) from neurosecretory cells in the hypothalamus to the anterior pituitary gland. GnRH regulates this gland's production of gonadotropins (gonad-stimulating hormones): *follicle-stimulating hormone* (FSH) and *luteinizing hormone* (LH).

The Ovarian Cycle

The gonadotropins (FSH and LH) produce cyclic changes in the ovaries (development of follicles, ovulation, and corpus luteum formation). Collectively, these changes constitute the ovarian cycle (Figs. 2–7 and 2–8). During each cycle FSH promotes growth of several primary follicles. Usually, however, only one of these develops into a mature follicle and ruptures through the surface of the ovary, expelling its oocyte (Fig. 2–8); hence, several follicles degenerate each month (i.e., they never mature).

FOLLICULAR DEVELOPMENT (Figs. 2–5 and 2–7). Development of an ovarian follicle is characterized by: (1) growth and differentiation of the primary oocyte, (2) proliferation of follicular cells, (3) formation of the zona pellucida, and (4) development of a connective tissue capsule, the *theca folliculi* (Gr. *theke*, box).

The ovarian follicle soon becomes oval in shape and the oocyte eccentric in position because the follicular cells proliferate more rapidly on one side. Subsequently, fluid-filled spaces appear around the follicular cells that soon coalesce to form a large, fluid-filled cavity called the *antrum*. When the antrum forms, the ovarian follicle is called a vesicular or *secondary follicle*. The primary oocyte is located at one side of the follicle where it is surrounded by a mound of follicular cells, the *cumulus oophorus*, that projects into the antrum (Fig. 2–7). The follicle continues to enlarge until it reaches maturity and produces a bulge on the surface of the ovary. It is now called a *mature follicle* (graafian follicle). The early development of ovarian follicles is induced by FSH, but final stages of maturation require LH as well. Growing follicles produce *estrogen*, a female sex hormone that

regulates development and function of the reproductive organs.

OVULATION (Fig. 2–8). Expulsion of an oocyte from the ovary usually occurs about two weeks before the next expected menstrual period, i.e., about 14 days after the first day of the menstrual period in the typical 28-day cycle (Fig. 2–7). Under FSH and LH influence, the follicle undergoes a sudden growth spurt, producing a swelling on the surface of the ovary. A small, oval, avascular spot called the *stigma* soon appears on this swelling (Fig. 2–8A). Soon the ovarian surface ruptures at the stigma, and the oocyte is expelled with the follicular fluid from the follicle and ovary. The released secondary oocyte is surrounded by the *zona pellucida* and follicular cells of the *corona radiata* (Figs. 2–4C and 2–8C).

Ovulation is triggered by a surge of LH production, which is induced by the high level of estrogen in the blood. Ovulation usually follows the LH peak by 12 to 24 hours. Some women do not ovulate due to an inadequate release of gonadotropins (FSH and LH); as a result, they are unable to become pregnant. In some of these patients *ovulation can be induced* by the administration of FSH and LH or drugs that stimulate their production. Multiple births frequently result from overstimulation of ovulation in these patients (see Chapter 8). The oral administration of estrogen, with or without progesterone, in the form of *birth control pills* suppresses ovulation by inhibiting the release of FSH and LH. As a result, the midcycle LH surge that triggers ovulation does not develop.

THE CORPUS LUTEUM (Figs. 2–7 and 2–8). Shortly after ovulation the walls of the ovarian follicle collapse and, under LH influence, develop into a glandular structure known as the corpus luteum. It secretes *progesterone* and estrogen. These hormones, particularly progesterone, cause the endometrial glands to secrete and prepare the endometrium for the implantation of a blastocyst (see Fig 3–4). If the ovum is fertilized, the corpus luteum enlarges to form a *corpus luteum of pregnancy* and increases its hormone production. If the ovum is not fertilized, the corpus luteum begins to degenerate 10 to 12 days after ovulation (Fig. 2–7).

The Menstrual Cycle

The hormones produced by the ovaries (estrogen and progesterone) produce changes in the **endometrium** (Fig. 2–7). These cyclic changes

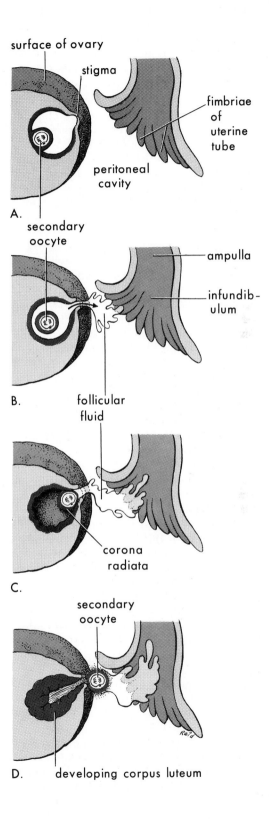

Figure 2–8. Diagrams illustrating ovulation. The stigma ruptures and the oocyte is expelled with the follicular fluid. Note that the mature follicle produces a bulge on the surface of the ovary. Increasing distention results in rupture of the follicle and the surface of the ovary at the stigma (an area of degeneration). As rupture occurs the secondary oocyte is expelled from the follicle and ovary with the follicular fluid.

constitute the endometrial or *uterine cycle,* commonly referred to as the menstrual cycle because menstruation is an obvious event. The length of the cycle illustrated in Figure 2–7 is 28 days, but the length of cycles varies from individual to individual (e.g., from 23 to 35 days in 90 per cent of healthy women).

Ovarian hormones cause cyclic changes in the structure of the reproductive tract, notably the endometrium. Although divided into phases (Fig. 2–7), it must be stressed that *the menstrual cycle is a continuous process* during which each phase gradually passes into the next one.

THE MENSTRUAL PHASE. The first day of menstruation is counted as the beginning of the menstrual cycle. The functional layer of the endometrium (Fig. 2–2B) is sloughed off and discarded during menstruation, which typically occurs at 28-day intervals and lasts four to five days.

THE PROLIFERATIVE PHASE. During the proliferative (estrogenic or follicular) phase, lasting about nine days, estrogen induces regeneration of the epithelium, lengthening of the glands, and multiplication of connective tissue cells. There is a two- to threefold *increase in the thickness of the endometrium* during this phase of repair and proliferation. Early during this phase, the surface epithelium reforms and covers the endometrium, the glands increase in number and length, and the spiral arteries elongate.

THE SECRETORY PHASE. During the secretory (progestational or luteal) phase, lasting about 13 days, progesterone induces the glands to become tortuous and secrete profusely, and the connective tissue to become edematous (a condition in which there are large amounts of fluid in the intercellular spaces). If fertilization does not occur, the secretory endometrium enters an *ischemic phase* during the last day of the menstrual cycle. The ischemia (localized deficiency of blood) results from intermittent constriction of the spiral arteries and gives the endometrium a pale appearance. The arterial constriction results from decreasing secretion of hormones by the degenerating corpus luteum.

Toward the end of the ischemic part of the secretory phase, the spiral arteries become constricted for longer periods. Blood eventually begins to seep through the ruptured walls of the spiral arteries into the surrounding connective tissue (stroma). Small pools of blood soon form and break through the endometrial surface, resulting in bleeding into the uterine lumen. This indicates the beginning of another menstrual phase.

As small pieces of the endometrium detach and pass into the uterine cavity, the ends of the spiral arteries tear and bleed into this cavity, resulting in an average loss of 20 to 80 ml of blood. Eventually, over three to five days, the entire compact layer and most of the spongy layer of the endometrium are discarded in the menstrual flow. The remnants of the spongy layer and the basal layer remain to undergo regeneration during the subsequent proliferative phase of the menstrual cycle. Consequently, the cyclic hormonal activity of the ovary is intimately linked with cyclic histological changes in the endometrium (Fig. 2–7).

If pregnancy does not occur, the menstrual cycles normally continue until the end of a woman's reproductive life, usually between the ages of 47 and 52. *Menstruation ceases at menopause.* If pregnancy occurs, the menstrual cycles stop and the endometrium passes into a *pregnancy phase.* With the termination of pregnancy,

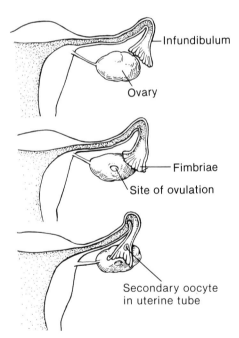

Figure 2–9. Schematic frontal sections of the uterus and uterine tubes, illustrating the movement of the uterine tubes that occurs during ovulation. Note that the funnel-shaped infundibulum of the tube becomes closely applied to the ovary and that its fingerlike fimbriae move back and forth over the ovary. They "sweep" the secondary oocyte into the infundibulum as soon as it is expelled from the ovarian follicle in the ovary (see Fig. 2–8).

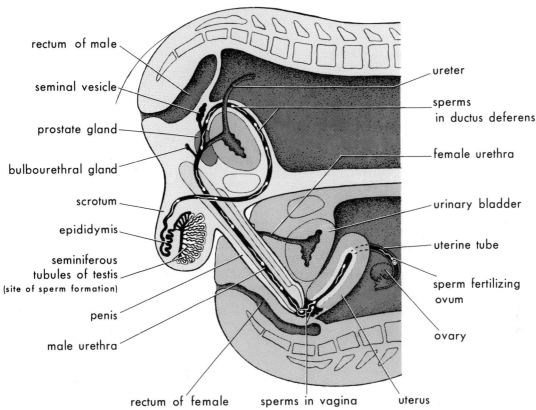

rectum of male

seminal vesicle

prostate gland

bulbourethral gland

scrotum

epididymis

seminiferous
tubules of testis
(site of sperm formation)

penis

male urethra

rectum of female   sperms in vagina   uterus

ureter

sperms
in ductus deferens

female urethra

urinary bladder

uterine tube

sperm fertilizing
ovum

ovary

Figure 2–10. Schematic sagittal section of male and female pelves, showing the penis in the vagina. The sperms are produced in the seminiferous tubules of the testis and stored in the epididymis. During ejaculation the sperms pass along the ductus deferens and ejaculatory duct and enter the urethra where they mix with secretions from the seminal vesicles, prostate, and bulbourethral glands. This mixture, called semen, is deposited in the superior portion of the vagina close to the external opening of the uterus. The sperms pass through the cervix and the cavity of the uterus into the uterine tubes, where fertilization usually occurs (see Figs. 3–1 and 3–2).

the ovarian and menstrual cycles resume after a variable period of time.

TRANSPORTATION OF GAMETES

OOCYTE TRANSPORT (Figs. 2–1, 2–8, and 2–9). At ovulation the secondary oocyte leaves the ovarian follicle and the ovary with the escaping follicular fluid. The fimbriated end of the uterine tube becomes closely applied to and partially covers the ovary at ovulation. The finger-like fimbriae of the tube move back and forth over the ovary and "sweep" the secondary oocyte into the tube. Due to movements of ciliated cells in the lining of the infundibulum and muscular contractions of the tube, the oocyte passes to the *ampulla* of the tube. Movement of the

oocyte results mainly from gentle *waves of peristalsis* that pass along the tube toward the uterus.

SPERM TRANSPORT. From 200 to 600 million of the sperms that are stored in the epididymis are deposited in the vagina during the process of *ejaculation* (Fig. 2–10). The sperms pass by movements of their tails into the cervical canal, but their passage through the remainder of the uterus and the uterine tubes results mainly from contractions of the walls of these organs. *Prostaglandins* in the semen are thought to stimulate uterine motility at the time of intercourse and assist in the movement of sperms through the uterus and into the tubes to the site of fertilization. It takes the sperms about five minutes to reach the fertilization site in the ampulla of the tube (Fig. 2–2A). Only about 200 sperms reach the fertilization site. Most sperms degenerate and are absorbed by the female genital tract. The main sites of reduction in the number of sperms are in the cervix and uterine tubes.

VIABILITY OF GAMETES

OOCYTES. Studies on early stages of development indicate that secondary oocytes are usually fertilized within 12 hours after their expulsion at ovulation (Fig. 2–8). Unfertilized oocytes die within 12 to 24 hours.

SPERMS. Most sperms probably do not survive for more than 48 hours in the female genital tract. Some sperms, however, retain their fertilizing power for two to three days. *Fructose* in the semen, secreted by the seminal vesicles (Fig. 2–10), is an energy source for the sperms (Barratt and Cooke, 1991).

SUMMARY

Fertilization (conception) involves the fusion of an ovum from a female and a sperm from a male. The reproductive system in both sexes is designed to ensure union of these gametes.

The secondary oocyte, developed in the ovary, is expelled from it at ovulation. It is carried into the infundibulum of the uterine tube by the sweeping motions of the fimbriae of the tube. Peristaltic waves in the tube move the oocyte to the fertilization site in the ampulla of the tube.

The sperms are produced in the seminiferous tubules of the testis and stored in the epididymis. During ejaculation, usually occurring during sexual intercourse, the semen is deposited in the vagina. Although there are several million sperms in the semen, only a few thousand pass through the cervical canal, uterine cavity, and along the uterine tube. Only about 200 sperms reach the ampulla where fertilization occurs if a secondary oocyte is present.

Commonly Asked Questions

1. Does a ruptured hymen indicate that a woman is not a virgin?
2. I have heard that a woman can have an erection. Is this true?
3. I know of a woman who claimed that she menstruated throughout her pregnancy. How could this happen?
4. If a woman forgets to take a birth control pill and then takes two, will she become pregnant?
5. What is *coitus interruptus?* I have heard that it is a safe method of birth control. Is this true?
6. I have been told that an IUD (intrauterine device) is a contraceptive. Is this correct?
7. I was told that a child of five can have a baby. Is this true?

The answers to these questions are given on page 326.

REFERENCES

Barratt CLR, Cooke ID: Sperm transport in the human female reproductive tract—a dynamic interaction. *Int J Androl 14:*394, 1991.

Beer E: Egg transport through the oviduct. *Am J Obstet Gynecol 165:*483, 1991.

Chandley AC: Meiosis in man. *Trends Genet 4:*79–83, 1988.

Clermont Y, Trott M: Kinetics of spermatogenesis in mammals: Seminiferous epithelium cycle and spermatogonial renewal. *Physiol Rev 52:*198, 1972.

Comhair FH, Huysse S, Hinting A, Vermeulen L, Schoonjans F: Objective semen analysis: has the target been reached? *Human Reprod. 7:*237, 1992.

Cormack DH: *Essential Histology.* Philadelphia, JB Lippincott Company, 1993.

Cumming DC, Cumming CE, Kieren DK: Menstrual mythology and sources of information about menstruation. *Am J Obstet Gynecol 164:*472, 1991.

Egarter C: The complex nature of egg transport through the oviduct. *Am J Obstet Gynecol 163:*687, 1990.

Hafez ESE: *Human Ovulation, Mechanisms, Prediction, Detection and Induction.* Amsterdam, North Holland Publishing Company, 1979.

Leeson CR, Leeson TS, Paparo A: *Text/Atlas of Histology.* Philadelphia, WB Saunders, 1988.

Moore KL: *Clinically Oriented Anatomy.* 3rd ed. Baltimore, Williams & Wilkins, 1992.

Moore KL, Persaud TVN: *The Developing Human: Clinically Oriented Embryology.* 5th ed. Philadelphia, WB Saunders, 1993.

Page EW, Villee CA, Villee DB: *Human Reproduction: Essentials of Reproductive and Perinatal Medicine.* 3rd ed. Philadelphia, WB Saunders, 1981.

Scott RT Jr, Hodgen GD: The ovarian follicle: life cycle of a pelvic clock. *Clin Obstet Gynecol 33:*551, 1990.

Settlage DSF, Motoshima M, Tredway DR: Sperm transport from the external cervical os to the fallopian tubes in women. *Fertil Steril 24:*655, 1973.

3

THE FIRST WEEK
OF
HUMAN DEVELOPMENT

THE BEGINNING OF HUMAN DEVELOPMENT

Human development begins at conception or fertilization[1] when a male gamete or sperm fuses with a female gamete or ovum to form a **zygote** (Gr. *zygōtos,* yoked together). This highly specialized, totipotent cell is the primordium of a new human being. By birth the zygote has given rise to millions of cells. Although large, the zygote is just visible to the unaided eye. It contains chromosomes and genes (units of genetic information) derived from the mother and father.

Fertilization

Freshly ejaculated sperms are unable to fertilize secondary oocytes. They must undergo an activation process, a seven-hour period of conditioning known as **capacitation.** During this process a glycoprotein coat and seminal proteins are removed from the surface of the acrosome (Fig. 3–1). Following capacitation, the sperms show no morphological changes, but they are more active and able to penetrate the corona radiata and zona pellucida surrounding the secondary

oocyte. Sperms are usually capacitated in the uterus and uterine tubes by substances in the secretions of these parts of the female genital tract.

When capacitated sperms contact the corona radiata surrounding a secondary oocyte (Fig. 3–1A), they undergo changes that result in the *development of perforations* in their acrosomes (Fig. 3–1B). These changes, known as the **acrosome reaction,** are associated with the release of enzymes (e.g., *hyaluronidase,* which causes dissociation of the follicular cells in the corona radiata). Later, other enzymes are released from the acrosome (e.g., *acrosin*), which produce a defect in the zona pellucida through which the sperm passes to the oocyte.

Fertilization is a sequence of events that begins with contact between a sperm and a secondary oocyte, and ends with the fusion of the nuclei of the sperm and ovum and the intermingling of maternal and paternal chromosomes during metaphase of the first mitotic division of the zygote (Fig. 3–2D and E). It is now believed that the oocyte sends a signal to the sperm even before they meet. Fertilization usually occurs in the dilated portion of the uterine tube called the *ampulla* (see Fig. 2–2A). The fertilization process takes about 24 hours.

Phases of Fertilization

1. The sperm passes through the corona radiata formed by follicular cells (Figs. 3–1 and

---

[1] Although development begins at conception (formation of the zygote), the stages and duration of pregnancy in clinical medicine are often calculated from the commencement of the mother's last normal menstrual period, which is about 14 days before conception.

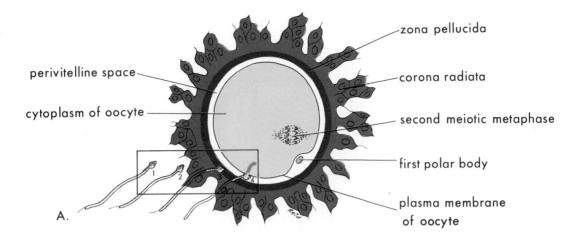

zona pellucida

perivitelline space

corona radiata

cytoplasm of oocyte

second meiotic metaphase

first polar body

plasma membrane
of oocyte

A.

sperm nucleus
containing
chromosomes

acrosome
containing
enzymes

perforations
in acrosome
wall

enzymes
breaking down
zona pellucida

sperm in cytoplasm
of oocyte without its
plasma membrane

plasma membrane
of sperm

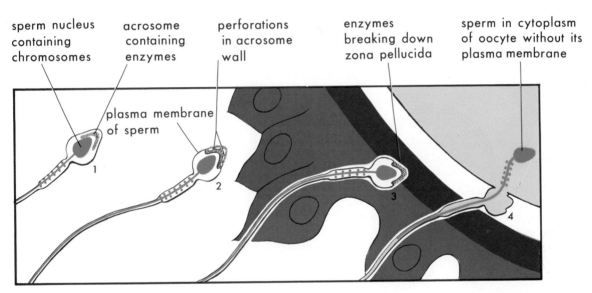

B.

Figure 3–1. Diagrams illustrating the early stages of fertilization. The acrosome reaction and penetration of a sperm into an ovum are shown. The details of the area outlined in *A* are given in *B*: (1) sperm during capacitation; (2) sperm undergoing the acrosome reaction; (3) sperm digesting a path for itself by the action of enzymes released from its acrosome; (4) sperm head fusing with ovum. Note that the sperm enters the oocyte but leaves its plasma membrane behind.

3–2). Dispersal of these cells results mainly from the action of enzymes, especially *hyaluronidase,* released from the acrosome of the sperm. Tubal mucosal enzymes also appear to be involved, and movements of the tail of the sperm also help it penetrate the corona radiata.

2. The sperm penetrates the zona pellucida following a pathway formed by other enzymes released from the acrosome (acrosin and neuraminidase).

3. The sperm head contacts the surface of the oocyte, and the plasma membranes of the two cells fuse. The membranes break down at the area of fusion, creating a defect through which the sperm can enter the oocyte.

4. The oocyte reacts to sperm contact in two ways: (a) the zona pellucida and the plasma membrane of the oocyte change so that the entry of more sperms is prevented, and (b) the oocyte completes the second meiotic division and expels the second polar body (Fig. 3–2*B*). The oocyte is now mature and its nucleus is called the *female pronucleus.* The reaction of the zona pellucida to sperm penetration is called the

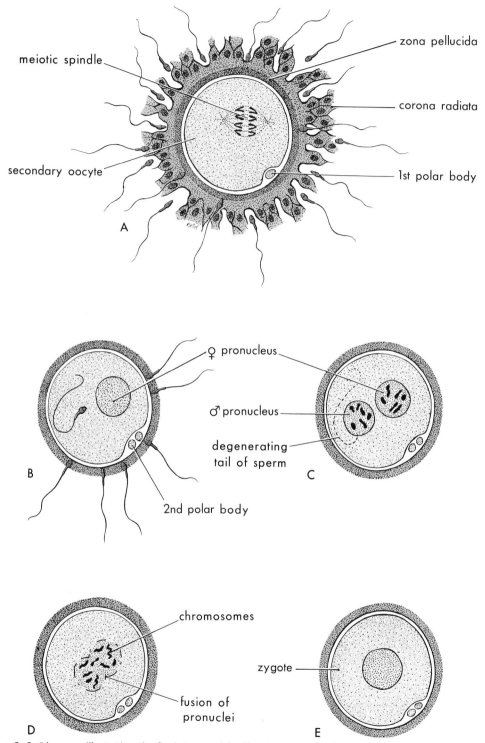

Figure 3–2. Diagrams illustrating the final stages of fertilization. *A,* Secondary oocyte about to be fertilized. (Only four of the 23 chromosome pairs are shown.) *B,* The corona radiata has disappeared, a sperm has entered the ovum, and the second meiotic division has occurred. The nucleus of the ovum is now called the female pronucleus. *C,* The sperm head has enlarged to form the male pronucleus. *D,* The pronuclei are fusing. *E,* The zygote has formed and is preparing for the first cleavage division (see Fig. 3–3*A*). The polar bodies are small, nonfunctional cells that soon degenerate.

zona reaction. The zonal changes result from the action of lysosomal enzymes released by cortical granules in the cytoplasm near the plasma membrane of the oocyte.

5. The sperm enters the cytoplasm of the ovum, but its plasma membrane is left behind on the surface of the oocyte (Fig. 3–1). The head of the sperm enlarges to form the *male pronucleus* as the tail of the sperm detaches and degenerates (Fig. 3–2C). Morphologically, the male and female pronuclei are indistinguishable. During formation of the pronuclei, they replicate their DNA.

6. The male and female pronuclei approach each other, lose their nuclear membranes, and fuse. The maternal and paternal chromosomes intermingle, forming a new diploid cell called a **zygote** (Fig. 3–2D and E), which is the primordium of a new human being. About four days after fertilization, an *early pregnancy factor* (EPF) appears in the maternal serum. EPF forms the basis of pregnancy tests during the first week of development (Nahhas and Barnea, 1990).

The Results of Fertilization

1. RESTORATION OF THE DIPLOID NUMBER OF CHROMOSOMES. Fusion of the nuclei of the two haploid germ cells (each with 23 chromosomes) produces a zygote, which is a diploid cell with 46 chromosomes, the normal number for the human species.

2. SPECIES VARIATION. Because half the chromosomes in the zygote come from the mother and the other half from the father, *the zygote contains a new combination of chromosomes* different from that of either parent; consequently, fertilization forms the basis of biparental inheritance and ensures variation of the human species. *Meiosis,* or reduction division of the developing gametes (see Fig. 2–5), allows independent assortment of maternal and paternal chromosomes among the germ cells. Furthermore, *crossing over of chromosomes* results in the relocation of segments of the maternal and paternal chromosomes and the "shuffling" of genes, which produces a recombination of genetic material.

3. PRIMARY SEX DETERMINATION. The embryo's chromosomal sex is determined at fertilization by the kind of sperm (X or Y) that fertilizes the ovum. Fertilization by an X-bearing sperm produces an XX zygote, which normally develops into a female; whereas, fertilization by a Y-bearing sperm produces an XY zygote, which nor-mally develops into a male. It is, therefore, the father rather than the mother whose gamete determines the sex of the embryo.

4. INITIATION OF CLEAVAGE OF THE ZYGOTE. Fertilization of the oocyte by a sperm also initiates early human development by stimulating the zygote to undergo *a series of rapid mitotic cell divisions* called cleavage (Fig. 3–3). Unfertilized oocytes degenerate about 24 hours after ovulation and are absorbed by the epithelium lining the uterine tubes.

In Vitro Fertilization (IVF) and "Embryo" Transfer

Fertilization of secondary oocytes *in vitro* (L. in glass) and transfer of the dividing zygotes ("cleaved embryos") into the uterus has provided an opportunity for many sterile women (e.g., due to tubal occlusion) to bear children. The first of these so-called *"test tube babies"* was born in 1978. Since then, several thousand pregnancies have occurred using this extracorporeal (outside the body) fertilization technique (Edwards, 1990).

The steps involved in in vitro fertilization and "embryo" transfer are as follows:

1. Ovarian follicles are stimulated to grow and mature by the administration of gonadotropins to the patient.

2. Several secondary oocytes are aspirated from mature ovarian follicles during *laparoscopy* (viewing the contents of the peritoneal cavity with a laparoscope) just prior to ovulation (see Fig. 2–8B).

3. The oocytes are placed in a test tube or Petri dish containing a special culture medium.

4. Sperms are added almost immediately.

5. Fertilization of the oocytes and cleavage of the zygotes are monitored microscopically.

6. Dividing zygotes ("cleaved embryos"), during the four- to eight-cell stage (Fig. 3–3), are inserted into the uterus via the cervical canal. The probability of a successful pregnancy is enhanced by implanting two or three dividing zygotes. Obviously, the chances of multiple pregnancies are higher than when pregnancy results from normal ovulation and passage of the morula into the uterus via the uterine tube. The incidence of spontaneous abortion of transferred embryos is also higher than normal.

Early dividing zygotes ("cleaved embryos") and blastocysts resulting from in vitro fertilization can be preserved for long periods by freezing them with a cryoprotective solution, such as glycerol (*cryopreservation*). After thawing, successful transfer of these dividing zygotes to the uterus is now common practice.

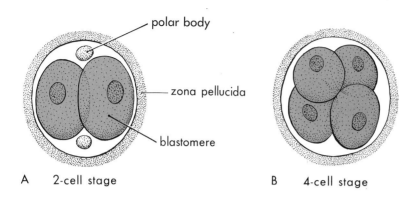

A   2-cell stage

B   4-cell stage

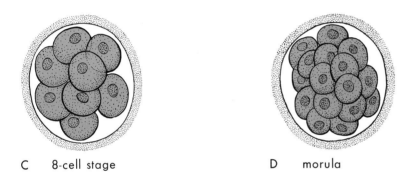

C   8-cell stage

D   morula

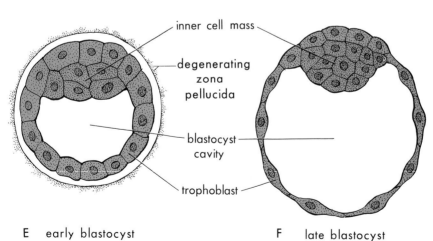

E   early blastocyst

F   late blastocyst

Figure 3–3. Drawings illustrating cleavage of the zygote and formation of the blastocyst. *E* and *F* are sections of blastocysts. Note that the zona pellucida has disappeared by the late blastocyst stage (about five days). The polar bodies shown in *A* are small, nonfunctional cells that soon degenerate. Cleavage of the zygote and formation of the morula occurs as the dividing zygote passes along the uterine tube. Blastocyst formation normally occurs in the uterus (see Fig. 3–5). Although cleavage increases the number of cells (blastomeres), note that each of the daughter cells is smaller than the parent cells. As a result, there is no increase in the size of the pre-embryo until the zona pellucida degenerates. The blastocyst then enlarges considerably (compare *E* and *F*).

CLEAVAGE OF THE ZYGOTE

Cleavage consists of repeated divisions of the zygote. As it passes down the uterine tube, the zygote undergoes rapid cell divisions within its zona pellucida. Mitotic division of the zygote into two daughter cells called **blastomeres** (Fig. 3–3A) begins shortly after fertilization. Subsequent divisions follow rapidly upon one another, forming progressively smaller blastomeres (Fig. 3–3B to D); hence, there is an increase in cells without an increase in cytoplasmic mass.

By the third day, a solid ball of 12 or more blastomeres has formed, which is called a **morula** (L. *morus,* mulberry). The blastomeres change their shape and tightly align themselves against each other to form a compact ball of cells. This process, called *compaction,* permits greater cell-to-cell interaction and is a prerequisite for the subsequent segregation of cells that will form the embryo. The morula, a mulberry-like cellular mass, enters the uterus and fluid passes into it from the uterine cavity. As the fluid increases and collects between the blastomeres, it separates these cells into two parts: (1) an outer cell layer (or "mass") called the **trophoblast,** and (2) a group of centrally located cells known as the *inner cell mass.* The inner cell mass (or **embryoblast**) subsequently differentiates into the embryo, whereas the trophoblast (Gr. *trophe,* nutrition) contributes to the formation of the placenta from which the embryo receives its nourishment (see Chapter 8).

By the fourth day after fertilization, the fluid-filled spaces between the blastomeres fuse to form a single large space known as the *blastocyst cavity.* This converts the morula into a **blastocyst** (Fig. 3–3E). The inner cell mass (embryoblast or future embryo) projects into the blastocyst cavity, and the trophoblast forms the wall of the

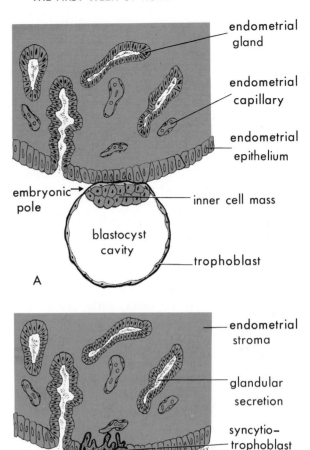

Figure 3–4. Drawings of sections illustrating the attachment of the blastocyst to the endometrial epithelium and the early stages of its implantation. *A,* Six days: the trophoblast is attached to the endometrial epithelium at the embryonic pole of the blastocyst. *B,* Seven days: the syncytiotrophoblast has formed from the trophoblast and has penetrated the endometrial epithelium and has started to invade the endometrial stroma (connective tissue).

blastocyst (Fig. 3–3F). The blastocyst lies free in the uterine secretions for about two days. These secretions provide the nutritional requirements of the blastocyst (pre-embryo).

On about the fifth day after fertilization, the *zona pellucida* degenerates and disappears (Fig. 3–3E and F). The blastocyst attaches to the endometrial epithelium on about the sixth day (day

20 of a 28-day menstrual cycle), usually at the *embryonic pole* (Fig. 3–4*A*). The trophoblast produces substances that destroy the adjacent endometrial epithelium (Fig. 3–4*B*). As invasion of the endometrium proceeds, two layers of trophoblast form: (1) an inner *cytotrophoblast* (cellular trophoblast), and (2) an outer *syncytio-trophoblast* (syncytial trophoblast). The syncytiotrophoblast is a multinucleated mass without recognizable cell boundaries. The fingerlike processes of the syncytiotrophoblast produce substances that erode the maternal tissues (blood vessels, glands, and connective tissue). This enables the blastocyst to penetrate the endometrium. By the end of the first week, the blastocyst is superficially implanted in the compact layer of the endometrium and is deriving its nourishment from the maternal blood and eroded endometrial tissues (Fig. 3–4*B*).

As the blastocyst implants, early differentiation of the inner cell mass or embryoblast occurs. At about seven days, a flattened layer of cells called the *hypoblast* (primitive embryonic endoderm) appears on the free surface of the inner cell mass or embryoblast (Fig. 3–4*B*). The hypoblast later forms the roof of the primary yolk sac (see Fig. 4–1*C*).

Abnormal Zygotes, Blastocysts, and Spontaneous Abortion

About 15 per cent of zygotes die and blastocysts abort, but this estimate is undoubtedly low because the loss of zygotes and blastocysts during the first two weeks is thought to be high. *Implantation of the blastocyst is a critical period of development* that may fail to occur due to the inadequate production of progesterone and estrogen by the corpus luteum (see Fig. 2–7). The actual rate of early spontaneous abortion is unknown because the women are unaware that they are pregnant at this early stage. Clinicians occasionally see a patient who states that her last menstrual period was delayed by several days and that her menstrual flow was then unusually profuse. Such patients have very likely had an early spontaneous abortion; thus, the overall early spontaneous abortion rate is thought to be about 45 per cent.

Early spontaneous abortions occur for a variety of reasons, one being the presence of chromosomal abnormalities in the zygote. This early loss of embryos, once called *pregnancy wastage,* appears to be a means of disposing of abnormal pre-embryos that could not have developed normally, i.e., in many cases spontaneous abortion is a *natural screening process.*

SUMMARY

Fertilization of the ovum usually occurs in the ampulla of the uterine tube. The process is complete when the haploid male and female pronuclei of the sperm and ovum, respectively, fuse to form a **zygote** (Fig. 3–5). This diploid cell is the beginning of a new human being. **The results of fertilization** are: (1) restoration of the diploid number of chromosomes, (2) variation of the species, (3) determination of sex, and (4) initiation of cleavage of the zygote.

As it passes down the uterine tube, the zygote undergoes *cleavage* into a number of smaller cells called *blastomeres.* About three days after fertilization, a ball of 12 or more blastomeres, called a *morula,* enters the uterus. A fluid-filled cavity soon forms in the morula, converting it into a *blastocyst* consisting of the inner cell mass or embryoblast, the trophoblast, and the blastocyst cavity.

The zona pellucida disappears about five days after fertilization, and the trophoblast of the blastocyst contacts the epithelium of the uterus. The syncytiotrophoblastic cells of the trophoblast invade the endometrial epithelium and underlying endometrial tissues. By the end of the first week, the blastocyst is superficially implanted in the endometrium. The *hypoblast* (primitive embryonic endoderm) appears on the free surface of the inner cell mass or embryoblast.

Commonly Asked Questions

Women do not commonly become pregnant after they are 48 years old, whereas men can impregnate women when they are very old. Why is this? Is there an increased risk of the Down syndrome or other severe congenital anomalies in the child when the father is over 50?

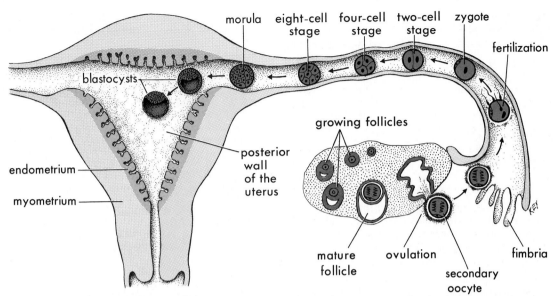

Figure 3–5. Diagrammatic summary of the ovarian cycle, fertilization, and human development during the first week. The secondary oocyte is released from the ovary at ovulation and passes to the ampulla of the uterine tube where it is met and fertilized by a sperm. The zygote divides repeatedly (i.e., undergoes cleavage) and becomes a morula as it passes down the uterine tube. The morula enters the uterus, develops a cavity, and becomes a blastocyst. The two blastocysts have been sectioned to show their internal structure. These stages are also illustrated in the timetable of development on page 2. By seven days the blastocyst begins to invade the endometrium, usually on the posterior wall of the uterus as shown in Figure 3–4B.

2. Are there contraceptive pills for men? If not, what is the reason?
3. Is a polar body ever fertilized? If so, does the fertilized polar body give rise to a viable embryo?
4. I have heard that a woman could have dissimilar twins resulting from one ovum being fertilized by a sperm from one man and another one being fertilized by a sperm from another man. Is this possible?
5. Are there differences in meaning between the terms impregnation, conception, and fertilization?
6. Do the terms cleavage and mitosis of the zygote mean the same thing?
7. How is the dividing zygote ("cleaved embryo") nourished during the first week? Do the blastomeres contain yolk?
8. Can one determine the sex of a dividing zygote ("early embryo") developing in vitro? If so, are there medical reasons for doing so?

The answers to these questions are given on page 327.

The answers to these questions are given on page 327.

REFERENCES

Carr DH, Gedeon M: Population cytogenetics of human abortuses. *In* Hook EB, Porter IH (eds): *Population Cytogenetics: Studies in Humans.* New York, Academic Press, 1977.

Chen CM, Sathananthan AH: Early penetration of human sperm through the vestments of human egg *in vitro. Arch Androl 16*:183, 1986.

Coulam CG: Epidemiology of recurrent spontaneous abortion. *Am J Reprod Immunol 26*:23, 1991.

Dooley M, Lim-Howe D, Savros M, Studd JWW: Early experience with gamete intrafallopian transfer (GIFT) and direct intraperitonal insemination (DIPT). *J Royal Soc Med 81*:637, 1988.

Edwards RG: Fertilization of human eggs in vitro: morals, ethics, and the law. *Q Rev Biol 49*:637, 1988.

Edwards RG: A decade of in vitro fertilization. *Research in Reprod 22*:1, 1990.

Fugger EP, Bustillo M, Dorfmann AD, Schulman JD:

Human preimplantation embryo cryopreservation: selected aspects. *Human Reprod 6*:131, 1991.

Gowchock S: Autoantibodies and fetal wastage. *Am J Reprod Immunol 26*:38, 1991.

Handyside AH, Kontogianni EH, Hardy K, Winston RML: Pregnancies from biopsied human preimplantation embryos sexed by Y-specific DNA amplification. *Nature 344*:768, 1990.

Harlap S: Gender of infants conceived on different days of the menstrual cycle. *New Eng J Med 300*:1445, 1979.

Hartshore GM, Elder K, Crow J, Dyson H, Edwards RG: The influence of in vitro development upon post-thaw survival and implantation of cryopreserved human blastocysts. *Human Reprod 6*:136, 1991.

Hertig AT, Adams EC, Menkin MC: Thirty-four fertilized human ova, good, bad and indifferent, recovered from 210 women of known fertility. *Pediatrics 23*:199, 1954.

Hertig AT, Adams EC, Mulligan WJ: On the preimplantation stages of the human ovum: A description of four normal and four abnormal specimens ranging from the second to the fifth day of development. *Contrib Embryol Carnegie Inst 35*:199, 1954.

Hertig AT, Rock J, Adams EC: A description of human ova within the first seventeen days of development. *Am J Anat 98*:435, 1956.

Moore KL, Persaud TVN: *The Developing Human: Clinically Oriented Embryology.* 5th ed. Philadelphia, WB Saunders, 1993.

Nahhas F, Barnea E: Human embryonic origin of early pregnancy factor before and after implantation. *Am J Reprod Immunol 22*:105, 1990.

O'Rahilly R, Müller F: *Developmental Stages in Human Embryos.* Washington, Carnegie Institute of Washington, 1987.

Oura C, Toshimori K: Ultrastructural studies on the fertilization of mammalian gametes. *Int Rev Cytol 122*:105, 1990.

Sidhu KS, Guraya SS: Current concepts in gamete receptors for fertilization in mammals. *In Rev Cytol 127*:253, 1991.

Steinkampf MP, Kretzer PA, McElroy E, Conway-Myers BA: A simplified approach to in vitro fertilization. *J Reprod Med 37*:253, 1991.

Talbot P: Sperm penetration through oocyte investments in mammals. *Am J Anat 174*:331, 1985.

Thompson MW, McInnes RR, Willard HF: *Thompson & Thompson Genetics in Medicine.* 5th ed. Philadelphia, WB Saunders, 1991.

Wassarman PM: The biology and chemistry of fertilization. *Science 235*:553, 1987.

Wood C, Trouson A (eds): *Clinical In Vitro Fertilization.* 2nd ed. New York, Springer-Verlag, 1989.

4

THE SECOND WEEK OF HUMAN DEVELOPMENT

FORMATION OF THE BILAMINAR EMBRYONIC DISC

Implantation or embedding of the blastocyst in the endometrium is completed during the second week of the pre-embryonic period (Fig. 4–1). As this important process takes place, changes occur in the inner cell mass or embryoblast that produce a thick, two-layered plate called the **embryonic disc** that will differentiate into the embryo. The amniotic cavity, amnion, yolk sac, connecting stalk, and chorionic sac also develop during the second week.

COMPLETION OF IMPLANTATION AND EARLY EMBRYONIC DEVELOPMENT

Implantation of the blastocyst begins at the end of the first week (see Fig. 3–4) and is completed by the end of the second week (Fig. 4–4B). The endometrium of the uterus is in the secretory phase at the time of implantation (see Fig. 2–7). The erosive *syncytiotrophoblast* of the blastocyst continues to invade the endometrium containing connective tissue, capillaries, and glands. As this occurs, the blastocyst slowly embeds itself in the endometrium.

As more trophoblast contacts the endometrium, it differentiates into two layers (Fig. 4–1A). The *cytotrophoblast* is mitotically active and forms new cells that migrate into the *syncy-tiotrophoblast*. The cells lose their cell membranes and form a thick, protoplasmic mass (i.e., a syncytium). The syncytiotrophoblast at the embryonic pole (adjacent to the embryonic disc) soon forms a thick, multinucleated layer (Fig. 4–1B). Isolated spaces, or *lacunae*, appear in the syncytiotrophoblast, which soon become filled with a mixture of blood from ruptured maternal capillaries and secretions from eroded endometrial glands (Fig. 4–1C). This nutritive fluid, or *embryotroph*, passes to the embryonic disc by diffusion.

The syncytiotrophoblast begins to produce a hormone, *human chorionic gonadotrophin* (hCG), which enters the maternal blood and forms the basis for **pregnancy tests** (Filly, 1988). Enough hCG is produced by the syncytiotrophoblast at the end of the second week to give a positive pregnancy test even though the woman is probably unaware she is pregnant. See also the discussion of the *early pregnancy factor* (EPF) on page 29.

Formation of the Amniotic Cavity, Amnion, Bilaminar Embryonic Disc, and Yolk Sac

As implantation progresses, a small space appears between the inner cell mass, or embryoblast, and the invading trophoblast. This space is the primordium of the *amniotic cavity*

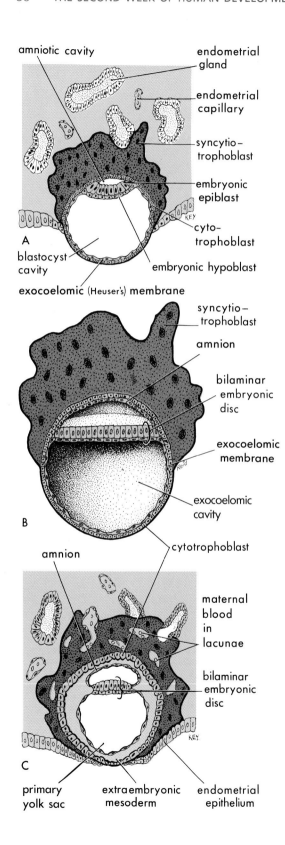

Figure 4–1. Drawings illustrating the implantation of a blastocyst into the endometrium. The size of the conceptus is about 0.1 mm. *A,* Drawing of a section through a blastocyst partially implanted in the endometrium (about eight days). Note the slitlike amniotic cavity. *B,* An enlarged, three-dimensional sketch of a slightly older blastocyst after removal from the endometrium. Note the extensive syncytiotrophoblast at the embryonic pole and the much larger amniotic cavity. *C,* Drawing of a section through a blastocyst of about nine days implanted in the endometrium. (Based on Hertig and Rock, 1945.) Note the lacunae (L. *lacus,* lake) appearing in the syncytiotrophoblast. These lacunae soon communicate with the endometrial blood vessels (Fig. 4–2B).

(Fig. 4–1A). As the amniotic cavity forms, changes occur in the inner cell mass which result in the formation of a flattened, essentially circular **embryonic disc**. It consists of two layers: (1) the *epiblast*, consisting of high columnar cells related to the amniotic cavity, and (2) the *hypoblast*, consisting of small cuboidal cells related to the blastocyst cavity.

As the amniotic cavity enlarges, a thin membrane called the **amnion** forms from *amnioblasts* that differentiate from the epiblast. The floor of the amniotic cavity is formed by the epiblast of the embryonic disc and is continuous peripherally with the amnion (Fig. 4–1B and C). Concurrently, other cells migrate from the hypoblast and form a thin, *exocoelomic membrane*, which encloses the exocoelomic cavity to form the primary yolk sac (primitive yolk sac). The embryonic disc (pre-embryo) now lies between the amniotic cavity and the primary yolk sac (Fig. 4–1C). The human yolk sac contains no yolk, but it is an essential structure for the early formation of blood (p. 55). Some cells, probably from the hypoblast, give rise to *extraembryonic mesoderm*. It forms a layer of loosely arranged mesenchymal tissue (connective tissue) around the amnion and primary yolk sac.

The ten-day human conceptus (embryo and its membranes) is completely embedded in the endometrium (Fig. 4–2). For a day or so, a small defect in the endometrial epithelium is indicated by a *closing plug* consisting of clotted blood and cellular debris (Figs. 4–2 and 4–3). By the eleventh day spaces are visible within the extraembryonic mesoderm; these spaces rapidly fuse to form a large cavity called the *extraembryonic coelom* (Figs. 4–2B, 4–3B, and 4–4). By day 13 the endometrial epithelium covers over the blastocyst, producing a minute, "wartlike" elevation of the endometrial surface (Fig. 4–3A).

By this time, adjacent syncytiotrophoblastic lacunae have fused to form intercommunicating **lacunar networks** (Figs. 4–2B and 4–3), the primordium of the *intervillous space of the placenta* (see Fig. 5–9). The endometrial capillaries around the implanted pre-embryo have become congested and dilated to form *sinusoids*, and some of them have been eroded by the syncytiotrophoblast. Maternal blood now seeps into the lacunar networks and begins to flow slowly through the lacunar networks, establishing a *primitive uteroplacental circulation*.

As maternal blood flows into the lacunae, its nutritive substances become available to the embryo. As both arterial and venous branches of

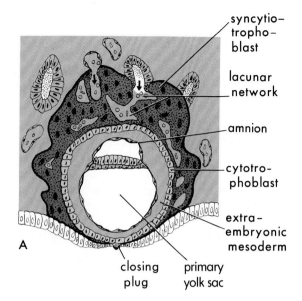

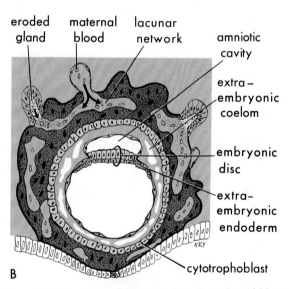

Figure 4–2. Drawings of sections through implanted blastocysts. *A*, 10 days, *B*, 12 days. (Based on Hertig and Rock, 1941.) This stage of development is characterized by the intercommunication of the lacunae that are filled with maternal blood. In *B*, note that large cavities have appeared in the extraembryonic mesoderm, forming the primordium of the extraembryonic coelom. Also note that extraembryonic endodermal cells have begun to form on the inside of the primary yolk sac.

the maternal blood vessels communicate with the lacunae, blood circulates through them. Oxygenated blood and nutrients pass into the lacunae from the *spiral arteries*, and deoxygenated blood and waste products are removed from them via the veins of the uterus (see Fig. 2–2B);

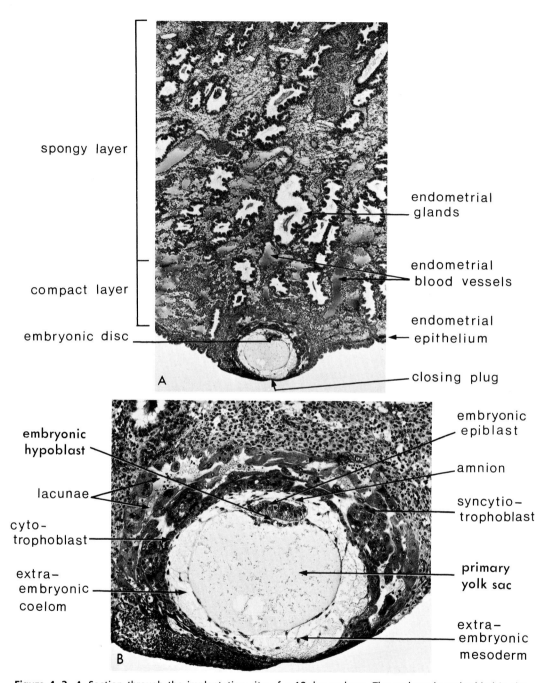

spongy layer

compact layer

embryonic disc

endometrial glands

endometrial blood vessels

endometrial epithelium

closing plug

A

embryonic hypoblast

lacunae

cyto-trophoblast

extra-embryonic coelom

embryonic epiblast

amnion

syncytio-trophoblast

primary yolk sac

extra-embryonic mesoderm

B

Figure 4–3. *A*, Section through the implantation site of a 12-day embryo. The embryo is embedded in the compact layer of the endometrium (× 30). *B*, Higher magnification of the conceptus and surrounding endometrium (× 100). (From Hertig AT, Rock J: *Contr Embryol Carneg Instn, Wash 29:*127, 1941. Courtesy of the Carnegie Institution of Washington.)

hence, the maternal blood supplies a rich source of materials for *embryonic nutrition* and serves as a disposal site for the embryo's waste products.

Development of the Chorionic Sac

By the end of the second week, *primary chorionic villi* (fingerlike projections of the chorion) have also formed (Figs. 4–4 and 4–5). These villi later differentiate into the vascularized chorionic villi of the placenta (see Fig. 5–9). The isolated coelomic spaces in the extraembryonic mesoderm have now fused to form a single, large, *extraembryonic coelom* (Fig. 4–4A and B). This fluid-filled cavity surrounds the amnion and yolk sac, except where the amnion is attached to the chorion by the *connecting stalk* (Fig. 4–4B). As the extraembryonic coelom forms, the primitive yolk sac decreases in size, resulting in a smaller, **secondary yolk sac** (Fig. 4–4B).

The extraembryonic coelom splits the extraembryonic mesoderm into two layers (Fig. 4–4B): (1) the *extraembryonic somatic mesoderm* lines the trophoblast and covers the amnion, and (2) the *extraembryonic splanchnic mesoderm* covers the yolk sac.[1] The extraembryonic somatic mesoderm and the two layers of trophoblast constitute the **chorion** (Fig. 4–5B). The chorion forms the *wall of the chorionic sac*, within which the embryo and its attached amniotic and yolk sacs are suspended by the *connecting stalk*. The extraembryonic coelom is now called the *chorionic cavity.*[2]

IMPLANTATION SITES OF THE BLASTOCYST

Implantation of a blastocyst usually occurs in the endometrium. Implantation of a blastocyst outside the uterus *(ectopic implantation)* gives rise to serious complications (Figs. 4–6 to 4–8).

Intrauterine Implantation Sites

The blastocyst usually implants in the midportion of the body of the uterus (Fig. 4–6), slightly more frequently on its posterior wall than on its anterior wall. Implantation of the blastocyst in the inferior segment of the uterus near the *internal ostium* (internal orifice of the cervix) results in *placenta previa*, a placenta that partially or completely covers the ostium (Fig. 4–6). This condition may cause bleeding during pregnancy and complications during delivery of the baby.

Extrauterine Implantation Sites

Implantation may occur *outside the cavity of the uterus* (Figs. 4–6 to 4–8). These are **ectopic pregnancies.** More than 95 *per cent of ectopic implantations occur in the uterine tube.* Most tubal pregnancies are in the ampulla or isthmus (see Figs. 2–2A, 4–6, and 4–8). The incidence of tubal pregnancy varies from 1 in 80 to 1 in 250 pregnancies, depending on the socioeconomic level of the population studied. *Endovaginal (transvaginal) sonography* is very helpful in detecting ectopic pregnancies (Ash et al., 1991).

There are several causes of ectopic tubal pregnancy, but they are usually related to factors that delay or prevent transport of the dividing zygote to the uterus (e.g., alterations resulting from *pelvic inflammatory disease*). In some cases the blockage results from a previous tubal infection that has damaged the mucosa, causing adhesions between its folds. Ectopic tubal pregnancies usually result in rupture of the uterine tube and hemorrhage into the peritoneal cavity during the first eight weeks followed by death of the embryo. *Tubal rupture and hemorrhage* constitute a threat to the mother's life and are therefore of major clinical importance. The affected tube and the conceptus are removed (Figs. 4–7 and 4–8).

Cervical implantations of the blastocyst are uncommon (Fig. 4–6). Some of these pregnancies are not recognized because the conceptus is expelled (spontaneously aborted) early in the gestation. In other cases, the placenta becomes firmly attached to the fibrous and muscular parts of the cervix, often resulting in bleeding and subsequent surgical intervention, e.g., *hysterectomy* (excision of the uterus).

Blastocysts expelled from the uterine tube ("early spontaneous abortions") may implant in the ovary (Fig. 4–6H) or in the abdominal cavity (Fig. 4–6G), but ovarian and abdominal pregnancies are extremely rare. In exceptional cases an *abdominal pregnancy* may progress to full term and the fetus may be delivered alive.

---

[1] *Splanchnic* refers to the viscera (Gr. *splanchnon*, viscus). Part of the yolk sac is incorporated into embryo (see Fig. 6–1) and forms viscera (plural of viscus). Knowing this helps one remember that splanchnic mesoderm surrounds viscera (e.g., the stomach and intestines).

[2] The amniotic sac (with the embryonic epiblast forming its "floor") and the yolk sac (with the embryonic hypoblast forming its "roof") are analogous to two balloons pressed together to form the bilaminar embryonic disc, which is suspended by a cord (the connecting stalk) from the inside of a larger balloon (the chorionic sac).

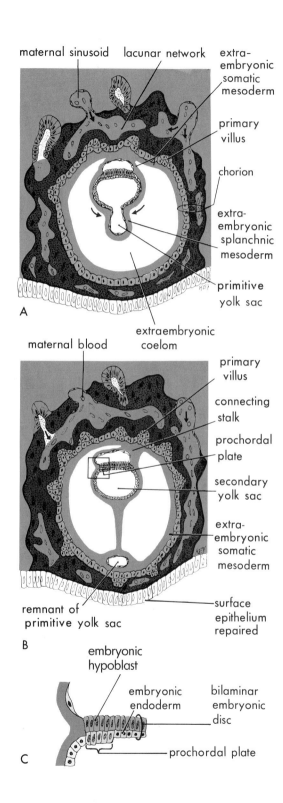

maternal sinusoid   lacunar network   extra-embryonic somatic mesoderm

primary villus

chorion

extra-embryonic splanchnic mesoderm

primitive yolk sac

A

extraembryonic coelom

maternal blood

primary villus

connecting stalk

prochordal plate

secondary yolk sac

extra-embryonic somatic mesoderm

remnant of primitive yolk sac

surface epithelium repaired

B

embryonic hypoblast

embryonic endoderm

bilaminar embryonic disc

prochordal plate

C

Figure 4–4. Drawings of sections through implanted human embryos. Note that (1) the defect in the surface epithelium of the endometrium has disappeared; (2) a small secondary yolk sac has formed inside the primary yolk sac as it is "pinched off;" (3) a large cavity, the extraembryonic coelom, now surrounds the yolk sac and amnion, except where the amnion is attached to the chorion by the connecting stalk; and (4) the extraembryonic coelom splits the extraembryonic mesoderm into two layers: extraembryonic somatic mesoderm lining the trophoblast and covering the amnion, and extraembryonic splanchnic mesoderm around the yolk sac. The trophoblast and extraembryonic somatic mesoderm together form the chorion, which eventually gives rise to the fetal part of the placenta. A, 13 days, illustrating the decrease in relative size of the primary yolk sac and the early appearance of primary chorionic villi at the embryonic pole. B, 14 days, showing the newly formed secondary yolk sac and the location of the prochordal plate (future site of mouth) in its roof. C, Detail of the prochordal plate area outlined in B.

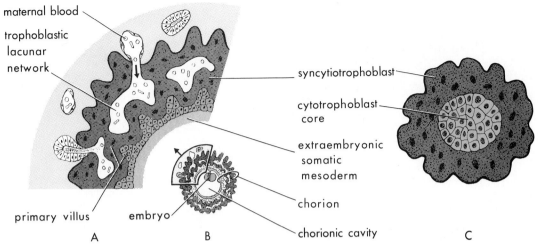

Figure 4–5. *A,* Detail of the section (outlined in *B*) of the wall of the chorionic sac. *B,* Sketch of a 14-day conceptus to illustrate its chorionic sac and the shaggy appearance of the primary villi (× 6). *C,* Drawing of a transverse section through a primary chorionic villus (× 300).

An abdominal pregnancy usually creates a serious condition because the placenta attaches to abdominal structures (e.g., the mesentery and spleen) and causes considerable postpartum (after childbirth) bleeding.

Inhibition of Implantation

The administration of relatively large doses of estrogen ("morning-after" pills) for several days after sexual intercourse usually interrupts pregnancy by preventing implantation of the blastocyst. Normally the endometrium progresses to the secretory phase of the menstrual cycle as the zygote forms, undergoes cleavage, and the blastocyst enters the uterus. The large amount of estrogen, usually administered as the synthetic estrogen *diethylstilbestrol* (DES), disturbs the normal balance between estrogen and

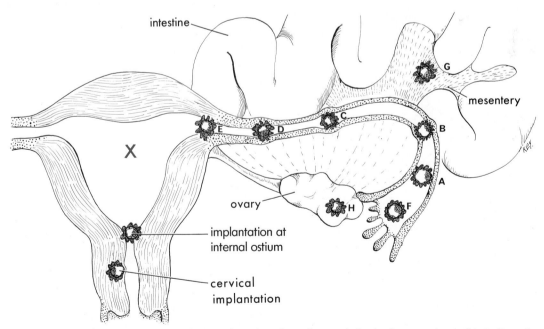

Figure 4–6. Drawing illustrating various implantation sites; the usual site in the posterior wall is indicated by an X. The approximate order of frequency of ectopic implantations is indicated alphabetically. *A* to *F,* Tubal pregnancies. *G,* Abdominal pregnancy. *H,* Ovarian pregnancy.

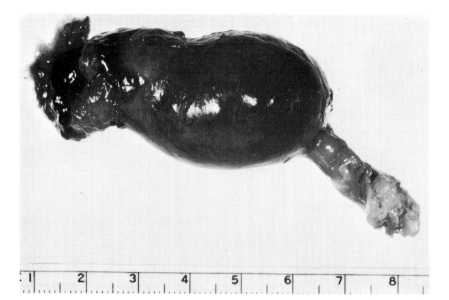

Figure 4–7. Photograph showing the gross appearance of an unruptured ectopic pregnancy located in the ampulla of a uterine tube that was surgically removed. When the chorionic sac distends the tube, partial separation of the placenta and rupture of the tube often occur. Spurts of blood escape from the tube and its infundibulum (shown at the left). Tubal rupture and the associated hemorrhage constitute a threat to the mother's life. (From Page EW, Villee CA, Villee DB: *Human Reproduction. Essentials of Reproductive and Perinatal Medicine.* 3rd ed. Philadelphia, WB Saunders, 1981.)

progesterone that is necessary for preparation of the endometrium for implantation of the blastocyst (see Fig. 2–7). When the secretory phase does not occur normally, implantation cannot take place and the blastocyst soon dies.

This hormone treatment results in the death of the blastocyst rather than in prevention of its formation; therefore, use of this method is largely restricted to special cases in which impregnation is not desired (e.g., after a sexual assault). Another reason this method is not routinely used for birth control is that the treatment is associated with a relatively high frequency of nausea, vomiting, and other adverse

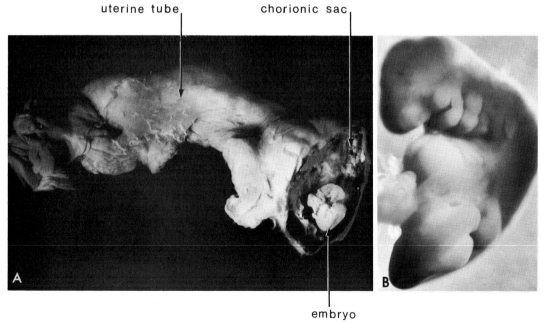

Figure 4–8. Photograph of a tubal pregnancy. *A,* The uterine tube has been sectioned to show the conceptus implanted in the mucous membrane (× 3). *B,* Enlarged photograph of the normal-appearing, four-week embryo (× 13). Ectopic pregnancies occur most often in the ampulla of the uterine tube. This serious condition may be caused by a delay in the passage of the dividing zygote along the tube. Ectopic tubal pregnancy results in death of the embryo and usually sudden massive bleeding from the ruptured tube. (Photographed by Professor Jean Hay, Department of Anatomy, University of Manitoba.)

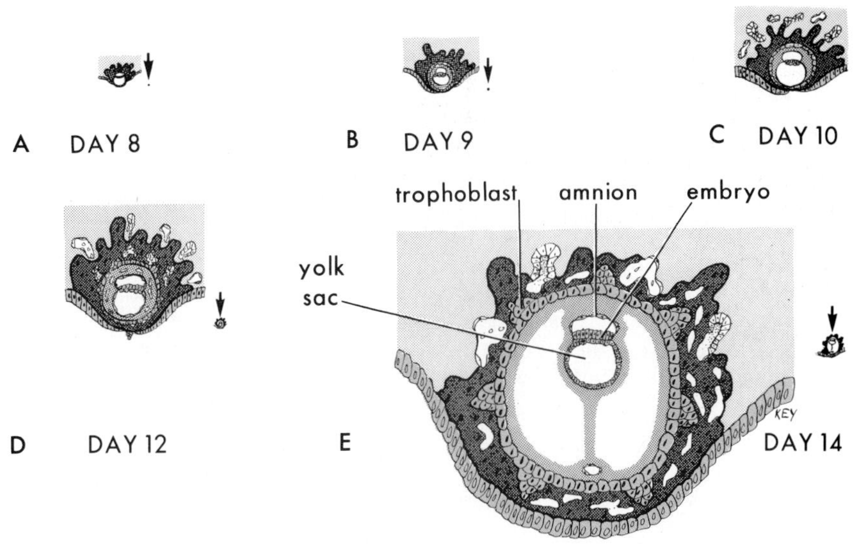

Figure 4–9. Drawings of sections of human blastocysts during the second week, illustrating the rapid expansion of the trophoblast and the relatively minute size of the embryos (× 25). The sketches indicated by the arrows show the actual size of the blastocysts. Obviously, an aborted conceptus would be difficult to detect in the menstrual fluid.

A   DAY 8

B   DAY 9

C   DAY 10

D   DAY 12

E   DAY 14

effects; consequently, contraception is preferable to contraimplantation. Various *intrauterine devices* (IUDs) also prevent implantation of the blastocyst, presumably by inducing a foreign-body response in the endometrium that inhibits implantation.

SPONTANEOUS ABORTION OF EARLY EMBRYOS

Abortion is usually defined as the termination of a pregnancy before 20 weeks' gestation, i.e., prior to the period of viability of an embryo or fetus (i.e., before it can survive when separated from its mother). *Almost all abortions that occur during the first three weeks occur spontaneously,* i.e., they are not induced. The frequency of early abortions is difficult to establish because they often occur before the woman is aware she is pregnant. An abortion that occurs a few days after the first missed menstrual period is very likely to be mistaken for a delayed menstruation. Detection of the conceptus in the menses

(menstrual blood) is very difficult because of its small size (Fig. 4–9).

The examination of most spontaneous abortions reveals abnormal conceptuses. A study of 34 early embryos recovered from women of known fertility revealed that 10 of them were so abnormal they probably would have aborted by the end of the second week (Hertig and Rock, 1956). *The incidence of chromosome abnormalities in early spontaneous abortions is high.* Summarizing the data of several studies, it has been estimated that about 50 per cent of all known spontaneous abortions result from chromosomal abnormalities. The higher incidence of early abortions in older women probably results from the increasing frequency of *nondisjunction* during oogenesis (see Chapters 2 and 9).

It has been estimated that from one third to one half of all zygotes never become blastocysts and implant. Failure of blastocysts to implant may result from a poorly developed endometrium, but in many cases there are probably lethal chromosomal abnormalities in the zygote (e.g., *monosomy* [p. 120]).

SUMMARY

Rapid proliferation of the trophoblast occurs during the second week (Fig. 4–9). The trophoblast consists of an internal cellular layer known as the *cytotrophoblast* and an external syncytial layer known as the *syncytiotrophoblast.* Lacunae develop in the syncytiotrophoblast and fuse to form *lacunar*

networks. The syncytiotrophoblast erodes maternal blood vessels, and blood seeps into the networks, forming a primitive *uteroplacental circulation.* Primary chorionic villi form on the external surface of the chorionic sac. Implantation is complete when the conceptus is completely embedded in the endometrium and the surface epithelium has grown over the embedded blastocyst.

Concurrently, *extraembryonic mesoderm* forms (probably arising from the hypoblast). This reduces the relative size of the blastocyst cavity and forms a *primary yolk sac*. As the extraembryonic coelom forms from spaces in the extraembryonic mesoderm, the primary yolk sac becomes smaller and is called the *secondary yolk sac*. The *amniotic cavity* appears as a slitlike space between the trophoblast and the inner cell mass, and the *amnion* forms from cells that arise from the cytotrophoblast.

Early in the second week, the inner cell mass or embryoblast differentiates into a **bilaminar embryonic disc** consisting of a layer of embryonic *epiblast* and a layer of embryonic *hypoblast*. At the end of the second week, a localized thickening of the hypoblast called the *prochordal plate* indicates the site of the future mouth. It is also an important organizer of the head region.

Commonly Asked Questions

1. What is meant by the term "implantation bleeding?" Is this menses (menstrual fluid)?
2. Can drugs taken during the first two weeks of pregnancy cause congenital anomalies of the embryo?
3. Recently I heard the term "interception" used in reference to birth control. What does it mean? Does this method prevent conception?
4. Can an ectopic pregnancy occur in a woman who has an intrauterine device (IUD)?
5. Can a blastocyst that implants in the abdomen *(abdominal pregnancy)* develop into a living, full-term fetus? How would it be delivered?

The answers to these questions are given on page 328.

REFERENCES

Alpin JD: Implantation, trophoblast differentiation and hemochorial placentation: mechanistic evidence *in vivo* and *in vitro*. *J Cell Sci* 99:681, 1991.

Ash KM, Lyons ES, Levi CS, Lindsay DJ: Endovaginal sonographic diagnosis of ectopic twin gestation. *J Ultrasound Med* 10:497, 1991.

Blandau RJ (ed): *The Biology of the Blastocyst*. Chicago, University of Chicago Press, 1971.

Chapman MG, Grudzinskas JG, Chard T (eds): *Implantation. Biological and Clinical Aspects*. Berlin, Springer-Verlag, 1988.

Coulam CB, Faulk WP, McIntyre JA: Spontaneous and recurrent abortions. *In* Quilligan EJ, Zuspan FP (eds): *Current Therapy in Obstetrics and Gynecology*, vol 3. Philadelphia, WB Saunders, 1990.

Enders AC, King BF: Formation and differentiation of extraembryonic mesoderm in the rhesus monkey. *Am J Anat* 181:327, 1988.

Filly RA: Ectopic pregnancy. *In* Callen PW (ed): *Ultrasonography in Obstetrics and Gynecology*, 2nd ed. Philadelphia, WB Saunders, 1988.

Hertig AT, Rock J: Two human ova of the pre-villous stage, having a developmental age of about eleven and twelve days respectively. *Contrib Embryol Carnegie Inst* 29:127, 1941.

Hertig AT, Rock J: Two human ova of the pre-villous stage, having a developmental age of about seven and nine days respectively. *Contrib Embryol Carnegie Inst* 29:127, 1945.

Hertig AT, Rock J: A description of 34 human ova within the first seventeen days of development. *Am J Anat* 98:435, 1956.

Li TC, Tristram A, Hill AS, Cooke ID: A review of 254 ectopic pregnancies in a teaching hospital in the Trent region, 1977–1990. *Human Reprod* 6:1002, 1991.

Lindenberg G, Hyttel P, Sjogren A, Greve T: A comparative study of attachment of human, bovine and mouse blastocysts to uterine epithelial monolayer. *Human Reprod* 4:446, 1989.

Moore KL, Persaud TVN: *The Developing Human: Clinically Oriented Embryology*, 5th ed. Philadelphia, WB Saunders, 1993.

Nahhas F, Barnea E: Human embryonic origin of early pregnancy factor before and after implantation. *Am J Reprod Immunol* 22:105, 1990.

Page EW, Villee CA, Villee DB: *Human Reproduction: Essentials of Reproductive and Perinatal Medicine*, 3rd ed. Philadelphia, WB Saunders, 1981.

Stander RW: Abdominal pregnancy. *Clin Obstet Gynecol* 5:1065, 1962.

Thom DH, Nelson LM, Vaughan TL: Spontaneous abortion and subsequent adverse birth outcomes. *Am J Obstet and Gynecol* 166:111, 1992.

5

THE THIRD WEEK OF HUMAN DEVELOPMENT

FORMATION OF THE TRILAMINAR EMBRYO

This is *the beginning of the embryonic period* (third to eighth weeks) during which rapid development of the embryo occurs from the bilaminar embryonic disc that formed during the second week. The third week follows the first missed menstrual period (see the *Timetable of Human Prenatal Development*, Fig. 1–1), and is characterized by the formation of the primitive streak, notochord, and *three germ layers* from which all embryonic tissues and organs develop.

Cessation of menstruation is usually the first sign that a woman may be pregnant. Relatively simple and rapid tests are now available for detecting pregnancy as early as the second week. These tests depend on the presence of an *early pregnancy factor* (EPF) in the maternal serum (Nahhas and Barnea, 1990) and *human chorionic gonadotropin* (hCG), a hormone produced by the syncytiotrophoblast and excreted in the mother's urine (see Chapter 8). A normal pregnancy can also be confirmed about three weeks after conception using *ultrasonography* (i.e., approximately five weeks after the last normal menstrual period [LNMP]).

Bleeding at the expected time of menstruation does not rule out pregnancy because, in some cases, there may be light bleeding from the implantation site of the blastocyst. This *implantation bleeding* is the result of leakage of blood into the uterine cavity from disrupted blood vessels around the implanted blastocyst. When such bleeding is interpreted as menstruation, an error occurs in determining the expected delivery date (EDD) of the baby.

The third week is important because three germ layers develop (primordia of the tissues and organs) and three important structures form (primitive streak, notochord, and neural tube).

GASTRULATION: FORMATION OF THE GERM LAYERS

The process by which the inner cell mass (embryoblast) is converted into a trilaminar embryonic disc is called gastrulation. The process begins at the end of the first week with the formation of the *hypoblast* (see Fig. 3–4). It continues during the second week with the formation of the *epiblast* (see Figs. 4–1 and 4–4), and is completed during the third week with the formation of three *primary germ layers:* ectoderm, mesoderm, and endoderm (Fig. 5–1). As development proceeds these layers give rise to the tissues and organs of the embryo (see Fig. 6–2).

The Primitive Streak

At the beginning of the third week, a thick linear band of embryonic epiblast known as the *primitive streak* appears caudally in the median

45

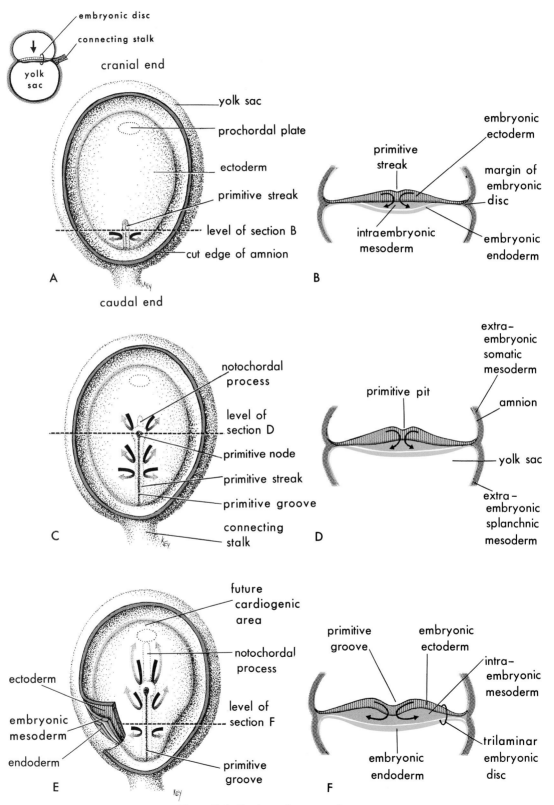

Figure 5-1. *See legend on opposite page*

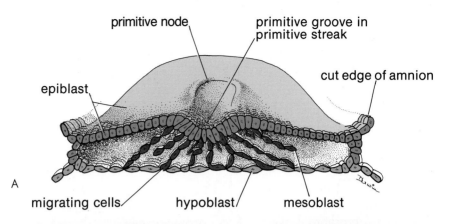

primitive node   primitive groove in
                  primitive streak

epiblast   cut edge of amnion

A

migrating cells   hypoblast   mesoblast

Figure 5–2. *A,* Drawing of the cranial half of the embryonic disc during the third week. The disc has been cut transversely to show the migration of mesenchymal cells from the primitive streak. This illustration also indicates that most of the definitive embryonic endoderm may also arise from the epiblast. Presumably, most hypoblastic cells are displaced to extraembryonic regions. *B,* Photograph of a human embryo of about 16 days. The primitive streak is clearly visible (Courtesy of Dr. Kohei Shiota, Professor of Anatomy and Chairman, Faculty of Medicine, Kyoto University, Kyoto, Japan).

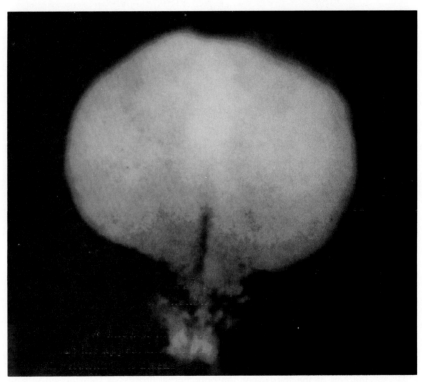

B

Figure 5–1. Drawings illustrating formation of the trilaminar embryonic disc (three-layered embryo). The small sketch at the upper left is for orientation; the arrow indicates the dorsal aspect of the embryonic disc shown in *A.* The arrows in all other drawings indicate migration of mesenchymal cells between the ectoderm and endoderm. *A, C,* and *E,* Dorsal views of the embryonic disc early in the third week, exposed by removal of the amnion. *B, D* and *F,* Transverse sections through the embryonic disc at the levels indicated. *The intraembryonic mesoderm forms as follows:* Cells of the epiblast move medially to the primitive streak and enter the primitive groove and pit. These cells lose their attachment to the epiblast and migrate between the epiblast and the hypoblast. These *mesoblastic cells* pass laterally and form a network of cells called the *mesoblast* (see Fig. 5–2). Some mesoblastic cells become organized into a layer called the intraembryonic mesoderm.

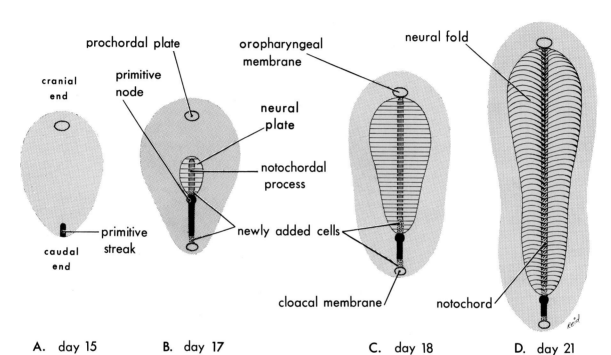

A. day 15　　　　**B. day 17**　　　　　　**C. day 18**　　　　**D. day 21**

Figure 5–3. Sketches of dorsal views of the embryonic disc, showing how it lengthens and changes shape during the third week. The primitive streak lengthens by addition of cells to its caudal end; the notochordal process lengthens by migration of cells from the primitive node. The notochordal process and adjacent mesoderm induce the overlying embryonic ectoderm to form the neural plate, the primordium of the central nervous system (CNS). Observe that, as the notochordal process elongates, the primitive streak shortens. At the end of the third week the notochordal process is transformed into the notochord (see Figs. 5–4 and 5–5). Note that the embryonic disc is originally egg-shaped but becomes pear-shaped and then slipperlike as the notochord develops.

plane of the dorsal aspect of the embryonic disc (Figs. 5–1 and 5–2). The primitive streak results from the "heaping up" of epiblastic cells that proliferate and migrate to the center of the embryonic disc. As the primitive streak elongates by addition of cells to its caudal end (Fig. 5–3), its cranial end enlarges to form a *primitive node* (knot).

The primitive streak gives rise to mesenchymal cells, which form loose embryonic connective tissue called *mesenchyme* or mesoblast (Fig. 5–2). The mesenchyme spreads laterally and cranially from the primitive streak, and some of it forms a layer between the epiblast and hypoblast known as the *intraembryonic mesoderm* (Fig. 5–1B). Some cells from the primitive streak invade the hypoblast and laterally displace most, if not all, of the hypoblastic cells. This newly formed germ layer is known as the intraembryonic or *embryonic endoderm.* The cells that remain in the epiblast form the intraembryonic or *embryonic ectoderm.*

Formation of the intraembryonic mesoderm converts the bilaminar embryonic disc into a trilaminar (three-layered) embryonic disc (Fig. 5–1E and F). The *embryonic ectoderm* gives rise to the epidermis and the nervous system (see Fig. 6–2). The *embryonic endoderm* forms the linings of the digestive and respiratory tracts. The *embryonic mesoderm* gives rise to muscle, connective tissues, cartilage, bone, and blood vessels.

FATE OF THE PRIMITIVE STREAK. The primitive streak continues to form mesenchyme until about the end of the fourth week; thereafter, mesenchyme production slows down. The primitive streak diminishes in relative size and becomes an insignificant structure in the sacrococcygeal region of the embryo (Fig. 5–3D). It normally undergoes degenerative changes and disappears, but primitive streak remnants may persist and give rise to a large tumor known as a *sacrococcygeal teratoma.* As primitive streak cells are pleuripotent, teratomas contain various types of tissue.

The Notochordal Process and Notochord

Cells migrate cranially from the primitive node of the primitive streak and form a median cellular cord known as the *notochordal process* (Figs. 5–1C and D and 5–3B). This cord grows cranially between the ectoderm and endoderm until it reaches the *prochordal plate,* a small circular area which indicates the *future site of the mouth.* The notochordal process can extend no further because the prochordal plate is firmly attached to the overlying ectoderm, forming the *oropharyngeal membrane* (Figs. 5–3C and 5–4C). Caudal to the primitive streak is another circular area known as the *cloacal membrane.* The embryonic disc remains bilaminar here also because the ectoderm and endoderm are fused (Figs. 5–3C and 5–4E). The cloacal membrane indicates the *future site of the anus.*

The **notochord** is a cellular rod that develops by transformation of the *notochordal process* (Fig. 5–4).[1] The notochord defines the *primitive axis of the embryo* and gives it some rigidity. In the lower chordate, *Amphioxus,* the notochord forms the skeleton of the adult animal. This cellular rod forms the mesenchymal axial skeleton in the human embryo and the basis of the adult bony *axial skeleton* (vertebral column, ribs, sternum, and skull). The notochord is the structure around which the vertebral column forms (see Chapter 16). It degenerates and disappears where it is surrounded by the vertebral bodies, but persists as the *nucleus pulposus* of each intervertebral disc.

The developing notochord induces the overlying ectoderm to form the **neural plate,** the primordium of the central nervous system (brain and spinal cord). By the end of the third week, the notochord is almost completely formed and extends cranially from the *oropharyngeal membrane* (derivative of the prochordal plate and associated ectoderm) to the primitive node caudally (Fig. 5–3C).

NEURULATION

The process of formation of the neural plate, the neural folds, and their closure to form the neural tube is called neurulation (Figs. 5–3 to 5–6). This process is completed by the end of the fourth week.

The Neural Plate

As the notochord develops, the embryonic ectoderm over it thickens to form the *neural plate* (Figs. 5–3, 5–4, and 5–6A). The neural plate gives rise to the *central nervous system* (see

---

[1] For details of notochord formation, see Moore and Persaud (1993).

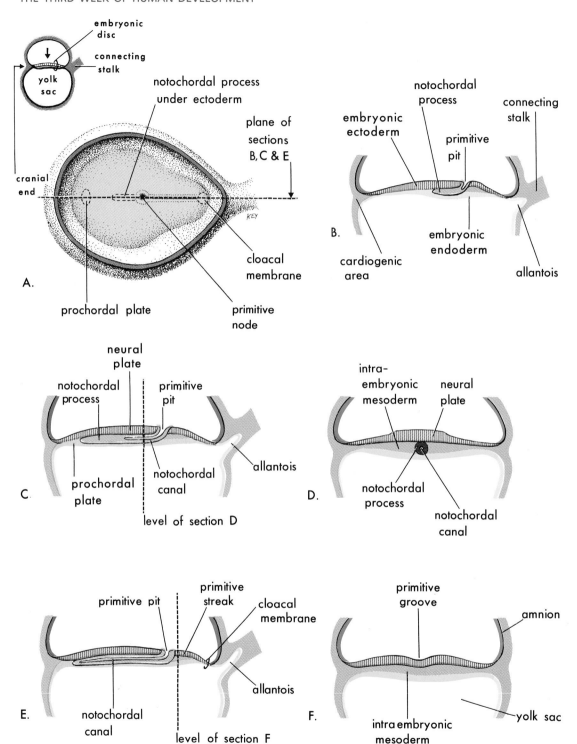

Figure 5–4. Drawings illustrating early stages of notochord development. The small sketch at the upper left is for orientation; the short arrow indicates the dorsal aspect of the embryonic disc. *A*, Dorsal view of the embryonic disc (about 16 days) exposed by removal of the amnion. The notochordal process is shown as if it were visible through the embryonic ectoderm. *B*, *C*, and *E*, Median sections, at the plane shown in *A*, illustrating successive stages in the development of the notochordal process and canal. Stages shown in *C* and *E* occur at about 18 days. *D* and *F*, Transverse sections through the embryonic disc at the levels shown.

Chapter 17). It first appears close to the primitive node; but, as the notochordal process elongates, the neural plate broadens cranially and eventually extends as far as the oropharyngeal membrane (Fig. 5–3C). On about the 18th day, the neural plate invaginates along its central axis to form a *neural groove* with neural folds on each side (Figs. 5–3D, 5–5, and 5–6).

The Neural Tube

By the end of the third week, the *neural folds* near the middle of the embryo have moved together and fused, converting the neural plate into a *neural tube* (Figs. 5–5F and 5–6D). Formation of this tube begins in the middle of the embryo and progresses toward the cranial and caudal ends. Progression of closure is more rapid toward the cranial end. Closure of the ends of the neural tube occurs by the end of the fourth week (see Chapter 6). The neural tube differentiates into the brain and spinal cord (see Chapter 17).

The Neural Crest

As the neural folds fuse to form the neural tube, some neuroectodermal cells lying along the crest of each fold lose their epithelial affinities and attachments to the neighboring cells. As the neural tube separates from the surface ectoderm (Fig. 5–6C and D), these neuroectodermal cells, called *neural crest cells,* migrate to the sides of the neural tube. Initially they form an irregular flattened mass called the *neural crest* (Fig. 5–6D) between the neural tube and the overlying surface ectoderm. The neural crest soon separates into right and left parts that migrate to the dorsolateral aspects of the neural tube where they give rise to the *sensory ganglia* of the spinal and cranial nerves. Many neural crest cells begin to migrate in lateral and ventral directions and disperse. Although these cells are difficult to identify, special tracer techniques have revealed that they disseminate widely and have important derivatives.

DERIVATIVES OF THE NEURAL CREST (see Figs. 6–2 and 17–8). Neural crest cells give rise to the spinal ganglia (dorsal root ganglia) and the ganglia of the autonomic nervous system. The ganglia of cranial nerves V, VII, IX, and X are also partly derived from the neural crest. In addition to forming ganglion cells, neural crest cells form the sheaths of nerves (Schwann cells)

and the meningeal covering of the brain and the spinal cord (see Chapter 17). They also contribute to the formation of pigment cells, the suprarenal (adrenal) medulla, and several skeletal and muscular components in the head (see Fig. 6–2 and Chapter 11).

Congenital Anomalies Resulting From Abnormal Neurulation

Because the primordium of the central nervous system (neural plate) appears during the third week and gives rise to neural folds and the primordium of the neural tube, disturbance of neurulation may result in severe abnormalities of the brain and spinal cord (see Chapter 17). Available evidence suggests that the primary disturbance (e.g., a teratogenic drug; see Chapter 9) affects the neuroectoderm, resulting in failure of closure of the neural tube (*neural tube defect*) in the brain and/or spinal cord regions. Extroversion (turning inside out) of the neural tissue then occurs and most of the exposed tissue degenerates. This results in meroanencephaly (anencephaly) and spina bifida cystica. In *meroanencephaly,* the brain is represented by a mass of mostly degenerated neural tissue exposed on the surface of the head (see Fig. 16–10).

THE ALLANTOIS

The allantois (Gr. *allas,* sausage) appears early in the third week as a relatively small, sausage-like outpouching or diverticulum from the caudal wall of the yolk sac (see Fig. 5–4B). The allantois remains very small in human embryos but is involved with early blood and blood vessel formation and *associated with development of the urinary bladder* (see Fig. 14–7). As the bladder enlarges, the allantois becomes the *urachus.* For a discussion of urachal anomalies see Moore and Persaud (1993).

DEVELOPMENT OF SOMITES

At the end of the third week as the notochord and neural tube form, the mesoderm beside them forms longitudinal columns called *paraxial mesoderm* (Fig. 5–5B). These mesodermal columns soon begin to divide into paired cuboidal bodies called *somites* (Fig. 5–5C and D). The first pair of somites (Gr. *soma,* body) develops a short distance caudal to the cranial end of the

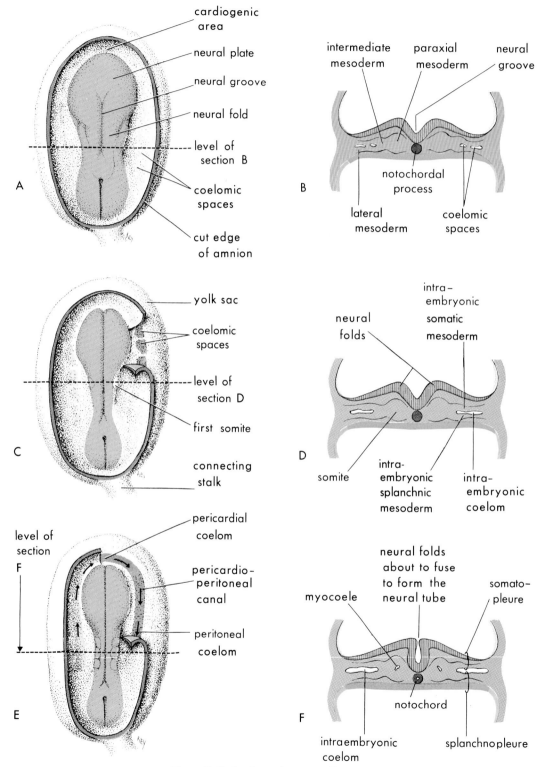

cardiogenic area

neural plate

neural groove

neural fold

level of section B

coelomic spaces

cut edge of amnion

A

intermediate mesoderm   paraxial mesoderm   neural groove

notochordal process

lateral mesoderm   coelomic spaces

B

yolk sac

coelomic spaces

level of section D

first somite

connecting stalk

C

intra-embryonic somatic mesoderm

neural folds

somite

intra-embryonic splanchnic mesoderm   intra-embryonic coelom

D

level of section F

pericardial coelom

pericardio-peritoneal canal

peritoneal coelom

E

neural folds about to fuse to form the neural tube

myocoele   somato-pleure

notochord

intraembryonic coelom   splanchnopleure

F

Figure 5–5. *See legend on opposite page*

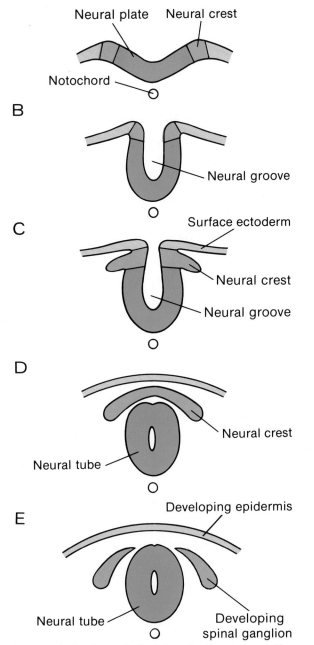

B

Neural plate   Neural crest

Notochord

C

Neural groove

Surface ectoderm

Neural crest

Neural groove

D

Neural crest

Neural tube

E

Developing epidermis

Neural tube

Developing spinal ganglion

Figure 5–6. Portions of diagrammatic transverse sections through progressively older embryos during the third and fourth weeks, illustrating formation of the neural groove, neural tube, and neural crest.

notochord. Subsequent pairs form in a craniocaudal sequence (see Fig. 6–3). About 38 pairs of somites form during the so-called somite period of development (days 20 to 30); eventually, 42 to 44 pairs develop. During the *somite period* the somites are used as one of the criteria for determining the embryo's age (see Table 6–1). The somites form distinct, surface elevations on the embryo (Fig. 5–5E; see also Fig. 6–3) and are somewhat triangular in transverse section. *The somites give rise to most of the axial skeleton* (vertebral column, ribs, sternum, and skull) and associated musculature, as well as the adjacent dermis of the skin (see Chapters 16 and 19).

DEVELOPMENT OF THE INTRAEMBRYONIC COELOM

The intraembryonic coelom (embryonic body cavity) first appears as isolated, coelomic spaces in the lateral mesoderm and the mesoderm that will form the heart called the *cardiogenic mesoderm* (Fig. 5–5A and B). These spaces soon coalesce to form a horseshoe-shaped cavity called the *intraembryonic coelom* (Fig. 5–5E). The intraembryonic coelom divides the lateral mesoderm into two layers (Fig. 5–5D): a *somatic or parietal layer* that is continuous with the extraembryonic mesoderm covering the amnion and a *splanchnic or visceral layer* that is continuous with the extraembryonic mesoderm covering the yolk sac. The somatic mesoderm and the overlying embryonic ectoderm form the body wall called the *somatopleure* (Fig. 5–5F), whereas the splanchnic mesoderm and the embryonic endoderm form the gut wall called the *splanchnopleure* (see Fig. 6–1).

During the second month, the intraembryonic coelom is divided into three body cavities: (1) the *pericardial cavity* containing the heart, (2) the *pleural cavities* containing the lungs, and (3) the *peritoneal cavity* containing the abdominal and pelvic viscera (see Chapter 10).

Figure 5–5. Drawings of embryos of 19 to 21 days, illustrating development of somites and the intraembryonic coelom. *A, C,* and *E,* Dorsal views of the embryonic disc exposed by removal of the amnion. *B, D,* and *F,* Transverse sections through the embryonic disc at the levels shown. Note the notochord in *F,* the cellular structure around which the vertebral column subsequently forms (see Chapter 16). *A,* Presomite embryo of about 19 days. *C,* An embryo of about 20 days showing the first pair of somites. A portion of the ectoderm and mesoderm on the right side has been removed to show the coelomic spaces in the lateral mesoderm. *E,* A three-somite embryo of about 21 days, showing the horseshoe-shaped intraembryonic coelom, exposed on the right by removal of the ectoderm and mesoderm of the embryo. The myocoele is an unimportant transitory cavity in the somite.

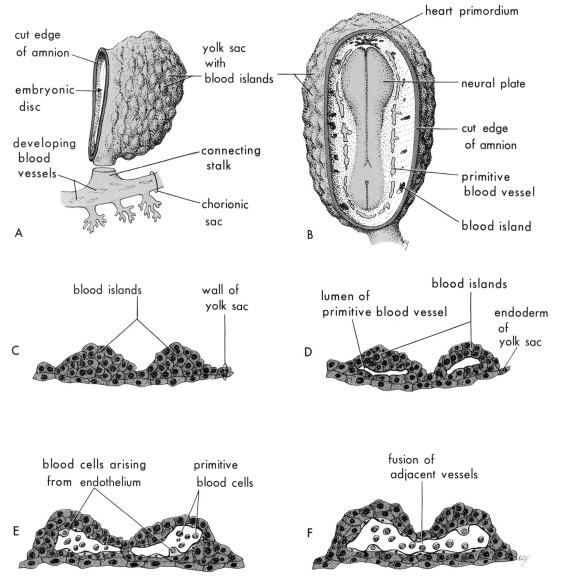

Figure 5–7. Successive stages in the development of blood and blood vessels. *A,* The yolk sac and a portion of the chorionic sac at about 18 days. *B,* Dorsal view of an embryo of about 19 days, exposed by removing the amnion. *C* to *F,* Sections of blood islands showing progressive stages of development of blood and blood vessels.

DEVELOPMENT OF THE PRIMITIVE CARDIOVASCULAR SYSTEM

At the beginning of the third week, blood and blood vessel formation *(angiogenesis)* begins in the extraembryonic mesoderm of the yolk sac, connecting stalk, and chorion (Fig. 5–7). Embryonic blood vessels begin to develop about two days later. The early formation of the cardiovascular system is correlated with the absence of a significant amount of yolk in the ovum and yolk sac. At the end of the second week embryonic nutrition is obtained from the maternal blood by diffusion across the extraembryonic coelom and yolk sac. As the embryo develops rapidly in the third week, there is a need for vessels to bring nourishment and oxygen to the embryo from the maternal circulation (Fig. 5–8).

Blood and blood vessel formation during the third week may be summarized as follows (Fig. 5–7): (1) mesenchymal cells known as *angio-*

blasts aggregate to form isolated masses and cords known as **blood islands,** (2) cavities appear within these islands, (3) angioblasts arrange themselves around each cavity to form a primitive *endothelium,* (4) the vessels fuse to form networks of endothelial channels, and (5) vessels extend into adjacent areas by fusing with other vessels.

Primitive plasma and blood cells develop from the endothelial cells of the vessels in the walls of the yolk sac and allantois (Fig. 5–7E). Blood formation does not begin in the embryo until the fifth week. It first occurs in the liver and later in the spleen, bone marrow, and lymph nodes. The mesenchymal cells surrounding the primitive endothelial blood vessels differentiate into the muscular and connective tissue elements of the vessels.

The *primitive heart* forms in a similar manner from mesenchymal cells in the cardiogenic area (Fig. 5–7B). Paired *endothelial heart tubes* de-

velop before the end of the third week and begin to fuse into a primitive heart tube (see Fig. 15–2). By the end of the third week, the endothelial heart tube has linked up with blood vessels in the embryo, connecting stalk, chorion, and yolk sac to form a primitive cardiovascular system (Fig. 5–8). The circulation of blood starts and the heart begins to beat. *The cardiovascular system is thus the first organ system to reach a functional state.*

DEVELOPMENT OF CHORIONIC VILLI

Shortly after the *primary chorionic villi* appear at the end of the second week (see Figs. 4–4 and 4–5), they begin to branch. Early in the third week mesenchyme grows into the primary chorionic villi, forming a core of loose connective tissue. The villi at this stage (called *secondary chorionic villi*) cover the entire surface of

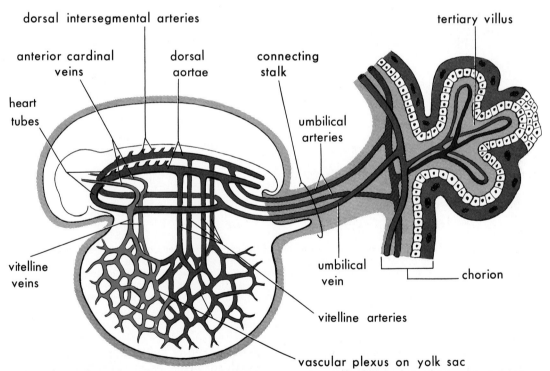

Figure 5–8. Diagram of the primitive cardiovascular system in a 20-day embryo, viewed from the left side. Observe the transitory stage of paired symmetrical vessels. Each endothelial heart tube continues dorsally into a *dorsal aorta,* which passes caudally. Branches of the aortae are: (1) *umbilical arteries* that connect with vessels in the chorion, (2) *vitelline arteries* that supply the yolk sac, and (3) *dorsal intersegmental arteries* that supply the body of the embryo. An umbilical vein returns blood from the chorion and divides into right and left umbilical veins within the embryo. Vessels on the yolk sac form a vascular plexus, which is connected to the heart tubes by *vitelline veins.* The anterior cardinal veins return blood from the head. The umbilical vein is shown in red to indicate that it carries oxygenated blood and nutrients from the chorion (embryonic part of the placenta) to the embryo.

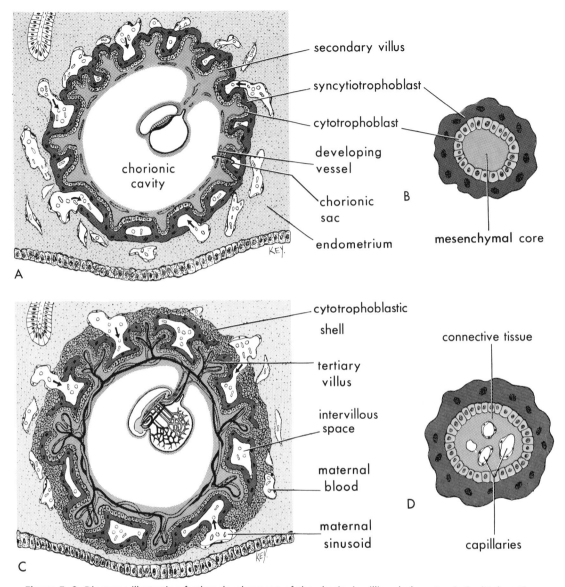

Figure 5–9. Diagrams illustrating further development of the chorionic villi and placenta. *A*, Sagittal section of an embryo (about 16 days). *B*, Section of a secondary chorionic villus. *C*, Section of an implanted embryo (about 21 days). *D*, Section of a tertiary or stem chorionic villus. The fetal blood in the capillaries is separated from the maternal blood surrounding the villus by the placental membrane composed of the endothelium of the capillary, mesenchyme, cytotrophoblast, and syncytiotrophoblast. For details about the placental membrane, see Chapter 8 and Figure 8–7.

the chorion (Fig. 5–9*A* and *B*). Soon, mesenchymal cells in the villi begin to differentiate into blood capillaries, which fuse to form *arteriocapillary venous networks*. After blood vessels have developed, the villi are called *tertiary chorionic villi* or **stem villi** (Fig. 5–9*D*; see also Fig. 8–5).

Vessels in these mature villi soon become connected with the embryonic heart via vessels that differentiate in the mesenchyme of the chorion and connecting stalk (Fig. 5–8). By the end of the third week, embryonic blood begins to circulate through the capillaries of the chorionic villi. *Oxygen and nutrients* in the maternal blood in the intervillous space diffuse through the walls of the villi and enter the fetal capillaries. *Carbon dioxide and waste products* diffuse from blood in the fetal capillaries through the walls of the villi into the maternal blood.

Concurrently, cytotrophoblast cells of the chorionic villi proliferate and extend through the syncytiotrophoblastic layer and join to form a *cytotrophoblastic shell* (Fig. 5–9C). It attaches the chorionic sac to the endometrium. Chorionic villi that are attached to the maternal tissues via the cytotrophoblastic shell are called *stem villi* (anchoring villi). The villi that grow from the sides of the stem villi are called *branch villi*. It is through these villi that the main exchange of material between the blood of the mother and the embryo takes place (see Figs. 8–5 to 8–7).

SUMMARY

Rapid development of the embryo occurs during the third week. This important period coincides with the week following the first missed menstrual period. As the primitive streak forms intraembryonic mesoderm, the bilaminar embryonic disc is converted into a trilaminar embryo composed of three primary germ layers (ectoderm, mesoderm, and endoderm). These layers will later give rise to all tissues and organs in the embryo (see Fig. 6–2).

The **primitive streak** appears at the beginning of the third week as a midline thickening of the embryonic *epiblast*. It gives rise to mesenchymal cells, which migrate laterally and cranially between the epiblast and hypoblast. As soon as the primitive streak begins to produce mesenchymal cells, the epiblast layer is known as the *embryonic ectoderm* and the hypoblast is known as the *embryonic endoderm*. The cells produced by the primitive streak soon organize into a third germ layer, the *intraembryonic mesoderm*.

Cells from the primitive node (knot) give rise to the *notochordal process*. This cellular cord soon develops a notochordal canal. When fully developed the notochordal process extends from the primitive node to the prochordal plate. The **notochord** develops from the notochordal process and forms the primitive skeletal support of the embryo around which the axial skeleton later forms.

The *neural plate* appears as a median thickening of the embryonic ectoderm, cranial to the primitive knot. Formation of the neural plate is induced by the developing notochord and the mesenchyme adjacent to it. A longitudinal *neural groove* develops in the neural plate which is flanked by *neural folds*. These folds meet and fuse to form the **neural tube**, the primordium of the central nervous system (CNS) As this process occurs, some cells migrate ventrolaterally to form the *neural crest*.

Neural crest cells give rise to spinal and autonomic ganglia, pigment cells, the suprarenal medulla, the meninges of the brain and spinal cord, and skeletal components of the head.

The mesoderm on each side of the notochord thickens to form longitudinal columns of *paraxial mesoderm*. Division of these columns into pairs of *somites* begins cranially by the end of the third week. The somites give rise to the vertebral column, ribs, and associated back muscles.

The *intraembryonic coelom* arises as isolated spaces in the lateral mesoderm and cardiogenic mesoderm. These coelomic spaces subsequently coalesce to form a single, horseshoe-shaped cavity, which eventually gives rise to the body cavities (e.g., the peritoneal cavity).

Blood vessels first appear on the yolk sac, around the allantois, and in the chorion. They develop within the embryo shortly thereafter. *Blood* and blood vessels develop as follows. Spaces appear within aggregations of mesenchyme *(blood islands)*, which soon become lined with endothelium derived from angioblasts which differentiate from mesenchymal cells. These primitive vessels unite with other vessels to form a *primitive cardiovascular system*. At the end of the third week, the heart is represented by *endothelial heart tubes*, which are connected to blood vessels in the extraembryonic membranes (yolk sac, umbilical cord, and chorionic sac). The primitive blood cells are derived mainly from the endothelial cells of blood vessels in the walls of the yolk sac and allantois. Blood begins to form in the embryo about two weeks later.

Primary chorionic villi become secondary chorionic villi as they acquire mesenchymal cores. Before the end of the third week, capillaries develop in the villi, transforming them into *tertiary or stem chorionic villi.* Cytotrophoblastic extensions from the chorionic villi mushroom out and join to form a *cytotrophoblastic shell* that anchors the stem villi and the chorionic sac to the endometrium.

The rapid development of chorionic villi during the third week greatly increases the surface area of the chorion for the exchange of nutrients and other substances between the maternal and embryonic circulations.

Commonly Asked Questions

1. Do women who have been taking contraceptive pills for many years have more early spontaneous abortions than women who have used other contraceptive methods?
2. Is the third week of development considered to be part of the embryonic period? What are the main embryonic structures that form?
3. What is meant by the term "menstrual extraction?" Is this the same as an early induced abortion?
4. Can drugs and other agents cause congenital anomalies of the embryo if they are present in the mother's blood during the third week? If so, what organs would be most susceptible?
5. Are there increased risks for the embryo associated with women over 40 having children? If so, what are they?

The answers to these questions are given on page 328.

REFERENCES

Beddington RSP: The origin of the foetal tissues during gastrulation in the rodent. *In* Johnson MH (ed): *Development In Mammals.* New York, Elsevier, 1983.

Boué J, Boué A, Lazar P: Retrospective and prospective epidemiological studies of 1500 karyotyped spontaneous abortions. *Teratology* 12:11, 1975.

Carr DH: Chromosomes and abortion. *Adv Hum Genet* 2:201, 1971.

Cook J: The early embryo and the formation of body pattern. *American Scientist* 76:35, 1988.

Depp R: How ultrasound is used by the perinatologist. *Clin Obstet Gynecol* 20:315, 1977.

Flint G: Embryology of the nervous system. *Br J Neurosurgery* 3:131, 1989.

Gilbert SF: *Developmental Biology.* Sunderland, Sinauer Associates, 1991.

Goodwin BC: Problems and prospects in morphogenesis. *Experientia* 44:633, 1988.

Hertig AT: Angiogenesis in the early human chorion and in the primary placenta of the macaque monkey. *Contrib Embryol Carnegie Inst* 25:37, 1935.

Holzgreve W, Flake AW, Langer JC: The fetus with sacrococcygeal teratoma. *In* Harrison MR, Golbus MS, Filly RA (eds): *The Unborn Patient. Prenatal Diagnosis and Treatment,* 2nd ed. Philadelphia, WB Saunders, 1991.

Horowitz T: *The Human Notochord. A Study of Its Development and Regression, Variations and Pathogenic Derivative, Chordoma.* Indianapolis, Limited Private Printing, 1977.

Jacobson AG, Sater AK: Features of embryonic induction. *Development* 104:341, 1988.

Jacobson M: *Developmental Neurobiology,* 2nd ed. New York, Plenum Press, 1989.

Keller R, Danichick M: Regional expression, pattern and timing of convergence and extension during gastrulation of *Xenopus laevis. Development* 103:193, 1988.

Kirby ML, Bockman DE: Neural crest and normal development: a new perspective. *Anat Rec* 209:1, 1984.

Kratochwil K: Embryonic Induction. *In* Yamada KM (ed): *Cell Interactions and Development.* New York, John Wiley & Sons, 1982.

Moore KL, Persaud TVN: *The Developing Human: Clinically Oriented Embryology,* 5th ed. Philadelphia, WB Saunders, 1993.

Nahhas F, Barnea E: Human embryonic origin of early pregnancy factor before and after implantation. *Am J Reprod Immunol* 22:105, 1990.

Navaratnam V: Organization and reorganization of blood vessels in embryonic development. *Eye* 5:(Pt.2)147, 1991.

O'Rahilly R: The manifestation of the axes of the human embryo. *Z Anat Entwicklungsgesch* 132:50, 1970.

Smith JL, Schoenwolf GC: Further evidence of extrinsic forces in bending of the neural plate. *J Comp Neurol* 307:225, 1991.

Weston JA: Regulation of neural crest cell migration and differentiation. *In* Yamada KM (ed): *Cell Interactions and Development.* New York, John Wiley & Sons, 1982.

Wilson KM: A normal human ovum of 16 days development, the Rochester ovum. *Contrib Embryol Carnegie Inst* 31:103, 1945.

6

THE FOURTH
TO EIGHTH WEEKS
OF HUMAN DEVELOPMENT

DEVELOPMENT OF TISSUES, ORGANS, AND BODY FORM

These five weeks constitute most of the **embryonic period** (third to eighth weeks). *This is a critical period of development* because the primordia of all major external and internal structures develop during this time. As the organs develop, the shape of the embryo gradually changes. By the end of the eighth week, the embryo has a remarkably human appearance.

PHASES OF DEVELOPMENT

Human development may be divided into three phases which, to some extent, are interrelated. The first of these is *growth* (increase in size), which involves cell division and the elaboration of cell products. The second process is *morphogenesis* (development of form), which includes mass cell movements. Morphogenesis is an elaborate process during which many complex interactions occur in an orderly sequence (Cooke, 1988). The movement of cells allows them to interact with each other during the formation of tissues and organs. *Differentiation* is the third phase of development (maturation of physiological processes). Completion of this process results in the formation of tissues and organs that are able to perform specialized functions. Because the organ systems develop during the fourth to eighth weeks, exposure of embryos to **teratogens** during this period (e.g., drugs and viruses) may induce or raise the incidence of congenital anomalies. They act during the stage of active differentiation of an organ or tissue (see Chapter 9).

FOLDING OF THE EMBRYO

A significant event in the establishment of general body form is the folding of the flat, trilaminar, embryonic disc into a somewhat cylindrical embryo (Fig. 6–1). During the fourth week the embryo grows rapidly, tripling its size. The gradual establishment of body form results from folding of the embryonic disc and the development of organs (e.g., the heart).

The folding in both the median and horizontal planes is mainly caused by rapid growth of the neural tube. The formation of these folds is a simultaneous process of constriction at the junction of the embryo and yolk sac and is not a separate sequence of events. Folding in the median plane produces head and tail folds that result in the cranial and caudal regions "swinging" ventrally as if on hinges (Fig. 6–1A_2 to D_2). During folding, part of the yolk sac is incorporated into the embryo.

The Head Fold

The developing brain grows cranially beyond the oropharyngeal membrane and soon overhangs the primitive heart (Fig. 6–1A_2 to D_2). As the head folds, the heart and oropharyngeal

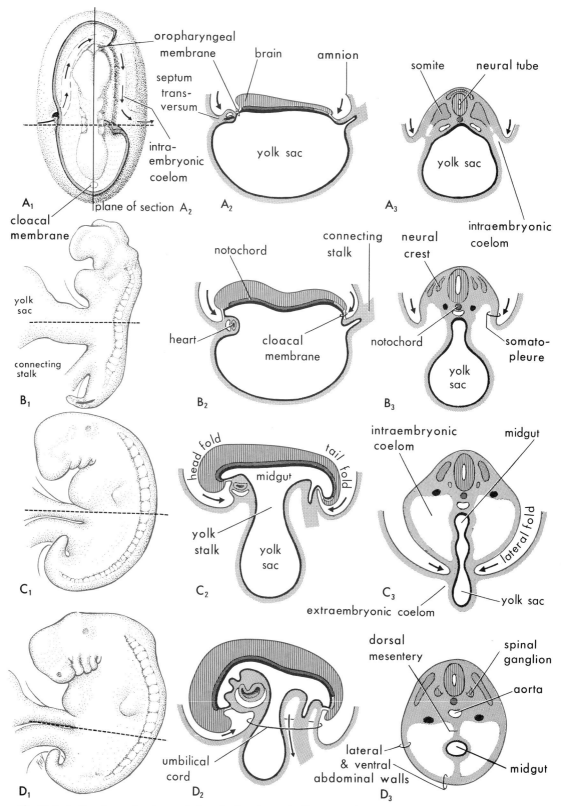

Figure 6–1. Drawings of embryos during the fourth week, illustrating folding in the median and horizontal planes. A_1, Dorsal view of a 22-day embryo. The continuity of the intraembryonic coelom and extraembryonic coelom is illustrated on the right side by removal of a portion of the embryonic ectoderm and mesoderm. B_1, C_1, and D_1, Lateral views of embryos of about 24, 26, and 28 days, respectively. A_2 to D_2, Longitudinal sections at the plane shown in A_1. A_3 to D_3, Transverse sections at the levels indicated in A_1 to D_1.

membrane move to the ventral surface. After folding, the mass of mesoderm cranial to the pericardial coelom, called the *septum transversum*, lies caudal to the heart. This septum subsequently develops into a major part of the diaphragm (see Chapter 10). During folding of the head, part of the yolk sac is incorporated into the embryo as the *foregut* (primordium of the pharynx, esophagus, etc.; see Chapter 13). It lies between the caudal part of the brain and the heart and ends blindly at the *oropharyngeal membrane*. This membrane separates the foregut from the *stomodeum* (primitive mouth or oral cavity).

The Tail Fold

Folding of the caudal end of the embryo occurs a little later than that of the cranial end (Fig. 6–1B_2 to D_2). As the embryo grows, the tail region projects over the *cloacal membrane* (future site of the anus). During folding of the tail region, part of the yolk sac is incorporated into the embryo as the *hindgut* (primordium of the descending colon, etc.; see Chapter 13). After folding, the *connecting stalk* (primordium of the *umbilical cord*) is attached to the ventral surface of the embryo (Fig. 6–1D_2).

The Lateral Folds

Folding of the embryo in the horizontal plane produces right and left *lateral folds* (Fig. 6–1A_3 to D_3). Each lateral body wall folds toward the median plane, rolling the edges of the embryonic disc ventrally and forming a roughly cylindrical embryo. As the lateral and ventral body walls form, part of the yolk sac is incorporated into the embryo as the *midgut* (primordium of the small intestine, etc.; see Chapter 13). Concurrently, the connection of the midgut with the yolk sac is reduced to a narrow *yolk stalk*. After folding, the region of the attachment of the amnion to the embryo is reduced to a relatively narrow region where the umbilical cord attaches to the ventral surface. As the midgut separates from the yolk sac, it becomes attached to the dorsal abdominal wall by a *dorsal mesentery* (Fig. 6–1D_3).

GERM LAYER DERIVATIVES

The three germ layers (embryonic ectoderm, mesoderm, and endoderm) formed during *gastrulation* (p. 45) from the inner cell mass or em-

bryoblast in the third week give rise to all the tissues and organs of the embryo (Fig. 6–2). The cells of each germ layer divide, migrate, aggregate, and differentiate in rather precise patterns as they form the various organ systems. Tissues that develop from the different germ layers are commonly associated in the formation of an organ (*organogenesis*). The main germ layer derivatives are as follows.

ECTODERM. This layer gives rise to the central nervous system (brain and spinal cord), the peripheral nervous system, the sensory epithelia of the eye, ear, and nose, the epidermis and its appendages (hair and nails), the mammary glands, the hypophysis cerebri (pituitary gland), the subcutaneous glands, and the enamel of teeth. *Neural crest cells* (Fig. 6–2), derived from neuroectoderm, give rise to the cells of the spinal, cranial (CNs V, VII, IX, and X), and autonomic ganglia; ensheathing cells of the peripheral nervous system; pigment cells of the dermis; muscle, connective tissues, and bone of branchial or pharyngeal arch origin (see Chapter 11); the *suprarenal (adrenal) medulla*, and the membranes covering the brain and spinal cord (meninges).

MESODERM. This layer gives rise to cartilage, bone, and connective tissue, striated and smooth muscles, the heart, blood and lymph vessels and cells, the kidneys, gonads (ovaries and testes), and the genital ducts, serous membranes lining the body cavities (pericardial, pleural, and peritoneal), the spleen, and the cortex of the suprarenal gland.

ENDODERM. This layer gives rise to the epithelial lining of the gastrointestinal and respiratory tracts, the parenchyma of the tonsils, thyroid gland, parathyroid glands, thymus, liver, and pancreas, the epithelial lining of the urinary bladder and most of the urethra, and the epithelial lining of the tympanic cavity, tympanic antrum, and auditory tube.

CONTROL OF EMBRYONIC DEVELOPMENT

Development results from genetic plans in the chromosomes. The individuality of each person is largely determined at fertilization by the genes contained in the chromosomes of the sperm and the ovum. These genes control the processes by which the body develops before and after birth. For a discussion of the molecular genetics of development, see Thompson et al. (1991).

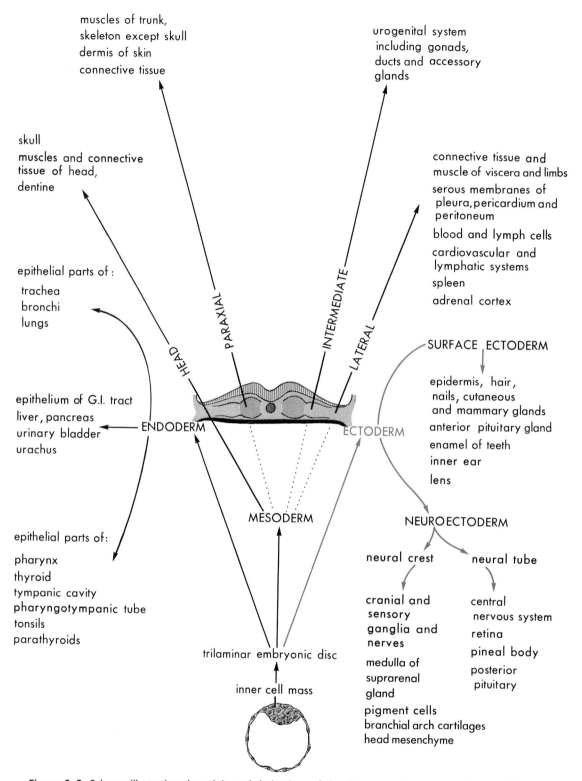

muscles of trunk,
skeleton except skull
dermis of skin
connective tissue

urogenital system
including gonads,
ducts and accessory
glands

skull
muscles and connective
tissue of head,
dentine

connective tissue and
muscle of viscera and limbs
serous membranes of
pleura, pericardium and
peritoneum
blood and lymph cells
cardiovascular and
lymphatic systems
spleen
adrenal cortex

epithelial parts of :
trachea
bronchi
lungs

SURFACE ECTODERM

epidermis, hair,
nails, cutaneous
and mammary glands
anterior pituitary gland
enamel of teeth
inner ear
lens

PARAXIAL

INTERMEDIATE

LATERAL

HEAD

epithelium of G.I. tract
liver, pancreas
urinary bladder
urachus

ENDODERM

ECTODERM

MESODERM

NEUROECTODERM

epithelial parts of:

pharynx
thyroid
tympanic cavity
pharyngotympanic tube
tonsils
parathyroids

neural crest

neural tube

cranial and
sensory
ganglia and
nerves
medulla of
suprarenal
gland
pigment cells
branchial arch cartilages
head mesenchyme

central
nervous system
retina
pineal body
posterior
pituitary

trilaminar embryonic disc

inner cell mass

Figure 6–2. Scheme illustrating the origin and derivatives of the three germ layers: ectoderm, endoderm, and mesoderm. Cells from these layers make contributions to the formation of the different tissues and organs; e.g., the endoderm forms the epithelial lining of the gastrointestinal tract, and the mesoderm gives rise to its connective tissues and muscles.

Most developmental processes depend upon a precisely coordinated interaction of genetic and environmental factors. There are control mechanisms that guide differentiation and ensure synchronized development, e.g., tissue interactions, regulated migrations of cells and cell colonies, controlled proliferations, and cell death. Each system of the body has its own developmental pattern, but most processes of morphogenesis are similar and relatively simple (Cooke, 1988).

> Defective genetic plans (e.g., an abnormal number of chromosomes or a gene mutation) result in congenital anomalies or *birth defects*. Abnormal development may also be caused by environmental factors (discussed in Chapter 9). Most developmental processes depend on a precisely coordinated interaction of genetic and environmental factors.

Induction

For a limited time during early development, certain embryonic tissues markedly influence the development of adjacent tissues. The tissues producing these influences or effects are called *inductors* or organizers. In order to induce, an inductor must be close to, but not necessarily in contact with, the tissue to be induced. During the development of the eye, for example, the optic vesicle induces the development of the lens from the surface ectoderm covering the head. In the absence of the optic vesicle, the lens fails to develop. Moreover, if the optic vesicle is removed and placed in association with surface ectoderm that is not usually involved in lens development, lens formation can be induced. Clearly then, development of a lens is dependent on the ectoderm acquiring an association with a second tissue.

Once the basic embryonic plan has been established by primary organizers, a chain of *secondary inductions* occurs. The nature of the inductive agents is not clearly understood, but it is generally accepted that some signal passes from the inducing tissue to the induced tissue. The precise nature of the signal is not known; however, the mechanism of the signal transfer appears to vary with the specific tissues involved. In some cases the signal appears to take the form of a diffusible molecule that passes from the inductor to the reacting tissue. In other cases the message is mediated through a nondiffusible, extracellular matrix secreted by the inductor and with which the reacting tissue comes

in contact. In still others, the signal appears to require that physical contacts occur between the inducing and the responding tissues. For a detailed discussion of induction, see Chapter 5 in Moore and Persaud (1993).

HIGHLIGHTS OF THE FOURTH TO EIGHTH WEEKS

The following descriptions summarize the main developmental events and changes in external form that occur during this period. The details of organ formation are given with discussions of the various systems (Chapters 12 to 19). Useful criteria for estimating developmental stages in human embryos are listed in Table 6–1.

The Fourth Week

Initially the embryo is almost straight, and the *somites* (primordia of the muscles and vertebrae) produce conspicuous surface elevations (Figs. 6–3 to 6–7). The *neural tube* is formed opposite the somites, but it is widely open at rostral and caudal openings called *neuropores*. By 24 days, the first or *mandibular arch* and the second or *hyoid arch* are visible (Fig. 6–3C). The major portion of the first branchial or pharyngeal arch, called the mandibular prominence, forms the mandible or lower jaw; and a rostral extension of it, the maxillary prominence, contributes to the maxilla or upper jaw (see Chapter 11).

A slight curve is produced in the embryo by the head and tail folds (Fig. 6–1), and the heart produces a large ventral prominence. Three pairs of branchial or pharyngeal arches are visible by 26 days (Figs. 6–3D and 6–6), and the forebrain produces a prominent swelling of the head. Longitudinal folding has given the embryo a characteristic C-shaped curvature.

Upper limb buds are recognizable as small swellings on the lateral body walls by 26 or 27 days (Figs. 6–3D and 6–7). The *otic pits*, the primordia of the internal ears, are also clearly visible. *Lower limb buds* appear as small swellings on the lateral body walls by 28 days (Fig. 6–3E). Lens placodes, ectodermal thickenings indicating the future lenses, are visible on the sides of the head. The fourth pair of branchial or pharyngeal arches is also visible by the end of the fourth week. The tail is a characteristic feature by the end of the fourth week.

Table 6–1. CRITERIA FOR ESTIMATING DEVELOPMENTAL STAGES IN HUMAN EMBRYOS

Age (Days)	Figure Reference	Carnegie Stage	No. of Somites	Length (mm)*	Main External Characteristics†
20–21	6–3A₁	9	1–3	1.5–3.0	*Flat embryonic disc. Deep neural groove and prominent neural folds. One to three pairs of somites present.* Head fold evident.
22–23	6–3A and B 6–4	10	4–12	2.0–3.5	*Embryo straight or slightly curved. Neural tube forming or formed opposite somites, but widely open at rostral and caudal neuropores.* First and second pairs of branchial arches visible.
24–25	6–3C 6–5	11	13–20	2.5–4.5	*Embryo curved owing to head and tail folds. Rostral neuropore closing.* Otic placodes present. Optic vesicles formed.
26–27	6–3D 6–6	12	21–29	3.0–5.0	*Upper limb buds appear. Rostral neuropore closed. Caudal neuropore closing.* Three pairs of branchial arches visible. Heart prominence distinct. Otic pits present.
28–30	6–3E 6–7	13	30–35	4.0–6.0	*Embryo has C-shaped curve. Caudal neuropore closed. Upper limb buds are flipper-like.* Four pairs of branchial arches visible. *Lower limb buds appear.* Otic vesicles present. Lens placodes distinct. Attenuated *tail* present.
31–32	6–8A	14	‡	5.0–7.0	*Upper limbs are paddle-shaped. Lens pits and nasal pits visible.* Optic cups present.
33–36	6–8B	15		7.0–9.0	*Hand plates formed; digital rays present.* Lens vesicles present. Nasal pits prominent. *Lower limbs are paddle-shaped.* Cervical sinuses visible.
37–40		16		8.0–11.0	*Foot plates formed.* Pigment visible in retina. Auricular hillocks developing.
41–43	6–8C 6–9	17		11.0–14.0	*Digital rays clearly visible in hand plates.* Auricular hillocks outline future auricle of external ear. Trunk beginning to straighten. Cerebral vesicles prominent.
44–46	6–10	18		13.0–17.0	*Digital rays clearly visible in foot plates.* Elbow region visible. Eyelids forming. Notches between the digital rays in the hands. Nipples visible.
47–48	6–11A	19		16.0–18.0	*Limbs extend ventrally.* Trunk elongating and straightening. Midgut herniation prominent.
49–51	6–11B 6–12	20		18.0–22.0	*Upper limbs longer and bent at elbows. Fingers distinct but webbed.* Notches between the digital rays in the feet. Scalp vascular plexus appears.
52–53	6–13A	21		22.0–24.0	*Hands and feet approach each other. Fingers are free and longer.* Toes distinct but webbed. Stubby tail present.
54–55		22		23.0–28.0	*Toes free and longer.* Eyelids and auricles of external ears more developed.
56	6–13B 6–14	23		27.0–31.0	*Head more rounded and shows human characteristics.* External genitalia still have sexless appearance. Distinct bulge still present in umbilical cord, caused by herniation of intestines. *Tail has disappeared.*

* The embryonic lengths indicate the usual range, but they do not indicate the full range within a given stage, especially when specimens of poor quality are included. In stages 10 and 11, the measurement is greatest length (GL); in subsequent stages crown-rump (CR) measurements are given (Fig. 6–16).

† Based on Nishimura et al. (1974), O'Rahilly and Müller (1987), and Shiota (1991).

‡ At this and subsequent stages, the number of somites is difficult to determine and so is not a useful criterion.

The Fifth Week

During this week, changes in body form are minor compared with the fourth week (Fig. 6–8A). *Extensive head growth* is mainly caused by rapid development of the brain. The face is in contact with the heart prominence. The second or hyoid arch has overgrown the third and fourth arches, forming an ectodermal depression known as the **cervical sinus.** The upper limbs are paddle-shaped, and the lens and nasal pits are visible. By the end of the fifth week, the *hand plates* have formed, and the lower limbs have become paddle-shaped. The primordia of the digits in the hands, called *digital rays*, begin to develop (see Fig. 16–12C). Development of the lower limb occurs a day or two later than that of the upper limb.

The Sixth Week

The head is now much larger relative to the trunk and is further bent over the *heart*

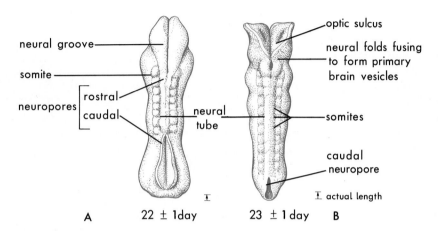

A   22 ± 1day   23 ± 1 day   B

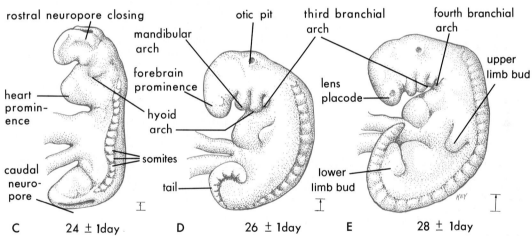

C   24 ± 1day   D   26 ± 1day   E   28 ± 1day

Figure 6–3. Drawings of four-week embryos. *A* and *B*, Dorsal views of embryos early in the fourth week with 8 and 12 somites, respectively. *C*, *D*, and *E*, Lateral views of older embryos with 16, 27, and 33 somites, respectively. The rostral neuropore is normally closed by 25 to 26 days, and the caudal neuropore is usually closed by the end of the fourth week.

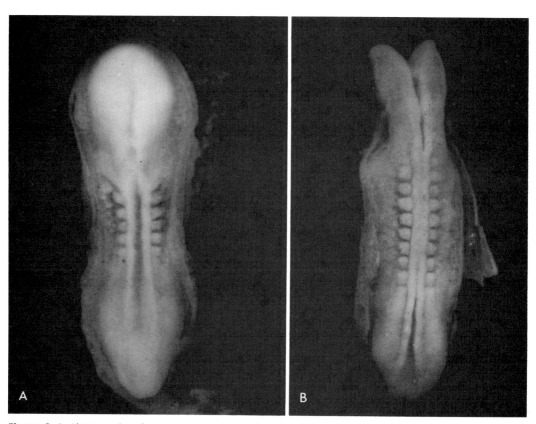

Figure 6–4. Photographs of embryos early in the fourth week. In *A*, the embryo is essentially straight; whereas, the embryo in *B* is slightly curved. In *A*, the neural groove is deep and open throughout its entire extent. In *B*, the neural tube has formed opposite the somites but is widely open at the rostral and caudal neuropores (see also Fig. 6–3*A*). The neural tube is the primordium of the central nervous system (brain and spinal cord). (Courtesy of Professor Hideo Nishimura, Kyoto University, Kyoto, Japan.)

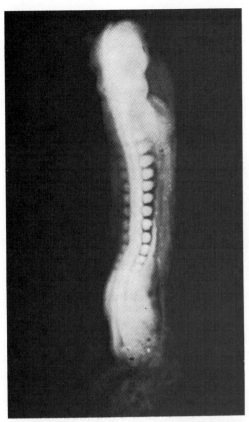

Figure 6–5. Photograph of an embryo during the fourth week (24 to 25 days). Ten of the 13 pairs of somites are easily recognized. The embryo is curved due to folding of the cranial and caudal ends. Observe the ventral prominence produced by the primitive heart (see also Fig. 6–3C). The rostral neuropore is almost closed, and the caudal neuropore is closing. (Courtesy of Professor Hideo Nishimura, Kyoto University, Kyoto, Japan.)

prominence (Figs. 6–8B and C and 6–9). This head position results from bending of the brain in the cervical region. The limbs now show considerable regional differentiation, especially the upper limbs. The elbow and wrist regions become identifiable, and the paddle-shaped hand plates have distinct *digital rays*. These rays indicate the future *digits* (fingers).

Several small swellings develop around the branchial or pharyngeal groove between the first two branchial or pharyngeal arches (Fig. 6–8C). This groove becomes the *external acoustic meatus* (L., a passage), and the swellings eventually fuse to form the auricle (pinna) of the external ear. Largely because retinal pigment begins to appear, the eye becomes more obvious. The somites are visible in the lumbosacral region until the middle of the week but are not useful criteria for estimating age at this time. By the end of the sixth week, the trunk and neck have begun to straighten.

The Seventh Week

The communication between the primitive gut and yolk sac has been reduced to a relatively small duct, the *yolk stalk* (Figs. 6–10 and 6–11A). The intestines have entered the extraembryonic coelom in the proximal portion of the umbilical cord. This process, called *umbilical herniation*, is a normal event in the embryo (Figs. 6–11B and 6–12B). The limbs undergo considerable change during the seventh week. Notches appear between the digital rays in the hand plates, clearly indicating the future digits (fingers). Digital rays are visible in the foot plates by the end of the seventh week (Fig. 6–11A).

The Eighth Week

At the beginning of the final week of the embryonic period, the digits of the hand are short and noticeably webbed (Figs. 6–11B, 6–12, and 6–13A). Notches are visible between the digital (toe) rays in the foot plates, and the tail is still visible but stubby. By the end of the eighth week, all regions of the limbs are apparent, the fingers have lengthened, and the toes are distinct. All evidence of the tail disappears by the end of the eighth week. The embryo now has unquestionably human characteristics (Figs. 6–13 and 6–14). The head is more round and erect but is still disproportionately large, constituting almost half of the embryo. The neck region has become established, and the eyelids are more obvious. The abdomen is less protuberant; however, the intestines are still in the proximal portion of the umbilical cord (Figs. 6–13 and 6–14).

Early in the eighth week the eyes are open; but, toward the end of the week, the eyelids begin to unite by epithelial fusion. The auricles of the external ears begin to assume their final shape but are still low-set on the head. Although sex differences exist in the appearance of the external genitalia, they are not distinct enough to permit accurate sexual identification by laypersons.

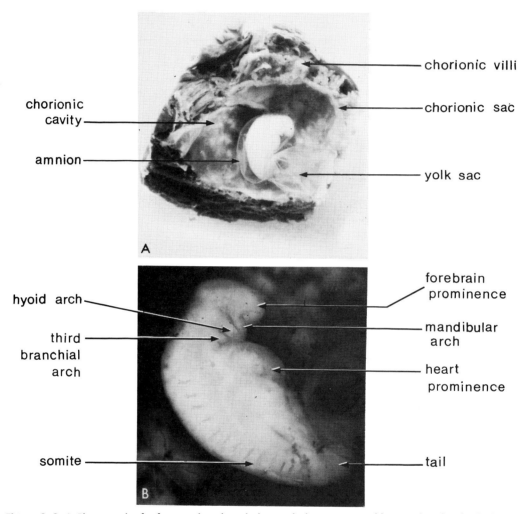

Figure 6–6. *A*, Photograph of a four-week embryo in its amniotic sac, exposed by opening the chorionic sac (× 5). *B*, Higher magnification of the embryo of 26 to 27 days (× 18). Although present, the upper limb bud is not visible in this photograph. (Photographed by Professor Jean Hay, Department of Anatomy, University of Manitoba.)

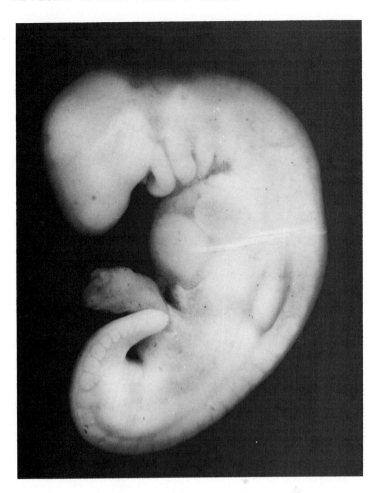

Figure 6–7. Photograph of a 28-day-old human embryo. It has a characteristic C-shaped curvature, four branchial or pharyngeal arches, and upper and lower limb buds. The lower limb bud is not recognizable in this photograph. The heart prominence is easily recognized. The curled tail with its somites is a characteristic feature of this stage. (Courtesy of Professor Hideo Nishimura, Kyoto University, Kyoto, Japan.)

ESTIMATION OF EMBRYONIC AGE

Information about the starting date of pregnancies may be difficult, partly because it is dependent on the mother's memory. Two reference points are commonly used for estimating gestational or embryonic age: (1) the onset of the *last normal menstrual period* (LNMP), and (2) the probable time of *fertilization* or conception (see Fig. 1–1). The probability of error in establishing the last normal menses is highest in women who become pregnant after discontinuing oral contraceptives. This is because the interval between stopping the hormones and ovulation is variable. In addition, slight uterine bleeding or "spotting" sometimes occurs after implantation of the blastocyst that may be incorrectly regarded as menstruation.

The zygote does not form until about two weeks after the onset of LNMP (see Fig. 1–1). Consequently, 14± two days must be deducted from the so-called gestational or "menstrual" age to obtain the actual or *fertilization* age of an embryo. The day fertilization occurs is the most accurate reference point for estimating age. This is commonly calculated from the estimated time of ovulation because the ovum is usually fertilized within 12 hours after ovulation.

Because it may be important to know the fertilization or *developmental age* of an embryo (e.g., for determining its sensitivity to drugs and viruses [Chapter 9]), all statements about age should indicate the reference point used, i.e., weeks after LNMP or the estimated time of fertilization. *Ultrasound assessment* of the size of the chorionic (gestational) sac and its contents (Fig. 6–15) enables physicians to obtain an accurate estimate of the date of conception (Callen, 1988).

Estimates of the age of recovered embryos (e.g., after a spontaneous abortion) are determined from external characteristics and

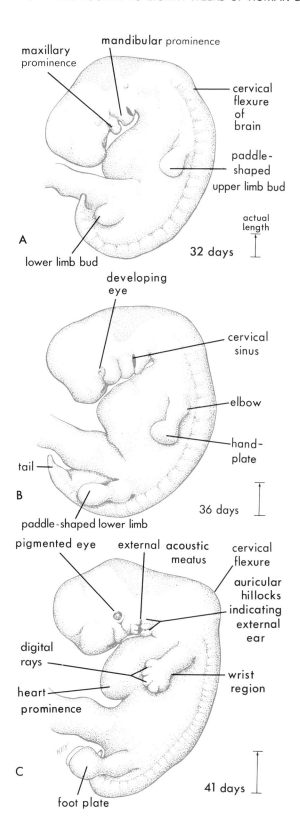

maxillary
prominence

mandibular prominence

cervical
flexure
of
brain

paddle-
shaped
upper limb bud

actual
length

A

32 days

lower limb bud

developing
eye

cervical
sinus

elbow

hand-
plate

tail

B

36 days

paddle-shaped lower limb

pigmented eye

external acoustic
meatus

cervical
flexure

auricular
hillocks
indicating
external
ear

digital
rays

wrist
region

heart
prominence

C

41 days

foot plate

Figure 6–8. Drawings of lateral views of embryos during the fifth and sixth weeks.

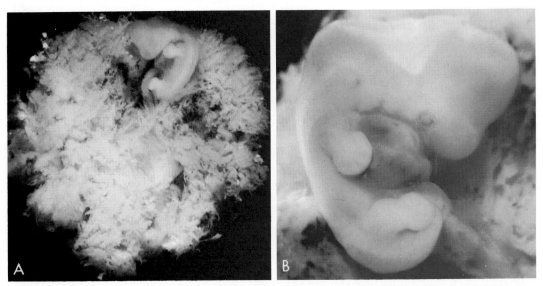

Figure 6–9. *A,* Photograph of a six-week embryo in its amniotic sac, exposed by opening the chorionic sac (× 2). *B,* Higher magnification of the embryo of about 41 days (× 6). Note the large size of the head compared with the rest of the body and the prominence of the cerebral vesicles, the primordia of the cerebral hemispheres of the brain. (Photographed by Professor Jean Hay, Department of Anatomy, University of Manitoba.)

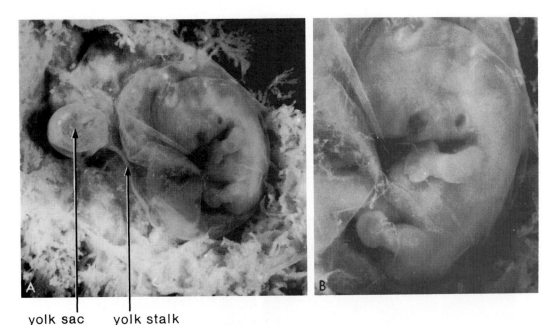

yolk sac   yolk stalk

Figure 6–10. *A,* Photograph of a seven-week embryo in its amniotic sac. It has been exposed by opening the chorionic sac (× 2.8). *B,* Higher magnification of the embryo of 44 to 46 days (× 5). Note the low position of its ear at this stage and the notches between the digital rays of its hand. Observe the yolk sac and its stalk which passes through the umbilical cord to the midgut (see Fig. 13–6).

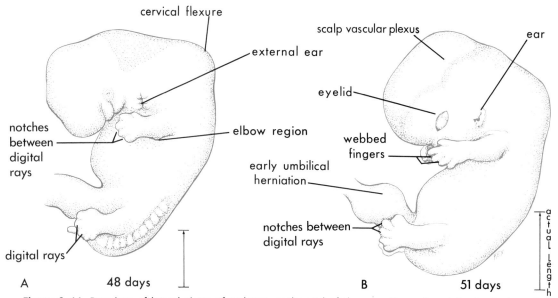

Figure 6–11. Drawings of lateral views of embryos at the end of the seventh week and the beginning of the eighth week. Note that the limbs now extend ventrally.

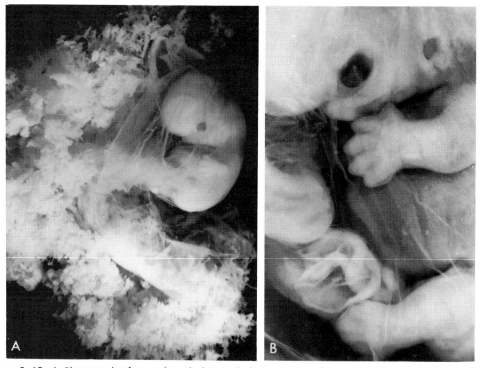

Figure 6–12. *A,* Photograph of an embryo in its amniotic sac, exposed by opening the chorionic sac (× 2). *B,* Higher magnification of this embryo of about 51 days (× 7). Note the large hand and the webbed fingers. (Photographed by Professor Jean Hay, Department of Anatomy, University of Manitoba.)

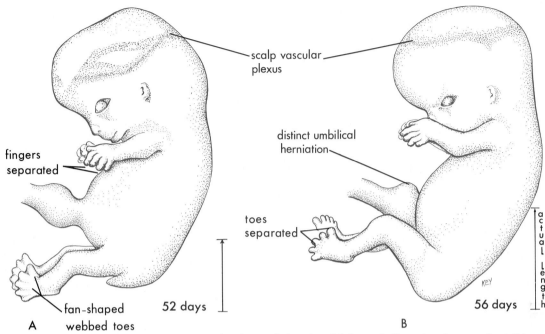

scalp vascular plexus

distinct umbilical herniation

fingers separated

toes separated

fan-shaped webbed toes

A

52 days

56 days

actual length

KEY

B

Figure 6–13. Drawings of lateral views of embryos during the eighth week. Note the absence of a tail in the mature embryo (*B*).

measurements of length (Table 6–1). The changing appearance of the developing limbs is a very useful criterion. Size alone may be an unreliable criterion because some embryos undergo a progressively slower rate of growth prior to death.

Methods of Measuring Embryos

Because embryos are straight early in the fourth week (Figs. 6–4 and 6–16), measurements indicate their *greatest length* (GL). The sitting height or *crown-rump length* (CRL) is used for most embryos, but standing height or crown-heel length (CHL) is sometimes used for embryos at the end of the eighth week (Figs. 6–14 and 6–16*D*).

The size of the embryo in a pregnant woman can also be estimated using ultrasound measurements (Fig. 6–15). *Transvaginal sonography* permits an early and accurate measurement of CRL (Lyons and Levi, 1991). At four weeks (six weeks after LNMP), the embryo, amnion, and yolk sac form a structure about 5 mm long that is detectable with careful scanning. After the fifth week (seven weeks after LNMP), discrete embryonic structures can be visualized (e.g., parts of the limbs), and CRL measurements can be made.

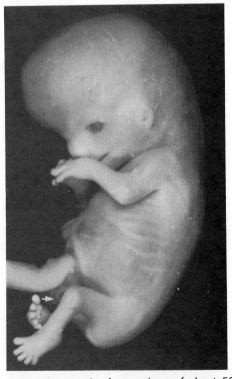

Figure 6–14. Photograph of an embryo of about 56 days (× 2). The intestines are still in the umbilical cord (*arrow*). The digits (fingers and toes) are clearly defined. Note the relatively large head and that the tail has disappeared. Its cartilaginous ribs are visible. (Photographed by Professor Jean Hay, Department of Anatomy, University of Manitoba.)

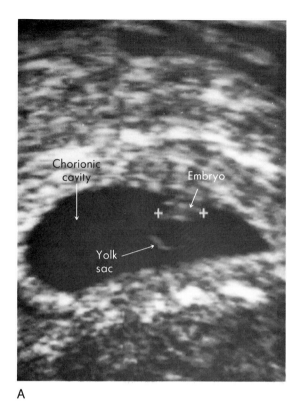

A

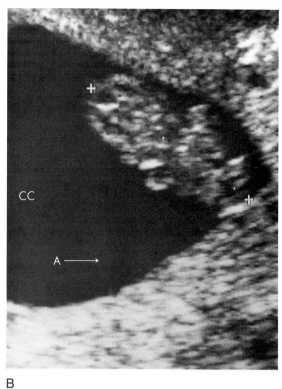

B

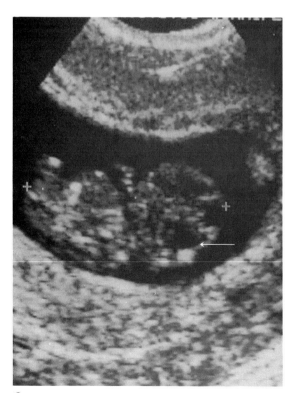

C

Figure 6–15. Ultrasound images of embryos. *A*, CRL 4.8 mm. The 4½-week-old embryo is indicated by the measurement cursors (+). Ventral to the embryo is the yolk sac. The chorionic cavity appears black (see also Fig. 5–1*B₂*). *B*, CRL 2.09 cm. Coronal scan of a 5-week-old embryo. The upper limbs are clearly shown. The embryo is surrounded by a thin amnion (*A*). The fluid in the chorionic cavity (CC) is more particulate than the amniotic fluid. *C*, CRL of 2.14 cm. Sagittal scan of a seven-week embryo demonstrating the eye, limbs, and the developing fourth ventricle of the brain *(arrow)*. (Courtesy of Dr. E.A. Lyons, Professor of Radiology and Obstetrics and Gynecology, Head of Radiology, Health Sciences Centre, University of Manitoba, Winnipeg, Manitoba, Canada.)

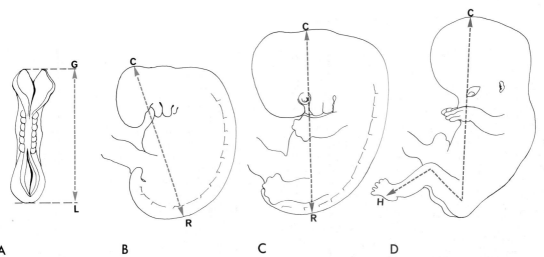

A   B   C   D

Figure 6–16. Sketches showing the methods used to measure the length of embryos. *A*, Greatest length. *A*, *B*, and *C*, Crown-rump length. *D*, Crown-heel length.

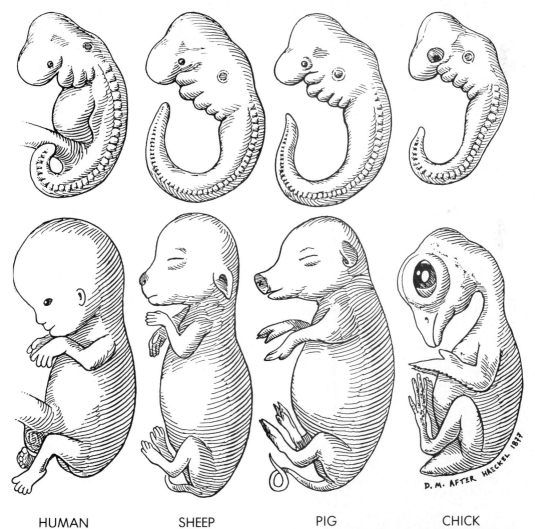

HUMAN   SHEEP   PIG   CHICK

Figure 6–17. Drawings of embryos of four species, showing how their early characteristics are similar. Observe the large prominence formed by the heart in the human embryo. By the eighth week, human embryos have distinctive characteristics. Note the absence of a tail.

SUMMARY

Early in the embryonic period, longitudinal and transverse folding converts the flat, trilaminar, embryonic disc into a C-shaped, cylindrical embryo. The dorsal part of the yolk sac is incorporated into the embryo during this folding and gives rise to the *primitive gut*. The gut becomes pinched off from the yolk sac but remains attached to it by the narrow yolk stalk. The head fold causes the large heart to lie ventrally and the brain to become the most cranial part of the embryo. The tail fold causes the connecting stalk (future umbilical cord) to move to the ventral surface of the embryo.

The three germ layers differentiate into various tissues and organs so that, by the end of the embryonic period, the primordia of all the main organ systems have been established. The external appearance of the embryo is greatly affected by the formation of the brain, heart, liver, somites, limbs, ears, nose, and eyes. As these structures develop, they produce characteristics that mark the embryo as unquestionably human. Because the primordia of all essential external and internal structures are developing during the fourth to eighth weeks, this is a critical period of development. Developmental disturbances during this period may give rise to major congenital anomalies (see Chapter 9).

Reasonable estimates of the age of embryos can be determined from: (1) the day of onset of the last normal menstrual period, (2) the estimated time of fertilization, (3) measurements of the chorionic sac and embryo, and (4) study of the embryo's external characteristics. The age of an embryo in utero can also be estimated by making ultrasound measurements (Fig. 6–15).

Commonly Asked Questions

1. I have heard that the early human embryo could be confused with the offspring of several other species, e.g., a pig, mouse, or chick. Is this true? What is the distinctive feature of early human embryos?
2. I cannot see a difference between an eight-week-old embryo and a nine-week-old fetus. Why do embryologists give them different names?
3. When does the embryo become a human being? What guidelines can be used?
4. Can the sex of embryos be determined by ultrasound study? What other methods can be used to diagnose sex?
5. What is the difference between the terms *primigravida* and *primipara*? I have also heard nurses refer to pregnant women as "primips." What does this mean?

The answers to these questions are given on page 328.

REFERENCES

Biggers JD: *Arbitrary Partitions of Prenatal Life. Human Reprod* 5:1, 1990.

Callen PW (ed): *Ultrasonography in Obstetrics and Gynecology,* 2nd ed. Philadelphia, WB Saunders, 1988.

Chapman MG, Grudzinskas JG, Chard T (eds): *The Embryo. Normal and Abnormal Development and Growth.* New York, Springer-Verlag, 1990.

Cooke J: The early embryo and the formation of body pattern. *American Scientist* 76:35, 1988.

Filly RA: The first trimester. *In* Callen PW (ed): *Ultrasonography in Obstetrics and Gynecology,* 2nd ed. Philadelphia, WB Saunders, 1988.

Guthrie S: Horizontal and vertical pathways in neural induction. *Trends in Neurosciences* 14:123, 1991.

Hinrichsen KV: The early development of morphology and patterns of the face in the human embryo. *Advances in Anatomy, Embryology and Cell Biology* 98:1. New York, Springer-Verlag, 1985.

Kalousek DK, Fitch N, Paradice BA: *Pathology of the Human Embryo and Previable Fetus. An Atlas.* New York, Springer-Verlag, 1990.

Kerner P: The rate of growth in young human embryos of Streeter's horizons XIII and XXIII. *Acta Anat* 66:176, 1967.

Kurtz AB, Needleman L: Ultrasound assessment of fetal age. *In* Callen PW (ed): *Ultrasonography in Obstetrics and Gynecology,* 2nd ed. Philadephia, WB Saunders, 1988.

Lyons EA, Levi CS: Ultrasound of the normal first trimester of pregnancy. Syllabus. Special Course. Ultrasound, Radiological Society of North America, 1991.

Moore KL, Persaud TVN: *The Developing Human. Clinically Oriented Embryology*, 5th ed. Philadelphia, WB Saunders, 1993.

Nieuwkoop PD, Johnen AG, Albers B: *The Epigenetic Nature of Early Chordate Development. Inductive Interaction and Competence*. London, Cambridge University Press, 1985.

Nishimura H, Takano K, Tanimura T, Yasuda M: Normal and abnormal development of human embryos. *Teratology 1*:281, 1968.

Nishimura H, Tanimura T, Semba R, Uwabe C: Normal development of early human embryos: Observation of 90 specimens at Carnegie stages 7 to 13. *Teratology 10*:1, 1974.

O'Rahilly R: Guide to the staging of human embryos. *Anat Anz 130*:556, 1972.

O'Rahilly R, Müller F: *Developmental Stages in Human Embryos*. Washington, Carnegie Institute of Washington, 1987.

Persaud TVN: *Environmental Causes of Human Birth Defects*. Springfield, Charles C Thomas, 1990.

Saxen L: Interactive mechanisms in morphogenesis. *In* Tarin D (ed): *Tissue Interactions in Carcinogenesis*. London, Academic Press, 1972.

Schats R, Van Os HC, Jansen CAM, Wladimiroff JW: The crown-rump length in early human pregnancy: a reappraisal. *Br J Obstet Gynaecol 98*:460, 1991.

Senterre J (ed): Intrauterine Growth Retardation: Nestle Nutrition Workshop Series, vol 18. New York, Raven Press, 1989.

Shiota K: Development and intrauterine fate of normal and abnormal human conceptuses. *Cong Anom 31*:67, 1991.

Thompson MW, McInnes RR, Willard HF: *Thompson & Thompson Genetics in Medicine*, 5th ed. Philadelphia, WB Saunders, 1991.

Wessels NK: *Tissue Interactions in Development*. Menlo Park, CA, WB Benjamin Incorporated, 1977.

7

THE NINTH
TO THIRTY-EIGHTH WEEKS
OF HUMAN DEVELOPMENT

THE FETAL PERIOD

The developmental period from the beginning of the **ninth week** after fertilization to **full term** (38 weeks after LNMP) is known as the fetal period (Fig. 7–1). It is characterized by maturation of the tissues and organs and rapid growth of the body. At nine weeks the human embryo is referred to as a *fetus* (L., offspring) to signify that it has developed into a recognizable human being. In addition, the fetus is less vulnerable than the embryo to the teratogenic effects of drugs, viruses, and radiation (see Chapter 9).

The transformation of an embryo to a fetus is not abrupt, but the name change is intended to signify the change from embryonic to fetal development. Development during the fetal period is primarily concerned with the growth and differentiation of tissues and organs that appeared during the embryonic period. Very few new structures appear during the fetal period. The rate of body growth during the fetal period is remarkable, especially between the ninth and sixteenth weeks (Figs. 7–1 and 7–4), and weight gain is phenomenal during the terminal months (Table 7–2; Fig. 7–10).

Fetuses weighing less than 500 gm at birth usually do not survive. The term *abortion* is applied to all pregnancies that terminate before the period of viability, i.e., before 22 weeks (Table 7–2). If given expert postnatal care, some fetuses weighing 500 to 1000 gm may survive if born prematurely; they are referred to as *immature infants*. Fetuses weighing between 1500 and 2500 gm are called *premature infants*. Although most of them survive, prematurity is one of the most common causes of morbidity (illness) and perinatal death (Behrman, 1992).

During a pregnant woman's first visit to a physician, the age of the embryo or fetus is estimated. The date of the last normal menstrual period (LNMP) is a time-honored guide to establishing *gestational age,* and it is reliable in most cases. To determine the *fertilization age* (developmental age) of the embryo, two weeks must be deducted from the gestational age because development does not begin until about two weeks after LNMP (see Fig. 1–1).

ESTIMATION OF FETAL AGE

If doubt arises about the age of a fetus, ultrasonic measurements can be taken to determine its size and probable age (Kurtz and Needleman, 1988). A pregnancy (gestational period) may be divided into days, weeks, or months (Table 7–1). Confusion arises if it is not stated whether a given time is calculated from: (1) the onset of the LNMP, or (2) the estimated day of fertilization. More uncertainty arises when months are used, particularly when it is not stated whether *calendar months* (28 to 31 days) or *lunar months*

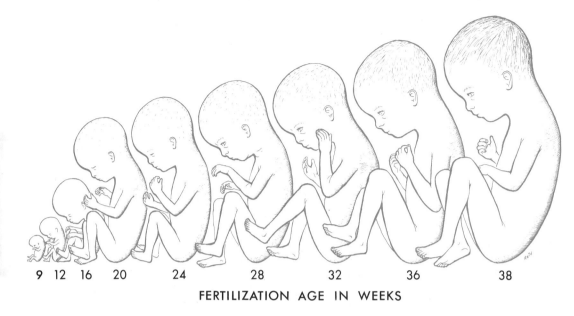

9 12 16 20   24   28   32   36   38

FERTILIZATION AGE IN WEEKS

Figure 7–1. Drawings of fetuses, about one-fifth actual size. Head hair begins to appear at about 20 weeks. Eyebrows and eyelashes are usually recognizable by 24 weeks, and the eyes are open by 26 weeks. The mean duration of pregnancy is 266 days (38 weeks) from fertilization, with a standard deviation of 12 days. In clinical practice it is customary to refer to full term as 40 weeks from the first day of the last normal menstrual period (LNMP). Thus, when a doctor refers to a pregnancy of 20 weeks, the actual age of the fetus is 18 weeks.

(28 days) are meant. Unless otherwise stated, fetal age in this book is calculated from the estimated time of fertilization, and months refer to calendar months. It is best to express the age of a fetus in weeks and to state whether the beginning or the end of a week is meant, because statements such as "in the tenth week" are nonspecific.

> Clinically, gestation in humans is divided into three periods or **trimesters,** each lasting three calendar months. By the end of the first trimester, all major systems are developed and the crown-rump length (CRL) of the fetus is about the width of one's palm (see Fig. 7–6*B*). At the end of the second trimester (26 weeks after LNMP), the fetus is usually too immature to survive if born prematurely, even though its length is nearly equal to the span of one's hand (see Fig. 7–8).

External Characteristics of Fetuses

Various measurements and external characteristics are useful in estimating fetal age (Table 7–2). *Foot length* correlates well with crown-rump length (CRL) and is particularly useful for estimating the age of incomplete or macerated fetuses. *Fetal weight* is often a useful criterion, but there may be a discrepancy between the fertilization age and the weight of a fetus, particularly when the mother has had metabolic disturbances during pregnancy; e.g., diabetes mellitus. In these cases, fetal weight often exceeds values considered normal for CRL.

Fetal dimensions obtained from measurements of fetuses using ultrasound closely approximate CRL measurements obtained from aborted fetuses (Table 7–2). In addition, the diameter of the head and the dimension of the trunk may be obtained. At nine to ten weeks, the head is still slightly larger than the trunk. Ultrasound CRL measurements of the fetus are predictive of fetal age with an accuracy of ± one to four days. Assessment of fetal size and age is enhanced when head and trunk dimensions are considered along with CRL measurements. Determination of the size of the fetus, especially of its head, is of great value to the obstetrician for the management of patients (e.g., those women with small pelves and/or those fetuses with intrauterine growth retardation (IUGR) and/or congenital anomalies).

Table 7–2. CRITERIA FOR ESTIMATING FERTILIZATION AGE DURING THE FETAL PERIOD

Age (weeks)	CR Length (mm)*	Foot Length (mm)*	Fetal Weight (gm)†	Main External Characteristics
Previable Fetuses				
9	50	7	8	*Eyes closing or closed.* Head more rounded. External genitalia still not distinguishable as male or female. Intestines in umbilical cord.
10	61	9	14	*Intestine in abdomen.* Early fingernail development.
12	87	14	45	*Sex distinguishable externally.* Well-defined neck.
14	120	20	110	*Head erect.* Lower limbs well developed. Early toenail development.
16	140	27	200	*Ears stand out from head.*
18	160	33	320	*Vernix caseosa covers skin.* Quickening (signs of life felt by mother).
20	190	39	460	*Head and body hair (lanugo) visible.*
Viable Fetuses‡				
22	210	45	630	*Skin wrinkled* and red.
24	230	50	820	*Fingernails present.* Lean body.
26	250	55	1000	*Eyes partially open.* Eyelashes present.
28	270	59	1300	*Eyes open.* Good head of hair. Skin slightly wrinkled.
30	280	63	1700	*Toenails present.* Body filling out. Testes descending.
32	300	68	2100	*Fingernails reach finger tips.* Skin pink and smooth.
36	340	79	2900	*Body usually plump.* Lanugo hairs almost absent. Toenails reach toe tips. Flexed limbs; firm grasp.
38	360	83	3400	*Prominent chest;* breasts protrude. Testes in scrotum or palpable in inguinal canals. Fingernails extend beyond finger tips.

* These measurements are averages and so may not apply to specific cases; dimensional variations increase with age. The method for taking CR (crown-rump) measurements is illustrated in Figure 6–16.

† These weights refer to fetuses that have been fixed for about two weeks in 10 per cent formalin. Fresh specimens usually weigh about 5 per cent less.

‡ There is no sharp limit of development, age, or weight at which a fetus automatically becomes viable or beyond which survival is ensured, but experience has shown that it is uncommon for a baby to survive whose weight is less than 500 gm or whose fertilization age or developmental age is less than 22 weeks. Even fetuses born during the 26- to 28-week period have difficulty surviving, mainly because the respiratory and central nervous systems are not completely differentiated. The term *abortion* refers to all pregnancies that terminate before the period of viability.

HIGHLIGHTS OF THE FETAL PERIOD

No formal system of staging is used for the fetal period, but it is useful to consider the changes that occur in periods of four to five weeks.

Table 7–1. COMPARISON OF GESTATIONAL TIME UNITS

Reference Point	Days	Weeks	Calendar Months	Lunar Months
Fertilization*	266	38	8¾	9½
LNMP	280	40	9	10

* The date of birth is calculated as about 266 days after the estimated day of fertilization, or 280 days after the onset of the last normal menstrual period (LNMP). From fertilization to the end of the embryonic period (8 weeks), age is best expressed in days; thereafter age is commonly given in weeks. Because ovulation and fertilization are usually separated by not more than 12 hours, these events are more or less interchangeable in expressing prenatal age. When stating age it is best to state the reference point used.

Nine to Twelve Weeks

At the beginning of the ninth week, the head constitutes one half the CRL of the fetus (Figs. 7–1 to 7–5); thereafter, growth in body length accelerates rapidly so that, by the end of 12 weeks, fetal length has more than doubled (Table 7–2). Growth of the head slows down considerably, however, compared with that of the rest of the body. The face is broad, the eyes widely separated, and the ears low-set. The eyes are usually closed during the ninth week. *Primary ossification centers* appear in the skeleton, especially in the skull and long bones (see Chapter 16).

Early in the ninth week, the legs are short and the thighs are relatively small (Fig. 7–3). At the end of 12 weeks, the upper limbs have almost reached their final relative lengths, but the

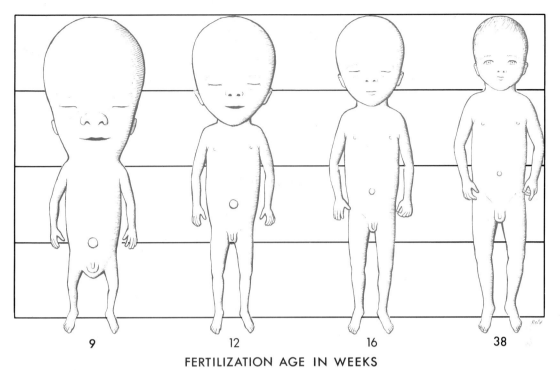

FERTILIZATION AGE IN WEEKS

Figure 7–2. Diagram illustrating the changing proportions of the body during the fetal period. By 36 weeks the circumferences of the head and the abdomen are approximately equal. After this, the circumference of the abdomen may be greater. All stages are drawn to the same total height.

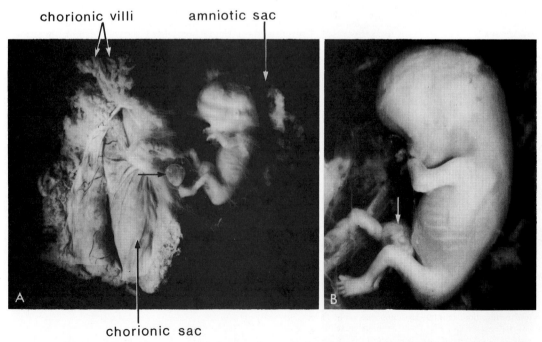

chorionic villi   amniotic sac

chorionic sac

Figure 7–3. Photographs of a nine-week fetus in its amniotic sac, exposed by removal from its chorionic sac. *A*, Actual size. The remnant of the yolk sac is indicated by an arrow. *B*, Enlarged photograph of the fetus (× 2). Note the following features: (1) large head, (2) cartilaginous ribs, and (3) intestines in the proximal part of the umbilical cord *(arrow)*. (Photographed by Professor Jean Hay, Department of Anatomy, University of Manitoba.)

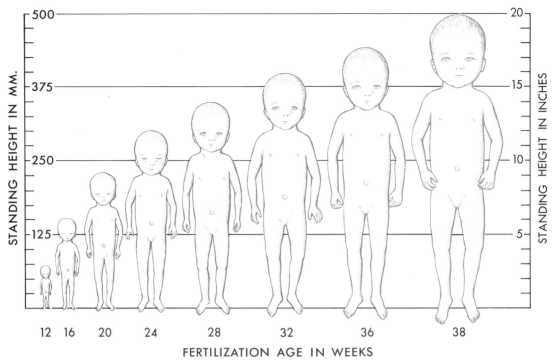

Figure 7–4. Diagram illustrating the changes in size of the human fetus when drawn to scale.

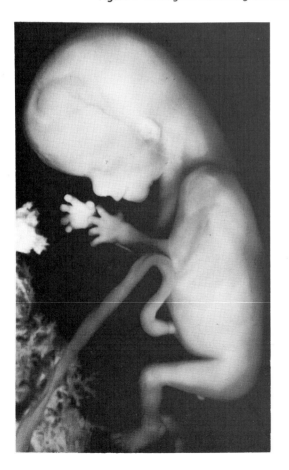

Figure 7–5. Photograph of an 11-week fetus exposed by removal from its chorionic and amniotic sacs (× 1.5). Note the relatively large head and that the intestine is no longer in the umbilical cord. Note that its head is still disproportionately large. (Photographed by Professor Jean Hay, Department of Anatomy, University of Manitoba.)

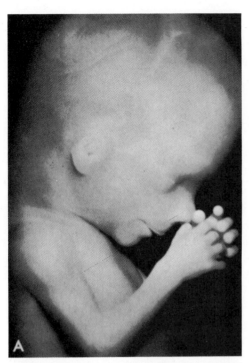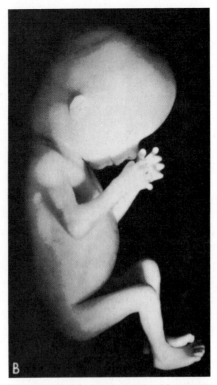

Figure 7–6. Photographs of a 13-week fetus. *A*, Enlarged photograph of its head and shoulders (× 2). Note that its eyes are closed due to adherence of the eyelids. *B*, Actual size. Note that its CRL is about the same as the width of the palm. (Photographed by Professor Jean Hay, Department of Anatomy, University of Manitoba.)

lower limbs are still not so well developed and are slightly shorter than their final relative lengths (Fig. 7–2). The external genitalia of males and females appear somewhat similar until the end of the ninth week. Their mature form is not established until the twelfth week (see Chapter 14).

Intestinal coils are visible in the proximal end of the umbilical cord (Fig. 7–3*B*) until the middle of the tenth week. By the eleventh week the intestines have usually returned to the abdomen. At the beginning of the ninth week, the liver is the major site of *erythropoiesis* (formation of blood cells). By the end of the twelfth week this activity has decreased in the liver and has begun in the spleen.

Urine starts to form between the ninth and twelfth weeks and is excreted into the amniotic fluid. The fetus reabsorbs some of this after swallowing it (p. 109). Waste products then pass into the maternal circulation by passage across the placental membrane (see Figs. 8–6 and 8–7). The fetus begins to move during the nine- to twelve-week period, but these movements cannot be detected by the mother.

Thirteen to Sixteen Weeks

Growth is very rapid during this period (Fig. 7–6; Table 7–2). Ultrasonography has revealed that slow *eye movements* occur at 14 weeks. By 16 weeks the head is relatively small compared with that of the 12-week fetus, and the lower limbs have lengthened. The skeleton shows clearly on radiographs (x-ray films) of the mother's abdomen toward the end of this period. At 16 weeks the appearance of the fetus is even more human because the eyes are facing anteriorly rather than laterally. In addition, the external ears are close to their definitive positions on the sides of the head.

Seventeen to Twenty Weeks

Growth slows down during this period (Fig. 7–7; Table 7–2). Fetal movements known as

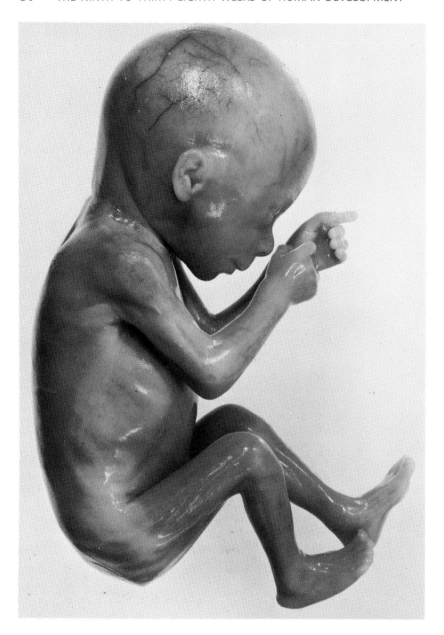

Figure 7–7. Photograph of a 17-week fetus. Actual size. Because there is very little subcutaneous fat and the skin is very thin, the underlying scalp vessels are clearly visible. Fetuses at this age are unable to survive if born prematurely, mainly because their respiratory systems are immature.

quickening are commonly recognized by the mother. The skin is covered with a greasy, cheeselike material known as *vernix caseosa*. It consists of a mixture of a fatty secretion from the fetal sebaceous glands of the skin and dead epidermal cells (see Chapter 19). The vernix caseosa protects the delicate fetal skin from abrasions, chapping, and hardening that could result from being bathed in amniotic fluid.

The bodies of 20-week fetuses are usually completely covered with fine downy hair called *lanugo;* this hair may help hold the vernix on the skin. Eyebrows and head hair are also visible at the end of this period. *Brown fat* forms during this time and is the site of heat production, particularly in the newborn infant. This specialized adipose tissue produces heat by oxidizing fatty acids. Brown fat is chiefly found at the root of the neck posterior to the sternum and in the perirenal area. Brown fat has a high content of mitochondria, giving it a definite brown hue.

Twenty-one to Twenty-five Weeks

There is a *substantial weight gain* during this period (Fig. 7–8). Although the body is still somewhat lean, it is better proportioned. Fingernails are present. The skin is usually wrinkled and is more translucent. The skin appears pink to red because blood in the capillaries is now visible. By 24 weeks the secretory epithelial cells (type II pneumocytes) of the lung have begun to produce *surfactant*, a surface-active lipid that maintains alveolar patency in the lungs (see Chapter 12). Although most organs and systems are rather well developed, a 22- to 25-week fetus often dies if born prematurely, mainly because its respiratory system is still immature.

Twenty-six to Twenty-nine Weeks

During this period a fetus often survives if born prematurely and given intensive care because its lungs are now capable of breathing air. The lungs and pulmonary vasculature have developed sufficiently to provide adequate gas exchange (see Fig. 12–7). In addition, the central nervous system has matured to the stage at which it can direct rhythmic breathing movements and control body temperature.

The eyes reopen at 26 weeks, and head and lanugo hair are well developed. Toenails become visible, and considerable subcutaneous fat has now formed under the skin, smoothing out many of the wrinkles. During this period the quantity of white fat in the body increases to about 3.5 per cent of body weight. *Erythropoiesis* in the spleen ends by 28 weeks, by which time the bone marrow has become the major site of formation of erythrocytes.

Thirty to Thirty-four Weeks

The *pupillary light reflex* of the eyes is present by 30 weeks. Usually by the end of this period, the skin is pink and smooth, and the upper and lower limbs have a chubby appearance. At this stage the quantity of white fat in the body is about eight per cent of body weight. Fetuses 32 weeks and older usually survive if born prematurely. The fetus usually assumes an upside-down position as the time of birth approaches; this positioning results partly from the shape of the uterus and partly because the head is heavier than the feet.

Thirty-five to Thirty-eight Weeks

Fetuses at 35 weeks have a firm grasp and exhibit a spontaneous orientation to light. Most fetuses during this "finishing period" are plump (Fig. 7–9). By 36 weeks the circumference of the head and the abdomen are approximately equal; after this, the circumference of the abdomen is greater than that of the head.

There is a *slowing of growth* as the time of birth approaches (Fig. 7–10). Normal fetuses usually reach a CRL of 360 mm and weigh about 3400 gm. By full term the amount of white fat in the body is about 16 per cent of body weight. A fetus lays down about 14 gm of fat a day during the last few weeks of gestation. In general, male fetuses grow faster than females, and male infants weigh more than female infants at birth.

By *full term* (38 weeks after fertilization; 40 weeks after LNMP), the skin is usually bluish-pink in color. The chest is prominent and the breasts protrude in both sexes. The testes are usually in the scrotum in full-term male infants; descent begins at about 28 to 32 weeks; thus, premature male infants commonly have undescended testes. The testes in these babies usually descend during early infancy.

The Time of Birth

The expected date of confinement (EDC) for the birth of a baby is roughly calculated as 266 days or 38 weeks after fertilization, or 280 days or 40 weeks from the onset of the last normal menstrual period (Table 7–1). Most fetuses are born within 10 to 15 days of this time. Prolongation of pregnancy beyond the EDC occurs in five to six per cent of women.

> The common clinical method of determining EDC is to count back three calendar months from the first day of the LNMP and then add a year and seven days. In women with regular menstrual cycles, this gives a reasonably accurate EDC. Ultrasound measurements of the CRL of fetuses are commonly used for obtaining a more precise prediction of EDC (Kurtz and Needleman, 1988).

FACTORS INFLUENCING FETAL GROWTH

The fetus requires substrates for growth and the production of energy. These substances pass

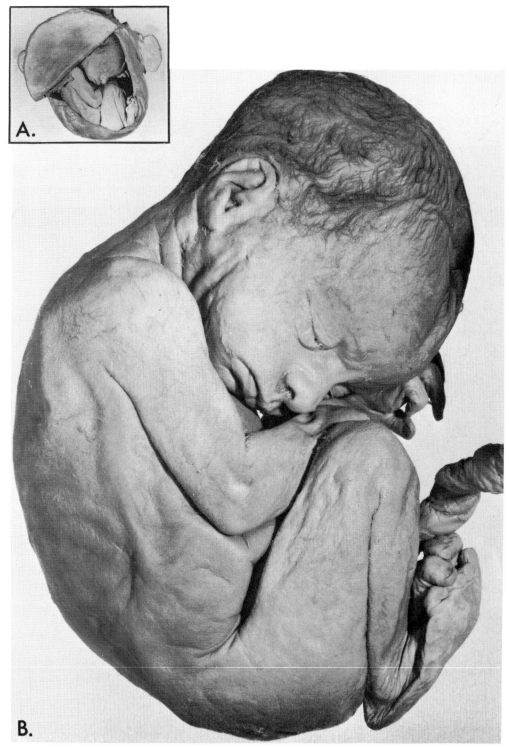

Figure 7–8. Photographs of a 25-week fetus. *A,* In the uterus. *B,* Actual size. Note the wrinkled skin and rather lean body caused by the scarcity of subcutaneous fat. Observe that the eyes are beginning to open. A fetus at this age might survive if born prematurely; hence, it is a viable fetus. The mother of this fetus was killed in an automobile accident and the fetus died before it could be removed by cesarean section.

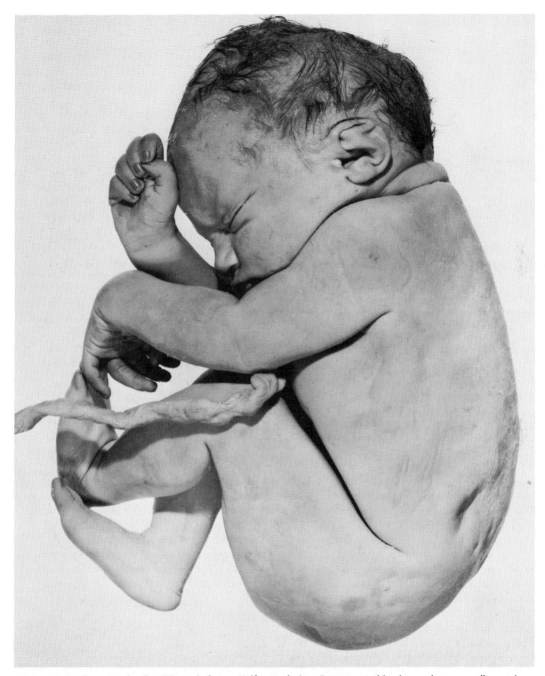

Figure 7-9. Photograph of a 36-week fetus. Half actual size. Fetuses at this size and age usually survive. Note the plump body resulting from the deposition of subcutaneous fat. This fetus' mother was killed in an automobile accident, and the fetus died before it could be delivered by cesarean section.

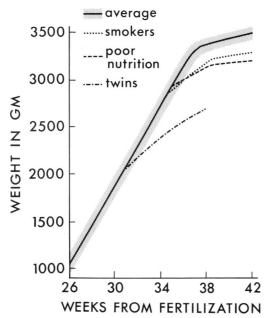

Figure 7–10. Graph showing the rate of fetal growth during the last trimester. Average refers to babies born in the United States. After 36 weeks the growth rate deviates from the straight line. The decline, particularly after full term (38 weeks), probably reflects inadequate fetal nutrition caused by degenerative placental changes. Note the adverse effect on fetal weight created by mothers who smoke heavily or eat a poor-quality diet. (Adapted from Gruenwald P: Growth of the human fetus. I. Normal growth and its variation. *Am J Obstet Gynecol 94*:1112, 1966.)

freely to the fetus from the mother via the placental membrane (see Figs. 8–5 to 8–7). *Glucose* is the primary source of energy for fetal metabolism and growth, but amino acids are also required. The *insulin* required for the metabolism of glucose is secreted mainly by the fetal pancreas. For a comprehensive account of fetal growth, see Bowie (1988).

Many factors may affect fetal growth: maternal, fetal, and environmental. In general, factors operating throughout pregnancy (e.g., *heavy cigarette smoking and consumption of alcohol*) tend to produce intrauterine growth retardation (IUGR) and small infants; whereas, factors operating during the last trimester (e.g., maternal malnutrition) usually produce underweight infants with normal length and head size. IUGR is usually defined as infant weight within the lowest tenth percentile for gestational age (Bowie, 1988).

MATERNAL MALNUTRITION. Severe maternal malnutrition resulting from a poor-quality diet is known to cause reduced fetal growth (Fig.

7–10). Poor nutrition and faulty food habits are common and are not restricted to mothers belonging to poverty groups.

CIGARETTE SMOKING. The growth rate of fetuses of mothers who smoke cigarettes is less than normal during the last six to eight weeks of pregnancy (Fig. 7–10). On average, the birth weight of infants whose mothers smoke heavily is 200 gm less than normal. The effect is greater on fetuses whose mothers also eat a poor-quality diet.

MULTIPLE PREGNANCY. Individuals of twins, triplets, and other multiple births usually weigh considerably less than infants resulting from a single pregnancy. It is evident that the total requirements of twins exceed the nutritional supply available from the placenta during the third trimester (Fig. 7–10).

SOCIAL DRUGS. Infants born to alcoholic mothers often exhibit IUGR as part of the *fetal alcohol syndrome* (see Chapter 9). Similarly, the use of marijuana and narcotic drugs (e.g., heroin) can cause IUGR and other obstetrical complications.

IMPAIRED UTEROPLACENTAL BLOOD FLOW. Maternal placental circulation may be reduced by a variety of conditions that decreases uterine blood flow (e.g., severe hypotension and renal disease). Chronic reduction of uterine blood flow can cause *fetal starvation* and IUGR.

PLACENTAL INSUFFICIENCY. Placental dysfunction or defects can also cause intrauterine fetal growth retardation. These placental changes reduce the total surface area available for exchange of nutrients between the fetal and maternal bloodstreams (see Chapter 8).

GENETIC FACTORS. It is well established that genetic factors can cause IUGR. In recent years structural and numerical chromosomal aberrations have also been associated with cases of retarded fetal growth (see Chapter 9). IUGR is pronounced in infants with Down syndrome and is characteristic of persons with trisomy 18 syndrome (see Fig. 9–5).

PERINATOLOGY

Perinatology is the branch of medicine concerned with the health of the fetus and newborn infant, generally covering the *perinatal period* from about 26 weeks after fertilization to about four weeks after birth. The subspecialty known as *perinatal medicine* combines certain aspects of obstetrics and pediatrics. A third trimester fetus is now regarded as an *unborn patient* on whom diagnostic and therapeutic procedures may be performed. Several techniques are now available for assessing the status of the human fetus and for providing prenatal treatment if required.

Fetal activity felt by the mother or palpated by the physician have been the classical clues for assessing fetal well-being. In the past, the fetal heartbeat was detected first by auscultation and later by electronic monitors; these techniques indicated fetal stress and distress. Later, gonadotropic hormones were detected in maternal blood. Many new procedures for assessing the status of the fetus have been developed in the last two decades. It is now possible to treat many fetuses whose lives are in jeopardy.

Procedures for Assessing the Status of the Fetus

DIAGNOSTIC AMNIOCENTESIS (Fig. 7–11*A*). Amniotic fluid is sampled by inserting a hollow needle through the mother's abdominal and uterine walls into the amniotic cavity. A syringe is then attached and amniotic fluid withdrawn. Because there is relatively little amniotic fluid prior to the fourteenth week, amniocentesis is difficult to perform prior to this time. Amniocentesis is relatively devoid of risk, especially when the procedure is performed by an experienced obstetrician who is guided by ultrasonog-

raphy for placental and fetal localization. Amniocentesis is the most common technique for detecting genetic disorders (e.g., **Down** syndrome) and is usually performed 13 to 14 weeks after the estimated time of fertilization.

The following are common *indications for amniocentesis:* (1) advanced maternal age (e.g., 38 years or older), (2) previous birth of a trisomic child (e.g., Down syndrome), (3) a chromosome abnormality in either parent (e.g., a chromosome translocation; see Chapter 9), (4) women who are carriers of X-linked recessive disorders (e.g., hemophilia), (5) a history of neural tube defects (NTDs) in the family (e.g., spina bifida; see Chapter 17), and (6) carriers of inborn errors of metabolism (Hobbins, 1991).

CHORIONIC VILLUS SAMPLING (CVS). Pieces of chorionic villi may be obtained by inserting a needle, guided by ultrasonography, through the mother's abdominal and uterine walls into the uterine cavity (Fig. 7–11*B*). CVS is commonly performed transcervically using ultrasound guidance (Hogge, 1991). Biopsies of chorionic villi are used for detecting chromosomal abnormalities, inborn errors of metabolism, and X-linked disorders. CVS can be performed between nine and eleven weeks of gestation (seven to nine weeks after fertilization). The rate of fetal loss is about one per cent, slightly more than the risk from amniocentesis (0.5 per cent). The major

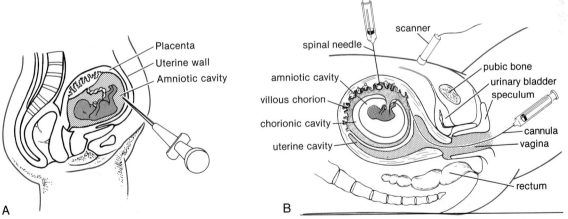

Figure 7–11. *A*, Drawing illustrating the technique of amniocentesis. A needle is inserted through the lower abdominal wall and uterine wall into the amniotic cavity. A syringe is attached and amniotic fluid withdrawn for diagnostic purposes (e.g., for cell cultures or alpha-fetoprotein studies). This technique is usually performed during the fourteenth to sixteenth weeks after the last normal menstrual period (LNMP). *B*, Drawing illustrating chorionic villus sampling (CVS). Two sampling approaches are illustrated: via the maternal anterior abdominal wall with a spinal needle, and via the vagina and cervical canal using a malleable cannula. This technique is usually performed around nine weeks after the LNMP (seven weeks after fertilization). Success and safety in both approaches depend upon use of a scanner (ultrasound imaging).

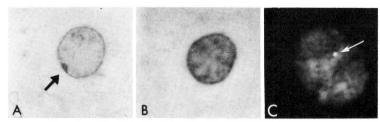

Figure 7–12. Nuclei of cells in amniotic fluid obtained by amniocentesis. *A,* Chromatin-positive nucleus indicating the presence of a female fetus; the sex chromatin is indicated by an arrow. *B,* Chromatin-negative nucleus indicating the presence of a male fetus. No sex chromatin is visible. Cresylecht violet stain (× 1000). *C,* Y-chromatin-positive nucleus indicating the presence of a male fetus. The arrow indicates the Y chromatin as an intensely fluorescent body obtained after staining the cell in quinacrine mustard. (*A* and *B* from Riis M, Fuchs F: Sex chromatin and antenatal sex diagnosis. *In* Moore KL [ed]: *The Sex Chromatin.* Philadelphia, WB Saunders, 1966. *C,* Courtesy of the late Dr. M. Ray, Department of Human Genetics and Department of Anatomy, University of Manitoba and Health Sciences Centre, Winnipeg, Canada.)

advantage of CVS over amniocentesis is that the results of chromosomal analysis are available several weeks earlier than when performed by amniocentesis.

SEX CHROMATIN PATTERNS. Fetal sex can be diagnosed by noting the presence or absence of sex chromatin in cells recovered from amniotic fluid (Fig. 7–12). By using a special staining technique, the Y chromosome can also be detected in cells obtained from amniotic fluid. Knowledge of *fetal sex* can be useful in diagnosing the presence of severe, sex-linked, hereditary diseases such as *hemophilia* or muscular dystrophy. These tests are not done to diagnose fetal sex for curious parents.

CELL CULTURES. Fetal sex and chromosomal abnormalities also can be determined by studying the sex chromosomes of cultured amniotic cells. These studies are commonly done when an autosomal abnormality is suspected, such as occurs in Down syndrome (see in Chapter 9). Inborn errors of metabolism and enzyme deficiencies in fetuses can also be detected by studying cell cultures. Cell cultures permit prenatal diagnosis of severe diseases for which there is no effective treatment and afford the opportunity to interrupt the pregnancy if desired.

ALPHA-FETOPROTEIN (AFP) ASSAY. AFP escapes from the circulation and enters the amniotic fluid from fetuses with open *neural tube defects* (see Chapter 17). The concentration of AFP in the amniotic fluid surrounding fetuses with spina bifida cystica and meroanencephaly (anencephaly) is very high. It is thus possible to detect the presence of these severe abnormalities by measuring the concentration of AFP in amniotic fluid. AFP concentration is also likely to be higher than normal in the maternal serum when these defects are present. The *maternal serum AFP* concentration is low when the fetus has Down syndrome and other chromosomal defects (Thompson et al., 1991).

Detection of an increased concentration of AFP in amniotic fluid is likely to be a useful diagnostic tool for detecting the presence or absence of *open neural tube defects,* e.g., meroanencephaly (partial absence of the brain) and other severe types of spina bifida in fetuses of mothers who have already had a child with a neural tube defect (see Fig. 17–10). The findings would help parents decide whether the pregnancy should be terminated (e.g., when the fetus lacks a complete brain and has no chance of survival).

INTRAUTERINE FETAL TRANSFUSION. Fetuses can be given intrauterine blood transfusions (e.g., for the treatment of erythroblastosis fetalis; also known as hemolytic disease of the newborn [HDN]). The blood is injected through a needle inserted into the fetal peritoneal cavity (Bowman, 1989). Over a period of five to six days, most of the cells pass into the fetal circulation via the lymphatics of the diaphragm. With recent advances in *percutaneous umbilical cord puncture,* blood can be transfused directly into the fetal vascular system.

FETOSCOPY. Using fiberoptic lighting instruments, parts of the fetal body may be directly visualized. It is possible to scan the entire fetus looking for congenital anomalies, such as cleft lip and limb defects. The fetoscope is usually introduced through the anterior abdominal and uterine walls into the amniotic cavity, similar to the way the needle is inserted during amniocen-

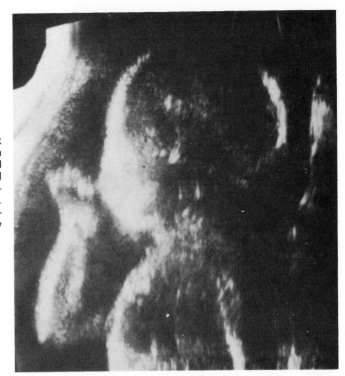

Figure 7–13. Ultrasound scan (sonogram) of a 30-week fetus that is sucking its thumb. Observe that its forearm bones are visible. The biparietal diameter of the head can be determined and compared with the abdominal diameter. Determination of these measurements facilitates estimation of the age and weight of the fetus. (From Thompson JS, Thompson MW: *Genetics in Medicine,* 3rd ed. Philadelphia. WB Saunders, 1980. Courtesy of Stuart Campbell.)

tesis (Fig. 7–11). Not only can the fetus be seen, but skin biopsies or blood samples can be taken.

Because of the risk to the fetus (estimated to be about 5 per cent) as compared with other prenatal diagnostic procedures as well as the poorer detail of the fetal anatomy that can be visualized, fetoscopy now has few indications for routine prenatal diagnosis or treatment of the fetus.

CORDOCENTESIS OR PERCUTANEOUS UMBILICAL CORD BLOOD SAMPLING (PUBS). Fetal blood samples may be obtained from umbilical vessels for chromosome analysis. Ultrasonographic scanning facilitates the procedure by outlining the location of the vessels. PUBS is often used about 20 weeks after LNMP for chromosome analysis when ultrasonographic or other examinations have shown a fetal anomaly.

ULTRASONOGRAPHY (Figs. 7–13 and 7–14; see also Fig. 6–15). Fetuses and chorionic sacs may be visualized during the embryonic period by using ultrasound techniques. Placental and fetal size, multiple births, and abnormal presentations can also be determined. *Ultrasound scans* give accurate measurements of the biparietal diameter of the fetal skull, from which close estimates of fetal length can be made. In most cases the male genitalia can be visualized by ultrasound.

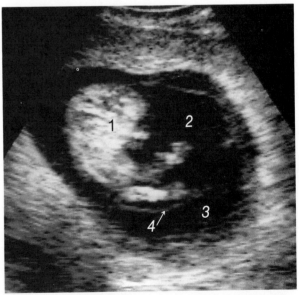

Figure 7–14. **Transvaginal** ultrasound scan of a fetus early in the ninth week (1) showing its relationship to the amniotic cavity (2), the extrafetal or chorionic cavity (3), and amnion (4). (From Wathen NC, Cass PL, Kitan MJ, Chard T: *Prenatal Diagnosis 11:*145, Copyright © 1991. Reprinted by permission of John Wiley and Sons, Ltd.).

Recent advances in ultrasonography have made this technique a major tool for prenatal diagnosis of fetal abnormalities, such as meroanencephaly, hydrocephaly, microcephaly, fetal ascites, and renal agenesis. Because of the cost, ultrasonography for estimation of gestational age and for the determination of congenital anomalies is not routine. It is indicated in *high-risk obstetrical patients* (e.g., when there is a medical indication for induction of labor).

SUMMARY

The fetal period begins nine weeks after fertilization (11 weeks after LNMP) and ends at birth. It is characterized by rapid body growth and differentiation of organ systems. An obvious change is the relative slowing of head growth compared with that of the rest of the body. By the beginning of the twelfth week, lanugo and head hair appear, and the skin is coated with *vernix caseosa*. The eyelids are closed during much of the fetal period but reopen at about 26 weeks. Until this time, the fetus is usually incapable of extrauterine existence, mainly because of the immaturity of its respiratory system. Fetuses born prematurely during the 26- to 36-week period usually survive, but full-term fetuses have the best chance of survival.

Until about 30 weeks the fetus appears reddish and wizened because of the thinness of its skin and the relative absence of subcutaneous fat. Fat usually develops rapidly during the last six to eight weeks, giving the fetus a smooth, plump appearance. This terminal ("finishing") period is devoted mainly to building up of tissues and preparation of systems involved in the transition from intrauterine to extrauterine environments, primarily the respiratory and cardiovascular systems.

Changes occurring during the fetal period are not so dramatic as those in the embryonic period, but they are very important. The fetus is less vulnerable to the teratogenic effects of drugs, viruses, and radiation, but these agents may interfere with normal functional development, especially of the brain and eyes (see Fig. 9–12).

Various techniques are available for assessing the status of the fetus and for diagnosing certain diseases and developmental abnormalities before birth (e.g., amniocentesis, chorionic villus sampling, and ultrasonography).

Commonly Asked Questions

1. I have heard that the mature embryo twitches and a first trimester fetus moves its limbs. Is this true? If so, can the mother feel her baby kicking at this time?
2. Some women have "morning sickness" during early pregnancy. What type of illness is this? How is it treated?
3. I have heard that the baby can cause cavities in the mother's teeth. Is this true?
4. I read in the paper that vitamin supplementation around the time of conception will prevent neural tube defects (NTDs), such as spina bifida. Is there scientific proof for this statement?
5. Can the fetus be injured by the needle during amniocentesis? Is there a risk of inducing a miscarriage or causing maternal or fetal infection?

The answers to these questions are given on page 329.

REFERENCES

Behrman RE: *Nelson Textbook of Pediatrics*, 14th ed. Philadelphia, WB Saunders, 1992.

Boehm CD, Kazazian Jr. HH: Prenatal diagnosis by DNA analysis. *In* Harrison MR, Golbus MS, Filly RA (eds): *The Unborn Patient. Prenatal Diagnosis and Treatment*, 2nd ed. Philadelphia, WB Saunders, 1991.

Bowie JF: Fetal Growth. *In* Callen PW (ed): *Ultrasonography in Obstetrics and Gynecology.* Philadelphia, WB Saunders, 1988.

Bowman JM: Hemolytic disease (Erythroblastosis fetalis). *In* Creasy RK, Resnik R (eds): *Maternal-Fetal Medicine: Principles and Practice,* 2nd ed. Philadelphia, WB Saunders, 1989.

Creasy RK, Resnik R: Intrauterine growth retardation. *In* Creasy RK, Resnik R (eds): *Maternal-Fetal Medicine: Principles and Practice,* 2nd ed. Philadelphia, WB Saunders, 1989.

England MA: *Color Atlas of Life Before Birth.* Chicago, Year Book Medical Publishers, 1983.

Filly RA: Sonographic anatomy of the normal fetus. *In* Harrison MR, Golbus MS, Filly RA (eds): *The Unborn Patient. Prenatal Diagnosis and Treatment,* 2nd ed. Philadelphia, WB Saunders, 1991.

Haddow JE: α-Fetoprotein. *In* Harrison MR, Golbus MS, Filly RA (eds): *The Unborn Patient. Prenatal Diagnosis and Treatment,* 2nd ed. Philadelphia, WB Saunders, 1991.

Hobbins JC: Amniocentesis. *In* Harrison MR, Golbus MS, Filly RA (eds): *The Unborn Patient. Prenatal Diagnosis and Treatment,* 2nd ed. Philadelphia, WB Saunders, 1991.

Hogge WA: Chorionic villus sampling. *In* Harrison MR, Golbus MS, Filly RA (eds): *The Unborn Patient. Prenatal Diagnosis and Treatment,* 2nd ed. Philadelphia, WB Saunders, 1991.

Illsley R, Mitchell RG: The developing concept of low birth weight and the present state of knowledge. *In* Illsley R, Mitchell RG (eds): *Low Birth Weight: A Medical Psychological and Social Study.* New York, John Wiley & Sons, 1984.

Kurtz AB, Needleman L: Ultrasound assessment of fetal age. *In* Callen PW (ed): *Ultrasonography in Obstetrics and Gynecology.* Philadelphia, WB Saunders, 1988.

Moore KL: *The Sex Chromatin.* Philadelphia, WB Saunders, 1966.

Nash JE, Persaud TVN: Embryopathic risks of cigarette smoking. *Exp Pathol* 33:65, 1988.

O'Rahilly R, Müller F: *Developmental Stages in Human Embryos. Publication 637.* Washington, Carnegie Institution of Washington, 1987.

Persaud TVN: Fetal alcohol syndrome. *CRC Critical Review in Anatomy & Cell Biology* 1:277, 1988.

Polin RA, Mennuti MT: Genetic disease and chromosomal abnormalities. *In* Fanaroff AA, Martin RJ (eds): *Neonatal-Perinatal Medicine. Diseases of the Fetus and Infant.* St. Louis, CV Mosby, 1987.

Senterre J (ed): *Intrauterine Growth Retardation. Nestle Nutrition Workshop Series,* vol. 18. New York, Raven Press, 1989.

Simpson JL, Elias S: Prenatal diagnosis of genetic disorders. *In* Creasy RK, Resnik R (eds): *Maternal-Fetal Medicine: Principles and Practice,* 2nd ed. Philadelphia, WB Saunders, 1989.

Spirt BA, Gordon LP, Oliphant M: *Prenatal Ultrasound: A Color Atlas with Anatomic and Pathologic Correlation.* New York, Churchill Livingstone, 1987.

Thompson MW, McInnes RR, Willard HF: *Thompson & Thompson Genetics in Medicine,* 5th ed. Philadelphia, WB Saunders, 1991.

Wald NJ, Cuckle HS: AFP screening in early pregnancy. *In* Spencer JAD (ed): *Fetal Monitoring.* Oxford, Oxford University Press, 1991.

Weaver DD: Inborn errors of metabolism. *In* Weaver DD (ed): *Catalogue of Prenatally Diagnosed Conditions.* Baltimore, The Johns Hopkins University Press, 1989.

8

THE PLACENTA AND FETAL MEMBRANES

The placenta is a *fetomaternal organ*, i.e., it consists of fetal and maternal components (Fig. 8–1*E* and *F*). The larger *fetal portion* develops from the chorionic sac, and the smaller *maternal portion* is derived from the endometrium. The placenta functions primarily as an organ that permits the exchange of materials carried in the blood streams of the mother and embryo/fetus (see Fig. 8–5). It allows nutritional materials and oxygen to reach the embryo/fetus and provides a route for the disposal of waste products and carbon dioxide.

The chorion, amnion, yolk sac, and allantois constitute the fetal membranes. They develop from the zygote but do not form parts of the embryo or fetus, except for the yolk sac and allantois. Part of the yolk sac is incorporated into the embryo and forms the primordium of the primitive gut (see Fig. 6–1). The allantois forms a fibrous cord called the *urachus* in the fetus and the *median umbilical ligament* in the adult (see Fig. 8–16).

THE PLACENTA

The placenta and fetal membranes perform the following *functions and activities:* protection, nutrition, respiration, excretion, and hormone production. At birth the placenta and fetal membranes are separated from the fetus; and, shortly after birth, the placenta and fetal membranes are expelled from the uterus as the *afterbirth* (see Figs. 8–9*F* and 8–11).

The Decidua

The term *decidua*[1] is applied to the functional layer of the gravid (pregnant) endometrium (see Fig. 2–2*B*) to indicate that its functional layer sheds or "falls off" at *parturition* (birth). For descriptive purposes, **three regions of the decidua** are named according to their relation to the implantation site (Fig. 8–1): (1) the part of the decidua deep to the conceptus that forms the maternal component of the placenta is the *decidua basalis*, (2) the superficial portion overlying the conceptus is known as the *decidua capsularis*, and (3) all the remaining endometrium lining the uterine wall is the *decidua parietalis* (L. *paries*, wall) or decidua vera. These decidual regions, clearly recognizable during *ultrasonography*, are important in diagnosing early pregnancy (Lyons and Levi, 1991).

As the conceptus enlarges, the decidua capsularis bulges into the uterine cavity (Fig. 8–1*A*) and eventually fuses with the decidua parietalis, thereby obliterating the uterine cavity (Fig. 8–1*F*). By about 22 weeks, the decidua capsularis degenerates and disappears. The decidua basalis forms the maternal part of the placenta.

---

[1] The Latin word *deciduus* means "a falling off," as occurs with leaves of deciduous trees in the autumn.

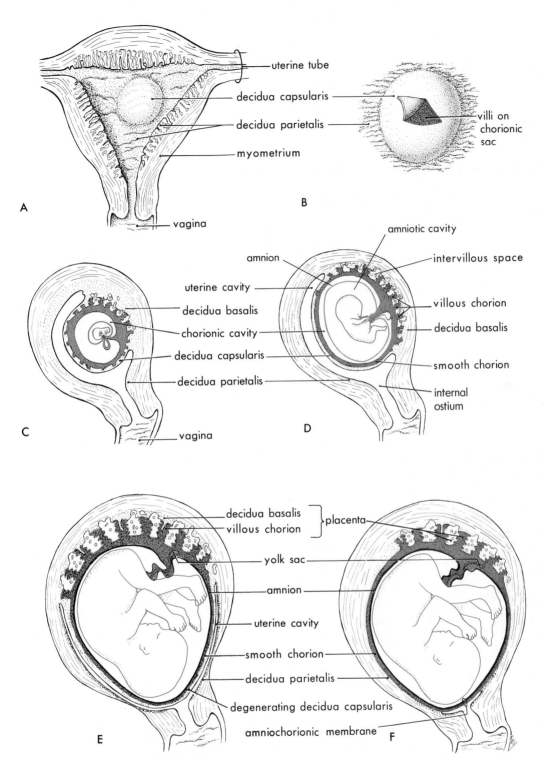

Figure 8–1. Drawings illustrating development of the human placenta and fetal membranes. *A,* Frontal section of the uterus, showing the elevation of the decidua capsularis caused by the expanding chorionic sac of an implanted four-week embryo. *B,* Enlarged drawing of the implantation site shown in *A.* The chorionic villi have been exposed by cutting an opening in the decidua capsularis. *C* to *F,* Sagittal sections of the gravid uterus from the fifth to twenty-second weeks, showing the changing relations of the fetal membranes to the decidua. In *F,* the amnion and chorion are fused with each other and the decidua parietalis, thereby obliterating the uterine cavity. Note that the chorionic villi persist only where the chorion is associated with the decidua basalis; here they form the villous chorion. Initially, the placenta is larger than the fetus; but, during the last half of pregnancy, the fetus grows faster than the placenta.

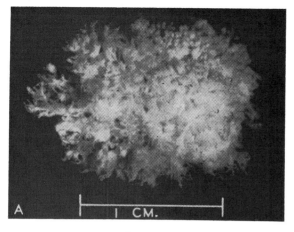

smooth
chorion

villous
chorion

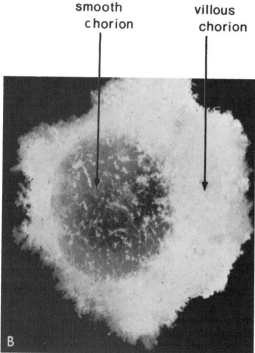

Figure 8–2. Photographs of spontaneously aborted human chorionic sacs containing embryos. *A*, 21 days. The entire sac is covered with chorionic villi (× 4). *B*, Eight weeks (actual size). Note that some villi have degenerated, leaving the chorion smooth. The remaining villous chorion forms the fetal contribution to the placenta. (Reproduced with permission from Potter EL, Craig JM: *Pathology of the Fetus and Infant*, 3rd ed. Copyright © 1975 by Year Book Medical Publishers, Chicago.)

Development of the Placenta

The rapid proliferation of the trophoblast and development of the chorionic sac were described in Chapters 4 and 5 (pp. 39 and 55). By the end of the third week, the anatomical arrangements necessary for physiological exchanges between the mother and embryo are established (see Figs. 5–9 and 8–1C). Until the eighth week, chorionic villi cover the entire surface of the chorionic sac (Figs. 8–1C and 8–2A). As this sac grows, the villi associated with the decidua capsularis are compressed, and the blood supply to them is reduced. These villi soon degenerate, producing an avascular, bare area known as the chorion laeve (L. *levis*, smooth) or **smooth chorion** (Figs. 8–1D and 8–2B). As these villi disappear, those associated with the decidua basalis rapidly increase in number, branch profusely, and enlarge (Figs. 8–2 to 8–5). This portion of the chorionic sac is known as the chorion frondosum (L. *frondosus*, leafy) or **villous chorion**. It forms the fetal component of the placenta (Figs. 8–1F and 8–3 to

8–5). The increase in the thickness of the placenta results from branching of the stem villi (Figs. 8–4 to 8–6).

The size of the chorionic sac is useful in determining *gestational age* (time elapsed since the LNMP) in patients with uncertain menstrual histories (Lyons and Levi, 1991). Growth of the chorionic sac is extremely rapid between the fifth and tenth weeks. Modern ultrasound equipment, especially instruments equipped with intravaginal transducers, enables ultrasonographers to detect the chorionic (gestational) sac when it has a *median sac diameter* (MSD) of 2 to 3 mm. Chorionic sacs with this MSD indicate that the gestational age is about 31 days (i.e., 16 to 17 days after fertilization). As the fetus grows, the uterus and placenta enlarge. Growth in the thickness of the placenta continues until the fetus is about 18 weeks old (20 weeks' gestation). The fully developed placenta covers 15 to 30 per cent of the decidua (lining of the pregnant uterus).

The fetal component of the placenta is formed by *villous chorion* (Figs. 8–1F, 8–3, and 8–4). The stem chorionic villi that arise from the *chorionic plate* project into the intervillous space containing maternal blood (Figs. 8–1D, 8–4, and 8–5).

The maternal component of the placenta is formed by the *decidua basalis* (Figs. 8–1E, 8–4, and 8–5). This constitutes all the endometrium that is related to the fetal component of the placenta. By the end of the fourth month, the decidua basalis is almost entirely replaced by the fetal component of the placenta (i.e., the fetal part of the placenta is larger than the maternal part).

THE FETOMATERNAL JUNCTION. The fetal portion of the placenta (villous chorion) is attached to the maternal portion of the placenta (decidua basalis) by the *cytotrophoblastic shell* (see Figs. 5–9 and 8–5). *Stem chorionic villi* ("anchoring villi") are attached firmly to the decidua basalis through the cytotrophoblastic shell. The stem

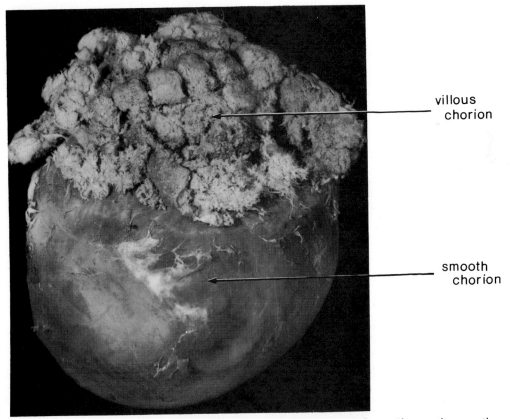

villous
chorion

smooth
chorion

Figure 8–3. Photograph of a human chorionic sac containing a 13-week fetus. Observe the smooth and villous areas of the chorion. Actual size. To visualize how this chorionic sac was situated in the uterus prior to its spontaneous abortion, see Figures 8–1E and 8–4. The irregular convex areas of the villous chorion are called cotyledons.

villi *anchor the chorionic sac* and placenta to the decidua basalis. Maternal arteries and veins pass freely through gaps in the cytotrophoblastic shell and open into the intervillous space (Fig. 8–5).

The shape of the placenta is determined by the form of the persistent area of chorionic villi (Fig. 8–1*F*). This is usually a circular area, giving the placenta a discoid shape (see Figs. 8–3 and 8–11). As the villi erode the decidua basalis to enlarge the intervillous space, they leave several wedge-shaped areas of decidual tissue called *placental septa*. They project toward the *chorionic plate* (Fig. 8–5) and divide the fetal part of the placenta into irregular convex areas called *cotyledons* (Figs. 8–3 and 8–11*A*). Each cotyledon, visible on the maternal surface of the

placenta (Figs. 8–3 and 8–11*A*), consists of two or more *stem villi* and their many branches called *branch villi*. By the end of the fourth month, the decidua basalis is almost entirely replaced by the cotyledons.

THE INTERVILLOUS SPACE (Figs. 8–1*D*, 8–4, and 8–5). The intervillous space, filled with maternal blood, is *derived from the lacunae* that developed in the syncytiotrophoblast during the second week (see Figs. 4–1*C*, 4–4, and 4–5). As the chorionic villi enlarge, the intervillous space enlarges. The lacunae fuse to form lacunar networks that coalesce to form a large, blood-filled space (sinus), the intervillous space. It is bounded by the chorionic plate and decidua basalis (Fig. 8–5). The intervillous space is divided into compartments by placental septa, but there is free communication between the intervillous spaces of different compartments because the septa do not reach the chorionic plate.

Maternal blood enters the intervillous space from the *spiral arteries* in the decidua basalis (Fig. 8–5; see also Fig. 2–2). These endometrial arteries pass through gaps in the cytotrophoblastic shell and discharge their blood into the intervillous space (Fig. 8–5). This large sinus is drained by endometrial veins that also penetrate the cytotrophoblastic shell. They are found over the entire surface of the decidua basalis. The *branch villi*[2] are continuously showered with well-oxygenated maternal blood that circulates through the intervillous space. The blood carries nutritional materials and oxygen that are necessary for fetal growth and development. Blood leaving the intervillous space takes away fetal waste products (e.g., carbon dioxide, excess water, salts, and products of protein metabolism).

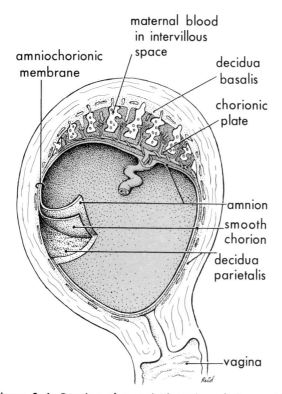

Figure 8–4. Drawing of a sagittal section of the gravid uterus at 22 weeks, showing the relation of the placenta and fetal membranes to each other and to the regions of the decidua. The fetus has been removed, and the amnion and smooth chorion have been cut and reflected to show their relationship to each other and the decidua parietalis. The fetal component of the placenta consists of the chorionic plate and the stem (chorionic) villi that arise from it and project into the intervillous space containing maternal blood. The maternal component of the placenta is formed by the decidua basalis. This comprises all the endometrium related to the fetal component of the placenta (Fig. 8–1*E* and *F*).

Labels in figure:
amniochorionic membrane
maternal blood in intervillous space
decidua basalis
chorionic plate
amnion
smooth chorion
decidua parietalis
vagina

Placental Circulation

The numerous branch villi of the placenta provide a large area where materials may be exchanged across the very thin *placental membrane* ("barrier") interposed between the fetal and maternal circulations (Figs. 8–6 and 8–7). The fetal blood acquires nutrients and oxygen from the maternal blood. Waste products formed within the embryo are carried by the umbilical arteries to the placenta where they are transferred to the maternal blood (Fig. 8–7). Within the placenta, the maternal and fetal

---

[2] Branches of the stem villi (Fig. 8–6*A*).

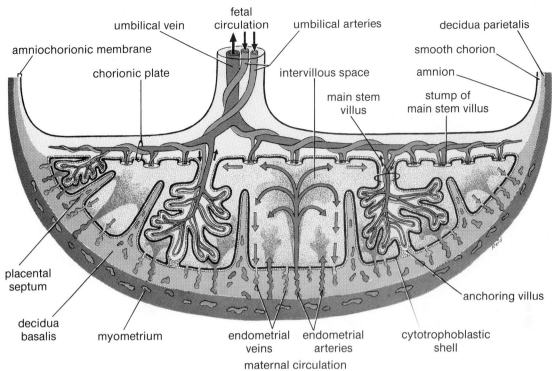

Figure 8–5. Schematic drawing of a section through a full-term placenta, showing: (1) the relation of the villous chorion (fetal part of the placenta) to the decidua basalis (maternal part of the placenta), (2) the fetal placental circulation, and (3) the maternal placental circulation. Maternal blood flows into the intervillous space from the spiral (endometrial) arteries in funnel-shaped spurts. Exchanges occur with the fetal blood (e.g., oxygen) as the maternal blood flows around the branch villi (Fig. 8–6A). The inflowing arterial blood pushes venous blood out into the endometrial veins, which are scattered over the entire surface of the decidua basalis. Note that the umbilical arteries carry poorly oxygenated fetal blood (blue) to the placenta and that the umbilical vein carries well-oxygenated blood (red) to the fetus. Note that the cotyledons are separated from each other by decidual septa, projections of the maternal portion of the placenta (decidua basalis). Each cotyledon consists of two or more main-stem villi and their many branches (branch villi). In this drawing, only one main-stem villus is shown in each cotyledon, but the stumps of those that have been removed are indicated. (See Figure 15–21 for a drawing of the fetal circulation and its relationship to the placenta.)

bloodstreams flow close to each other but they do not normally mix. The fetal and maternal circulations are separated by a very thin layer of tissues known as the placental membrane. It is through the placental membranes of the many branch villi that the main exchange of material between the mother and fetus takes place (Fig. 8–6A to C).

The Placental Membrane ("Barrier")

This composite membrane consists of *extrafetal tissues* separating the maternal and fetal blood (Figs. 8–6 and 8–7). Until about 20 weeks, it consists of four layers (Fig. 8–6B): (1) syncytiotrophoblast, (2) cytotrophoblast, (3) connective tissue in the chorionic villus, and (4) endothelium of the fetal capillaries. Although the placental membrane is often called the "placental barrier," this term is inappropriate because there are few compounds, endogenous or exogenous, that are unable to cross the placental membrane in detectable amounts. The placental membrane acts as a true barrier only when the molecule has a certain size, configuration, and charge (e.g., heparin).

As pregnancy advances, the placental membrane becomes progressively thinner, and many capillaries come to lie very close to the syncytiotrophoblast (Fig. 8–6C). Most drugs and other substances present in the maternal plasma will also be found in the fetal plasma. At some sites nuclei in the syncytiotrophoblast form nuclear aggregations or *syncytial knots* (Fig. 8–6C).

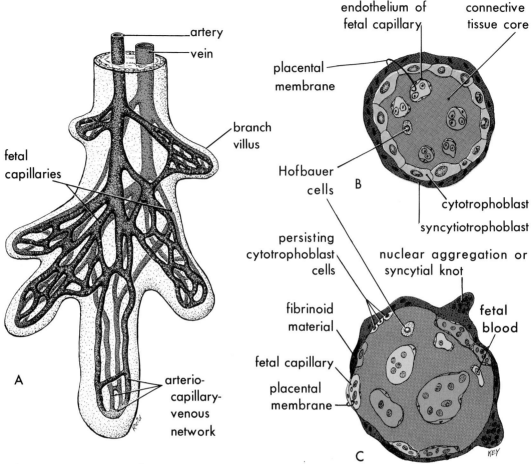

Figure 8–6. *A,* Drawing of a stem (chorionic) villus, showing its branch villi and arteriocapillary-venous system carrying fetal blood. The artery carries poorly oxygenated blood and waste products from the fetus; whereas, the vein carries well-oxygenated blood and nutrients to the fetus. *B* and *C,* Drawings of sections through a branch villus at 10 weeks and at full term, respectively. The branch villi are bathed externally by maternal blood in the intervillous space. The placental membrane, composed of extrafetal tissues, separates the maternal blood from the fetal blood (see also Fig. 8–7). Hofbauer cells have the general qualities of phagocytic (scavenger) cells.

Syncytial knots continually break off and are carried from the intervillous space into the maternal circulation. Some of them lodge in capillaries of the maternal lung where they are rapidly destroyed by local enzyme action. Toward the end of pregnancy, *fibrinoid material* forms on the surfaces of villi (Fig. 8–6C); it consists of fibrin and other unidentified substances. Fibrinoid material results mainly from placental aging and appears to reduce placental functions.

Fetal Placental Circulation

Poorly oxygenated blood leaves the fetus and passes in the *umbilical arteries* to the placenta (Figs. 8–5, 8–6, and 8–11). The blood vessels form an extensive *arteriocapillary-venous system* within the chorionic villus, bringing the fetal blood very close to the maternal blood. The well-oxygenated fetal blood passes into thin-walled veins, which converge to form the large *umbilical vein* (see Fig. 8–12A). This large vessel carries the oxygenated blood to the fetus (see Fig. 15–21).

Maternal Placental Circulation

The blood in the intervillous space is temporarily outside the maternal circulatory system (Fig. 8–5). It enters the intervillous space through 80 to 100 *spiral (endometrial) arteries* in the decidua basalis (see Figs. 2–2*B* and 8–5). The blood is propelled in jetlike streams by the maternal blood pressure and spurts toward the *chorionic plate*, forming the "roof" of the inter-villous space. The blood slowly flows around and over the surface of the branch villi, allowing an exchange of metabolic and gaseous products with the fetal blood. The maternal blood eventually reaches the "floor" of the intervillous space, where it enters the endometrial veins and the maternal circulation.

The welfare of the embryo and fetus depends more on the adequate bathing of the branch villi with maternal blood than on any other factor. Reductions of uteroplacental circulation result in *fetal hypoxia*. Prolapse of the umbilical cord may cause fetal hypoxia and anoxia. Chronic reductions of uteroplacental circulation (e.g., caused by the effects of nicotine in cigarette smoke [p. 88]) result in *fetal hypoxia* and disturbances of growth known as intrauterine growth retardation (IUGR); see Chapter 7.

Placental Functions and Activities

The placenta has *three main functions and activities:* (1) *metabolism*, (2) *transport of substances* (e.g., oxygen and carbon dioxide), and (3) *endocrine secretion*. These comprehensive activities are essential for maintaining pregnancy and promoting normal embryonic/fetal development.

PLACENTAL METABOLISM. The placenta, particularly during early pregnancy, synthesizes glycogen, cholesterol and, fatty acids, which serve as sources of nutrients and energy for the embryo/fetus. Many of the placenta's metabolic activities are undoubtedly critical for its other two major placental activities (transport and endocrine secretion).

PLACENTAL TRANSPORT OF SUBSTANCES. Almost all materials are transported across the placental membrane by one of the following *four main transport mechanisms:* (1) simple diffusion, (2) facilitated diffusion, (3) active transport, and (4) pinocytosis. Passive transport by *simple diffusion* is usually characteristic of substances

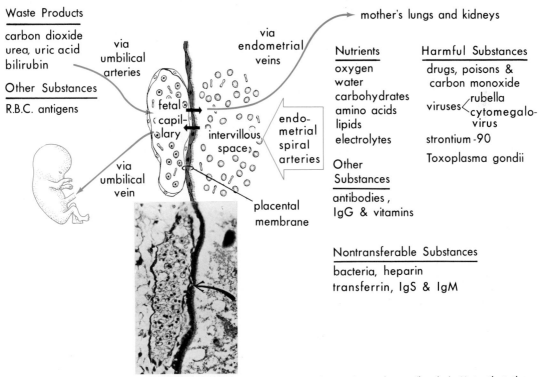

Figure 8–7. Diagrammatic illustration of transfer across the placental membrane (barrier). Note that the intervillous space contains maternal blood and the placental membrane is composed of extrafetal tissues. (Inset photomicrograph from Javert CT: *Spontaneous and Habitual Abortion*, Copyright © 1957 by McGraw-Hill. Used by permission of McGraw-Hill Book Company.)

moving from areas of higher to lower concentration until equilibrium is established. In *facilitated diffusion* there is transport through electronic charges. *Active transport* against a concentration gradient requires energy. Such systems may involve enzymes that temporarily combine with the substances concerned. *Pinocytosis* (Gr. *pinein*, to drink) is a form of endocytosis in which the material being engulfed is a small sample of extracellular fluid. This method of transport is usually reserved for large molecules. For other methods that substances use to cross the placental membrane, see Moore and Persaud (1993).

GASES. Oxygen, carbon dioxide, and carbon monoxide cross the placental membrane by *simple diffusion.* Interruption of oxygen transport for even a few minutes will endanger embryonic/fetal survival. The placental membrane approaches the efficiency of the lungs for gas exchange.

NUTRITIONAL SUBSTANCES. Water is rapidly and freely exchanged between the mother and her fetus by simple diffusion and in increasing amounts as pregnancy advances. There is little or no transfer of maternal cholesterol, triglycerides, or phospholipids. There is transport of free fatty acids, but the amount transferred appears to be relatively small. *Vitamins* cross the placenta and are essential for normal development. Water-soluble vitamins cross the placental membrane more quickly than fat-soluble ones. *Glucose* from the mother, and produced by the placenta, is quickly transferred to the embryo/fetus by diffusion.

HORMONES. Protein hormones do not reach the embryo/fetus in significant amounts except for a slow transfer of thyroxine and triiodothyronine. Unconjugated steroid hormones pass the placental membrane rather freely. *Testosterone* and certain synthetic progestins cross the placenta and may cause external masculinization of female fetuses (see Fig. 9–14; Table 9–5).

ELECTROLYTES. These are freely exchanged across the placenta in significant quantities, each at its own rate. When a mother receives *intravenous fluids,* they also pass to the fetus and affect its water and electrolyte status.

ANTIBODIES. Some passive immunity is conferred upon the fetus by transplacental transfer of maternal antibodies. The alpha and beta globulins reach the fetus in very small quantities; but many of the gamma globulins, notably the IgG (7S) class, are readily transported to the fetus.

Maternal antibodies confer fetal immunity to such diseases as diphtheria, smallpox, and measles, but no immunity is acquired to pertussis (whooping cough) or chickenpox. The fetus has a poor capacity to produce antibodies until well after birth.

OTHER TRANSFERABLE SUBSTANCES. Although the placental membrane separates the maternal and fetal circulations, small amounts of blood may pass from the fetus to the mother through microscopic breaks in the placental membrane. If the fetus is Rh-positive and the mother Rh-negative, the fetal cells may stimulate the formation of anti-Rh antibody by the mother. This passes to the fetal blood stream and causes hemolysis of fetal Rh-positive blood cells and anemia in the fetus.

Some fetuses with this condition, known as *hemolytic disease of the newborn* (HDN), fail to make a satisfactory intrauterine adjustment and may die unless delivered early or given intrauterine blood transfusions (see Chapter 7, p. 90). Exchange transfusions of blood are also performed after birth using the umbilical vein. Most of the infant's blood is replaced with Rh-negative donor blood. This technique prevents death of babies with HDN who are very anemic. It also avoids brain damage by preventing or controlling hyperbilirubinemia. HDN is relatively uncommon because Rh immunoglobulin given to the mother usually prevents development of this disease in the fetus (Thompson et al., 1991).

When the placenta separates at birth (see Fig. 8–9F), the mother often receives a small transfusion of fetal blood into her circulation from ruptured fetal chorionic vessels. If she is Rh-negative and the infant Rh-positive, the fetal red cells can stimulate a permanent antibody response in the mother. These fetal red blood cells can be destroyed rapidly by giving the mother high-titer, anti-Rh antibody. In this way she does not become sensitized.

WASTE PRODUCTS. Carbon dioxide, the major waste product, diffuses across the placenta even more rapidly than oxygen. Urea and uric acid pass the placental membrane by simple diffusion, and bilirubin is quickly cleared.

DRUGS. Most drugs and their metabolites cross the placenta freely. As pregnancy advances, *thinning of the placental membrane facilitates the passage of drugs.* Some drugs cause congenital anomalies (see Table 9–5). *Fetal drug addiction* may occur following maternal use of drugs such as heroin, and newborns may experience withdrawal symptoms[3]. Except for muscle relaxants, such as succinylcholine and curare, most agents used for the management of labor (p. 104) readily cross the placenta. These drugs may cause respiratory depression in the newborn infant. All sedatives and analgesics affect the fetus to some degree.

INFECTIOUS AGENTS. Rubella virus, cytomegalovirus, Coxsackie viruses and those associated with variola, varicella, measles, encephalitis, and poliomyelitis may pass through the placental membrane and cause *fetal infection.* In some cases (e.g., **rubella virus**), congenital anomalies may be produced (see Table 9–5).

PLACENTAL ENDOCRINE SECRETION. Using precursors derived from the fetus and/or the mother, the *syncytiotrophoblast of the placenta synthesizes various hormones.*

Protein Hormones. The two well-documented protein hormone products of the placenta are: (1) *human chorionic gonadotropin* (hCG), and (2) human chorionic somatomammotropin (hCS), also known as human placental lactogen (hPL). The glycoprotein hCG, similar to LH, is first secreted by the syncytiotrophoblast during the second week (p. 35). *HCG maintains the corpus luteum* in the ovary, preventing the onset of menstruation (see Chapter 2). In addition to hCG and hPL, *human chorionic thyrotropin* (hCT) and *human chorionic adrenocorticotropin* (hCACTH) are formed by the placenta.

Steroid Hormones. Estrogens and progesterones are the only steroid hormones known to be secreted by the placenta. *Progesterone* can be obtained from the placenta at all stages of pregnancy, indicating that it is important for the *maintenance of pregnancy.*

UTERINE GROWTH DURING PREGNANCY

The uterus normally lies entirely in the pelvis minor (Fig. 8–8A). It expands during pregnancy as the fetus grows and rises out of the pelvic cavity to the level of the umbilicus (navel) by about 20 weeks (Fig. 8–8B). By 28 to 30 weeks, the uterus occupies a large part of the abdominopelvic cavity and reaches the epigastric region[4] (Fig. 8–8C). As the uterus increases in size and weight, its walls become thinner.

---

[3] Because psychic dependence on these drugs is not developed during the fetal period, no liability to subsequent narcotic addiction exists in the infant after withdrawal is complete.

[4] The area inferior to the xiphoid process of the sternum and superior to the umbilicus.

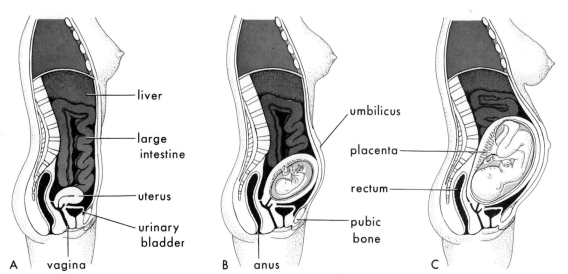

Figure 8–8. Drawings of sagittal sections of a woman's body. *A,* Not pregnant. *B,* 20 weeks' pregnant. *C,* 30 weeks' pregnant. Note that, as the fetus enlarges, the uterus increases in size, and its fundic part rises in the abdominal cavity to accommodate the rapidly growing fetus. The mother's abdominal viscera are displaced by the growth of the fetus and uterus, and her abdominal skin and muscles are greatly stretched.

PARTURITION (CHILDBIRTH)

The *birth process*, during which the fetus, placenta, umbilical cord, and fetal membranes are expelled from the mother's reproductive tract (Figs. 8–9 and 8–10) is called *parturition* (L. *parturitio*, childbirth). The onset of labor (L., toil) is caused mainly by hormones (e.g., oxytocin). **Labor** is the sequence of *involuntary uterine contractions* that results in the dilation of the cervix of the uterus and delivery of the fetus, placenta, umbilical cord, and fetal membranes from the uterus. The peristaltic contractions of the uterine smooth muscle are elicited by **oxytocin** that is released from the pituitary gland. Oxytocin also stimulates release of *prostaglandins*. Estrogens also increase myometrial activity and stimulate the release of oxytocin and prostaglandins. Although occurring in a continuous sequence, labor is divided into four stages for convenience of description.

The Four Stages of Labor

The *first stage of labor* is the dilation stage. The amnion and chorion are forced into the cervical canal by contractions of the uterus (Fig. 8–9A). The cervix dilates slowly; and, when it is fully dilated or even before, the amniotic and chorionic sacs rupture, allowing the amniotic fluid to escape. The duration of this stage is about 12 hours for first pregnancies; however, there are wide variations.

The *second stage of labor* is the expulsion stage. It begins when the cervix is fully dilated and ends when the baby is delivered (Fig. 8–9). As the contractions of the uterus become stronger, they are aided by voluntary contractions of the maternal abdominal muscles. The baby is forced through the cervical canal and vagina (Figs. 8–9B to E and 8–10). As soon as the fetus is outside the mother, it is called a newborn infant (baby). The average duration of this stage is 50 minutes for first pregnancies.

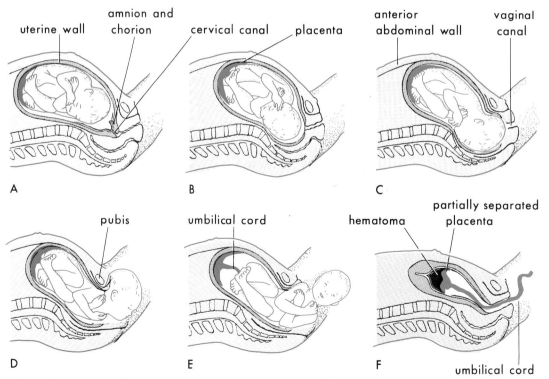

Figure 8–9. Drawings illustrating parturition, the process of childbirth. *A* and *B*, The cervix is dilating during the first stage of labor. *C* to *E*, The fetus passes through the cervix and vagina during the second stage of labor. *F*, As the uterus contracts during the third stage of labor, the placenta folds and pulls away from the uterine wall. Separation of the placenta results in bleeding, forming a large hematoma (mass of blood). Later, the placenta and its associated membranes are expelled from the uterus (not shown) by further uterine contractions. The lay term for the expelled placenta and membranes is "afterbirth."

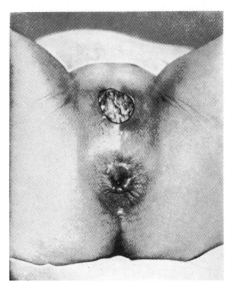

Figure 8–10. Photographs illustrating delivery of the baby's head during the second stage of labor. *A*, The head distends the mother's perineum, and its crown becomes visible. This is called "crowning." *B*, The perineum slips back over the head and face. *C*, The head is delivered; subsequently, the body of the fetus is expelled. (From Greenhill JB, Friedman EA: *Biological Principles and Modern Practice of Obstetrics.* Philadelphia, WB Saunders, 1974.)

A

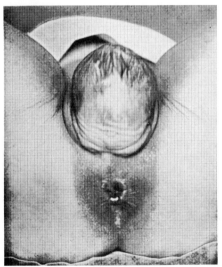

B

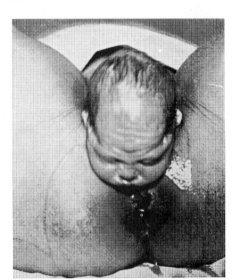

C

The *third stage of labor* (placental stage) begins as soon as the baby is born and ends when the placenta and membranes ("afterbirth") are expelled from the uterus. The placenta separates through the spongy layer of the decidua basalis (see Fig. 2–2*B*). After delivery of the baby, the uterus continues to contract. A *hematoma* (collection of blood) forms behind the placenta (Fig. 8–9*F*) and separates it from the decidua basalis. The duration of the third stage is about 15 minutes in 90 per cent of pregnancies. Retraction of the uterus reduces the area of placental attachment (Fig. 8–9*F*); thus, the placenta and fetal membranes soon separate from the wall of the uterus and are expelled through the vagina and pudendal cleft[5].

The *fourth stage of labor*, the recovery stage, begins as soon as the placenta and membranes are expelled and ends when the mother's condition has stabilized. The myometrial contractions constrict the spiral endometrial arteries that formerly supplied the intervillous space (Fig. 8–5). These contractions prevent excessive maternal bleeding. This stage lasts about two hours.

THE PLACENTA, UMBILICAL CORD, AND FETAL MEMBRANES AFTER BIRTH

The placenta (Gr. *plakuos*, a flat cake) commonly has the form of a flat, circular or oval disc (Fig. 8–11), with a diameter of 15 to 20 cm and a thickness of 2 to 3 cm. The placenta weighs 500 to 600 gm, usually about one sixth the weight of the fetus. The margins of the placenta are continuous with the ruptured amniotic and chorionic sacs (Figs. 8–5 and 8–11*A* and *C*). Several variations in placental shape occur (e.g., bidiscoid placenta).

Although there are many variations in the size and shape of the placenta, most of them are of little physiological or clinical significance. *Ultrasonography* is now widely used for identification and clinical assessment of placental abnormalities. For illustrations of the variations in placental shape and a discussion of their possible clinical implications, see Moore and Persaud (1993).

THE MATERNAL SURFACE OF THE PLACENTA (Figs. 8–3 and 8–11*A*). The characteristic cobblestone appearance of this surface is produced by the

cotyledons, which are separated by grooves that were formerly occupied by the *placental septa* (Fig. 8–5). The surface of the cotyledons is usually covered by thin, grayish shreds of decidua basalis that separated with the placenta. Most of the decidua is temporarily retained in the uterus and shed with subsequent uterine bleeding.

THE FETAL SURFACE OF THE PLACENTA (Fig. 8–11*B*). The umbilical cord attaches to this surface, and its amniotic covering is continuous with the amnion adherent to this surface of the placenta (see Fig. 8–15). The *chorionic vessels* radiating from the *umbilical cord* are clearly visible through the smooth, transparent amnion. The umbilical vessels branch on the fetal surface.

The Umbilical Cord

The umbilical cord is a vascular cable that connects the embryo or fetus to the placenta (see Fig. 8–15). The attachment of the umbilical cord is usually near the center of the placenta (Fig. 8–11*B*), but it may be located anywhere (e.g., at the edge [Fig. 8–11*D*]). The cord is usually 1 to 2 cm in diameter and 30 to 90 cm in length (average 55 cm).

The umbilical cord usually has two arteries and one vein that are surrounded by mucoid connective tissue often called *Wharton's jelly* (Fig. 8–12*A*). Because the umbilical vein is longer than the arteries and the vessels are longer than the cord, twisting and bending of the vessels is common. The vessels frequently form loops, producing so-called *false knots*, which are of no clinical significance.

True knots in the umbilical cord may be hazardous to the fetus (Fig. 8–13). Simple looping of the cord around the fetus occasionally occurs (Fig. 8–14). In about one fifth of all deliveries, the cord is looped once around the neck. If the cord becomes tightly looped around the neck or a limb, the circulation of blood to and from the embryo or fetus will be impeded. If the circulation is cut off, the embryo or fetus will die. In about one in 200 newborns, only one umbilical artery is present (Fig. 8–12*B*). This condition is associated with a 15 to 20 per cent incidence of cardiovascular anomalies.

The Amnion and Amniotic Fluid

The amnion forms a membranous *amniotic sac* that contains amniotic fluid. It surrounds the embryo and later the fetus (Figs. 8–14 and

---

[5] The slit between the labia majora into which the vestibule of the vagina opens (see Figs. 2–1 and 2–3).

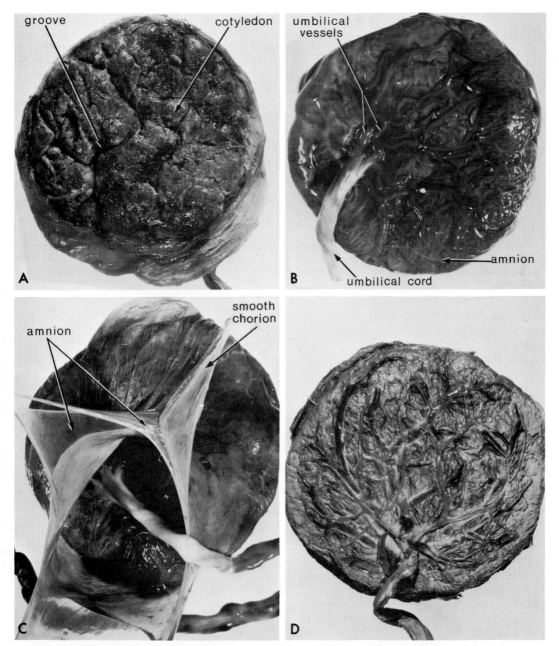

Figure 8–11. Photographs of placentas after birth, about one third actual size. *A,* Maternal surface showing many cotyledons and the grooves around them. *B,* Fetal surface showing the blood vessels running under the amnion and converging to form the umbilical vessels at the attachment of the umbilical cord. *C,* The amnion and smooth chorion are arranged to show that they are fused and continuous with the margins of the placenta. *D,* Placenta with a marginal attachment of the cord, often called a battledore placenta because of its resemblance to the bat used in the medieval game of battledore and shuttlecock.

mucoid connective tissue

umbilical arteries   umbilical vein   umbilical artery   umbilical vein

amnion

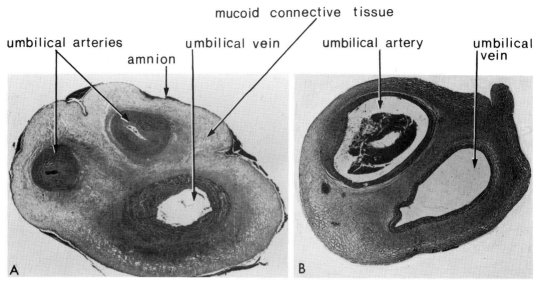

Figure 8–12. Transverse sections through full-term umbilical cords. *A,* Normal. *B,* Abnormal, showing only one artery. About 15 per cent of fetuses that have only one umbilical artery have cardiovascular anomalies (× 3). (From Javert CT: *Spontaneous and Habitual Abortion.* Copyright © 1957 by McGraw-Hill. Used by permission of McGraw-Hill Book Company.)

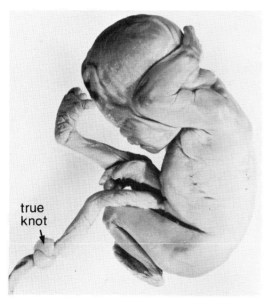

true knot

Figure 8–13. Photograph of a 20-week fetus with a true knot *(arrow)* in the umbilical cord. Half actual size. The diameter of the cord is greater in the portion closest to the fetus, indicating that there was obstruction of blood flow in the umbilical arteries. The fetus died due to lack of oxygen. It was retained in the uterus for about four weeks. The patient then went into labor and delivered this dead (stillborn) fetus.

8–15). Formation of the amniotic cavity and early development of the amnion are described in Chapter 4 (p. 35). Because the amnion is attached to the margins of the embryonic disc (Fig. 8–15*A*), its junction with the embryo (future umbilicus) becomes located on the ventral surface as a result of the folding of the embryo (see Chapter 6). As the amniotic sac enlarges, it gradually obliterates the chorionic cavity (Fig. 8–1) and enfolds the umbilical cord, forming its epithelial covering (Fig. 8–15*C* and *D*).

RUPTURE OF THE AMNIOTIC SAC. If the amnion ruptures or is torn, it may cause various fetal anomalies that constitute the *amniotic band disruption complex* (ABDC). These anomalies vary from digital constriction to major scalp, craniofacial, and visceral defects. The cause of these anomalies is probably related to constriction of the embryo by encircling amniotic bands. The incidence of the *amniotic band syndrome* (ABS) is about one in every 1200 live births. Prenatal ultrasound diagnosis of ABS is now possible.

ORIGIN OF AMNIOTIC FLUID. Most fluid is derived from the maternal tissue (interstitial) fluid by diffusion across the amniochorionic mem-

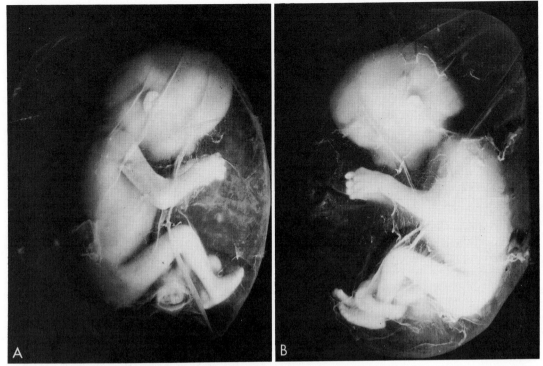

Figure 8–14. Photographs of a 12-week fetus in its amniotic sac. Actual size. This fetus and its membranes aborted spontaneously. It was then removed from its chorionic sac with its amniotic sac intact. In *B*, note that the umbilical cord is looped around the left ankle of the fetus. Coiling of the cord around parts of the fetus affects their development when the coils are so tight that the circulation to those parts is affected.

brane from the decidua parietalis (Fig. 8–1*F* and 8–5). Other sources of amniotic fluid are the fetal respiratory tract and through the fetal skin. Later, the fetus makes a major contribution by excreting urine into the amniotic fluid (about a half liter daily during late pregnancy).

Amniotic fluid is swallowed by the fetus and absorbed by its respiratory and gastrointestinal tracts. In fetal conditions such as *renal agenesis* (absence of kidneys) or urethral obstruction, the volume of amniotic fluid may be abnormally small *(oligohydramnios)*. An excess of amniotic fluid *(polyhydramnios)* may occur when the fetus does not drink the usual amount of fluid. This condition is often associated with anomalies of the central nervous system, e.g., *meroanencephaly* (anencephaly) and hydrocephalus (see Chapter 17). In other anomalies, such as esophageal or duodenal atresia (see Chapter 13), amniotic fluid accumulates because it is unable to pass to the intestine for absorption. *Ultrasonography* has become the technique of choice for diagnosing polyhydramnios.

EXCHANGE OF AMNIOTIC FLUID. Large volumes of fluid move in both directions between the fetal and maternal circulations, mainly via the *placental membrane*. Fetal swallowing of amniotic fluid is also a normal occurrence. Most of the fluid passes into the gastrointestinal tract, but some of it also enters the lungs. In either case, the fluid is absorbed and enters the fetal circulation. It then passes into the maternal circulation via the placental membrane (Figs. 8–5 to 8–7).

COMPOSITION OF AMNIOTIC FLUID. About 99 per cent of the fluid in the amniotic cavity is water. Amniotic fluid is a solution in which undissolved material is suspended (e.g., desquamated fetal epithelial cells and approximately equal portions of organic and inorganic salts). Half the organic constituents are protein; the other half consists of carbohydrates, fats, enzymes, hormones, and pigments. As pregnancy advances, the composition of the amniotic fluid changes as fetal excreta (*meconium* [fetal feces] and urine) are added.

SIGNIFICANCE OF AMNIOTIC FLUID. The embryo, suspended by the umbilical cord, floats freely in the amniotic fluid. This buoyant medium: (1) permits symmetrical external growth and devel-

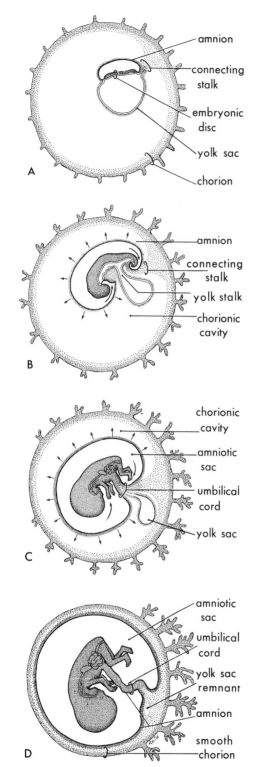

opment of the embryo, (2) prevents adherence of the amnion to the embryo, (3) cushions the embryo against jolts by distributing impacts the mother may receive, (4) helps to control the embryo's body temperature by maintaining a relatively constant temperature, (5) enables the fetus to move freely, thus aiding musculoskeletal development, (6) protects the fetus from infection because it has an antibacterial activity, and (7) influences fetal lung development (see Chapter 12).

THE YOLK SAC

Early development of the yolk sac is described in Chapters 4 and 5 (pp. 35 and 54). By nine weeks the yolk sac has shrunk to a pear-shaped remnant, about 5 mm in diameter. It is connected to the midgut by a narrow *yolk stalk* (Fig. 8–15C). Although the human yolk sac is nonfunctional as far as storing yolk is concerned, its development is essential for several reasons: (1) It has a role in transferring nutrients to the embryo during the second and third weeks, during the period when the uteroplacental circulation is being established. (2) Blood develops in the walls of the yolk sac beginning in the third week (see Fig. 5–7) and continues to form there until *hemopoietic (hematopoietic) activity* begins in the liver during the sixth week. (3) During the fourth week the dorsal part of the yolk sac is incorporated into the embryo as the *primitive gut* (see Fig. 6–1). Its endoderm gives rise to the epithelium of the trachea, bronchi, and lungs, and of the digestive tract. (4) *Primordial germ cells* appear in the wall of the yolk sac early in the third week and subsequently migrate to the developing sex glands or gonads, where they become the primitive germ cells (spermatogonia in males or oogonia in females; see Chapter 14).

FATE OF THE YOLK SAC (Fig. 8–15). The yolk sac shrinks as pregnancy advances and eventually becomes very small. The yolk stalk usually detaches from the gut by the end of the fifth week. In about two per cent of adults, the intraabdominal part of the yolk stalk persists as an *ileal diverticulum* known clinically as *Meckel's diverticulum* (see Chapter 13).

Figure 8–15. Drawings illustrating how the amnion enlarges until it fills the chorionic sac. Also shown is how: (1) the amnion enfolds on the umbilical cord and forms its epithelial covering, and (2) the yolk sac is partially incorporated into the embryo as the primitive gut. *A,* Three weeks. *B,* Four weeks. *C,* Ten weeks, *D,* 20 weeks.

THE ALLANTOIS

The early development of the allantois is described in Chapter 5 (p. 51). Although the allantois is nonfunctional in human embryos, it is important for four reasons: (1) blood formation occurs in its walls during the first two months, (2) its blood vessels become the umbilical vessels (Fig. 8–16A and B), (3) fluid from the amniotic cavity diffuses through the epithelial covering of the umbilical cord into the umbilical vein for transport to the placenta (Figs. 8–12 and 8–15), and (4) the intraembryonic portion of the allantois runs from the umbilicus to the urinary bladder. As the bladder enlarges, the allantois involutes to form a thick tube called the urachus (see Fig. 14–8).

> During the second month, the extraembryonic portion of the allantois degenerates. Its intraembryonic portion runs from the umbilicus to the urinary bladder with which it is continuous (Fig. 8–16B). As the bladder enlarges, the allantois involutes to form a thick tube called the *urachus*. After birth, the urachus becomes a fibrous cord called the *median umbilical ligament* (Fig. 8–16D).

TWIN AND OTHER MULTIPLE PREGNANCIES

Multiple births are more common now due to the stimulation of ovulation that occurs when human gonadotropins or other ovulation-inducing drugs are administered to women with *ovulatory failure* (failure of ovulation). See the discussion of *in vitro fertilization* on page 29.

> In North America, twins normally occur about once in every 90 pregnancies, triplets once in 90^2 pregnancies, quadruplets about once in 90^3, and quintuplets about once in 90^4 pregnancies. These estimates increase when ovulations have

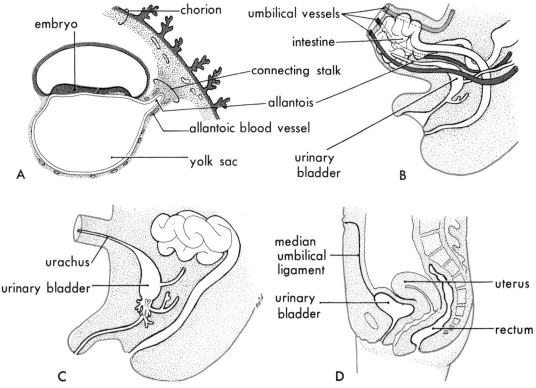

Figure 8–16. Drawings illustrating the development and usual fate of the allantois. *A,* Three weeks. *B,* Nine weeks. *C,* Three months. *D,* Woman. This nonfunctional structure forms the urachus in the fetus and the median umbilical ligament in the adult.

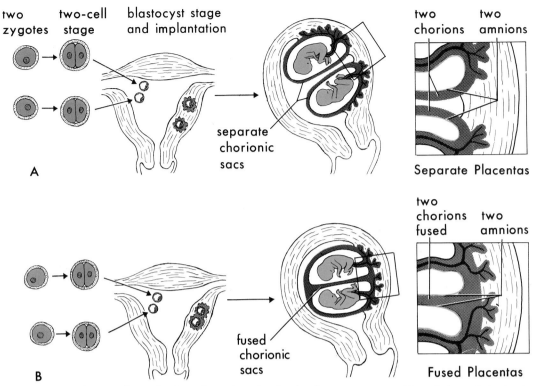

Figure 8–17. Diagrams illustrating how dizygotic twins develop from two zygotes. The relations of the fetal membranes and placentas are shown for instances in which, *A*, The blastocysts implant separately, and *B*, The blastocysts implant close together. In both cases there are two amnions and two chorions, and the placentas may be separate or fused.

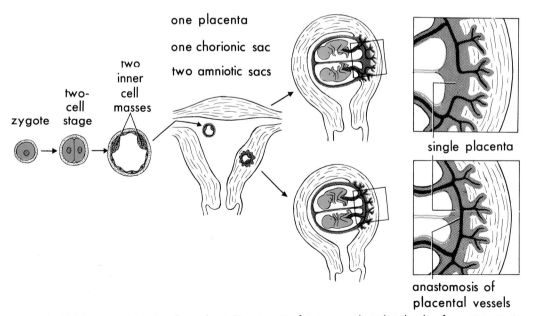

Figure 8–18. Diagrams illustrating how about 65 per cent of monozygotic twins develop from one zygote by division of the inner cell mass (embryoblast) toward the end of the first week of development. Such twins always have separate amnions, a single chorion, and a common placenta.

been primed with hormones, a technique that is in general use for women who are sterile because of occlusion of the uterine tubes.

Twins (MZ and DZ)

Twins may originate from two zygotes (Fig. 8–17), in which case they are *dizygotic* (DZ) *twins* (also called nonidentical or fraternal twins). About one third of twins are derived from one zygote (Fig. 8–18); they are called *monozygotic* (MZ) *twins* or identical twins. Twins occur about once in 90 pregnancies; about two thirds of the total number are DZ twins. In addition, the rate of MZ twinning shows little variation with the mother's age; whereas, *DZ twinning increases with maternal age*.

There is a tendency for DZ but not MZ twins to repeat in families. It has also been found that, if the firstborn are twins, a repetition of twinning or some other form of multiple birth is about five times more likely to occur at the next

pregnancy than it is in the general population. The study of twins is important in human genetics because of their usefulness for comparing the effects of genes and environment on development. If an abnormal condition does not show a simple genetic pattern, comparison of its incidence in MZ and DZ twins can reveal that heredity is involved (Thompson et al., 1991).

DIZYGOTIC (DZ) TWINS (Fig. 8–17). Because they result from the fertilization of two ova by different sperms, *DZ twins may be of the same sex or different sexes*. For the same reason, they are no more alike genetically than brothers or sisters born at different times. Dizygotic twins always have two amnions and two chorions, but the chorions and placentas may be fused.

MONOZYGOTIC (MZ) TWINS (Figs. 8–18 and 8–19). Because they result from the fertilization of one ovum, MZ twins are: (1) of the same sex, (2) genetically identical, and (3) very similar in physical appearance. Physical differences between identical twins are caused by

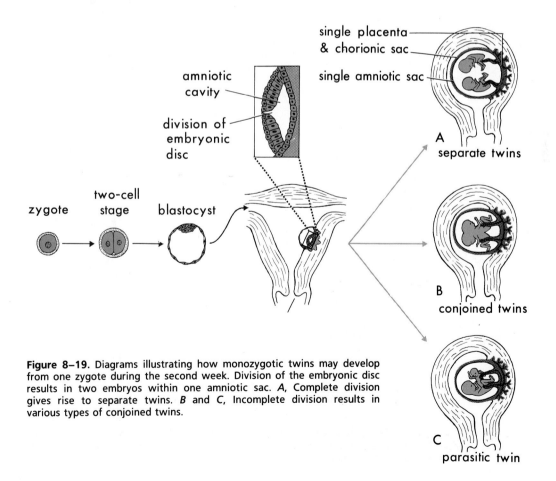

Figure 8–19. Diagrams illustrating how monozygotic twins may develop from one zygote during the second week. Division of the embryonic disc results in two embryos within one amniotic sac. *A,* Complete division gives rise to separate twins. *B* and *C,* Incomplete division results in various types of conjoined twins.

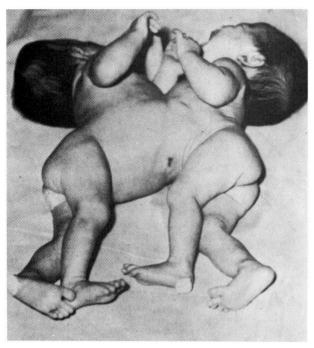

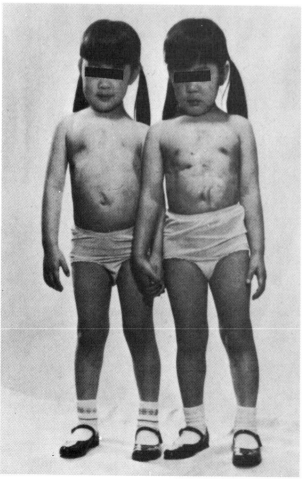

Figure 8–20. *A*, Photograph of newborn monozygotic conjoined twins, showing union in the thoracic regions (thoracopagus). During the twinning process there was incomplete division of the embryonic disc (see Fig. 8–19*B*). *B*, The twins about four years after separation. (From de Vries PA: Case history–the San Francisco twins. *In* Bergsma D [ed]: *Conjoined Twins. Birth Defects. Original Article Series,* vol. III, No. 1, 1967. © The National Foundation, New York.)

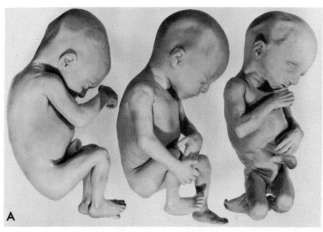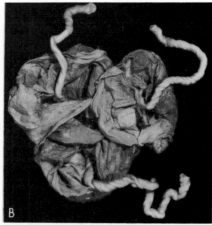

Figure 8–21. *A,* Photograph of 20-week triplets: monozygotic male twins (left) and a single female (right). *B,* Photograph of their fused placentas shows the twin placenta with two amnions (left) and the single placenta (upper right). These triplets obviously developed from two zygotes.

environmental factors (e.g., anastomosis of placental vessels resulting in differences in blood supply from the placenta).

About 35 per cent of MZ twins begin to develop early in the first week and result from the separation of the blastomeres at two-, four-, or eight-cell stages (see Fig. 3–3). Each blastomere or group of blastomeres gives rise to a blastocyst that implants separately in the endometrium and develops its own placenta. The placentas may remain separate or they may fuse in the same manner as DZ twins (see Fig. 8–17).

About 65 per cent of MZ twins begin to develop around the end of the first week and result from early division of the inner cell mass or embryoblast into two embryonic primordia. Two identical embryos, each in its own amniotic sac, subsequently develop within one chorionic sac. The twins have a common placenta and often some placental vessels join (see Fig. 8–18).

In unusual cases, abnormal division of the embryonic cells occurs in the second week, after the amniotic sac has formed. As a result, both embryos develop within the same amniotic cavity. These MZ twins are in one amniotic sac and one chorionic sac (Fig. 8–19A). Such twins are rarely delivered alive because the umbilical cords are frequently entangled; as a result, the circulation ceases and one or both fetuses die.

MZ twins may sometimes be discordant for a variety of birth defects and genetic disorders despite their origin from a single zygote. In addition to environmental differences and chance variation, various reasons for discordance are recognized (see Thompson et al., 1991).

CONJOINED TWINS (Figs. 8–19B and C and 8–20). If the embryoblast or embryonic disc does not divide completely, various types of conjoined twins ("siamese twins") may form. These are named according to the regions that are attached, e.g., thoracopagus indicates that there is anterior union of the thoracic regions.

Most twins (DZ and MZ) are born prematurely because the uterus becomes overdistended and the twins become crowded within the uterus. This overcrowding interferes with the growth of the twins during the late stages of pregnancy. In addition, the placenta ceases to provide sufficient nutrition; hence, a twin is always smaller than a single infant at a comparable stage of gestation (see Fig. 7–10). Birth defects are also more common in twins than in singletons.

Other Types of Multiple Birth

Triplets occur once in about 8100 pregnancies and may be derived from: (1) one zygote and be identical, (2) two zygotes and consist of identical twins and a single infant (Fig. 8–21), or (3) three zygotes and be of the same sex or different sexes. In the last case, the infants are no more similar than those from three separate pregnancies. Similar possible combinations occur in quadruplets, quintuplets, sextuplets, and septuplets. Multiple births higher than triplets are uncommon, but they have occurred more often in recent years following the administration of gonadotropins to women with ovulatory failure.

SUMMARY

In addition to the embryo, the fetal membranes and most of the placenta originate from the zygote. The chorion, amnion, yolk sac, and allantois constitute the fetal membranes. The placenta consists of two parts: (1) a larger fetal portion derived from the *villous chorion*, and (2) a maternal portion formed by the *decidua basalis*. The two parts are held together by stem villi that anchor the fetal part to the cytotrophoblastic shell which adheres to the decidua basalis.

The fetal circulation is separated from the maternal circulation by a thin layer of extrafetal tissues known as the *placental membrane* ("barrier"). It is a permeable membrane that allows water, oxygen, nutrient substances, hormones, and noxious agents (e.g., drugs) to pass from the mother to the embryo or fetus. Excretory products pass from the embryo/fetus through the placental membrane to the mother.

The principal *activities of the placenta* are: (1) metabolism, (2) transfer, and (3) endocrine secretion. All three activities are essential for the maintenance of pregnancy and the normal growth and development of the embryo and fetus.

The fetal membranes and placenta(s) in multiple pregnancies vary considerably depending on the derivation of the embryos and the time when division of embryonic cells occurs. The common type of twins is *dizygotic* (DZ) *twins*, with two amnions, two chorions, and two placentas that may or may not be fused. *Monozygotic* (MZ) *twins* represent about a third of all twins; they are derived from one zygote. MZ twins commonly have two amnions, one chorion, and one placenta. Other types of multiple birth (*triplets*, etc.) may be derived from one or more zygotes.

Although the yolk sac and allantois are vestigial structures, their formation is essential for normal embryonic development. Both are important early sites of blood formation, and parts of them are incorporated into the embryo. Part of the yolk sac forms the primitive gut, and the allantois forms the urachus which later forms the median umbilical ligament.

The amnion forms a sac for amniotic fluid and provides a covering for the umbilical cord. The amniotic fluid provides: (1) a protective buffer for the embryo, (2) room for fetal movements, and (3) assistance in the regulation of fetal body temperature.

Commonly Asked Questions

1. What is meant by the term "stillbirth?" Do older women have more stillborn infants? I have heard that more males than females are born dead. Is this true?
2. My sister's baby was born dead due to a "cord accident." What does this mean? Do these accidents always kill the baby? If not, what defects may be present?
3. What is the scientific basis of the pregnancy test kits that are sold in drug stores? Are they accurate?
4. What is the proper name for what laypeople refer to as the "bag of waters?" What is meant by a "dry birth?" Does premature rupture of this "bag" induce the birth of the baby and/or cause fetal distress?
5. What does the term "fetal distress" mean? How is the condition recognized? What causes fetal stress and distress?
6. I have heard that twins are born more commonly to older mothers. Is this true? I have also heard that twinning is hereditary. Is this correct?
7. Can pregnant women with AIDS pass the virus to their babies? If so, does it affect their development?

The answers to these questions are given on page 330.

REFERENCES

Bassett JM: Current perspectives on placental development and its integration with fetal growth. *Proc Nutr Soc 50*:311, 1991.

Behrman RE (ed): *Nelson's Textbook of Pediatrics,* 14th ed. Philadelphia, WB Saunders, 1992.

Bernischke K, Kaufman P: *The Pathology of the Human Placenta.* Berlin, Springer-Verlag, 1990.

Bulmer MG: *The Biology of Twinning in Man.* Oxford, Clarendon Press, 1970.

Creasy RK, Resnik R (eds): *Maternal-Fetal Medicine. Principles and Practice,* 2nd ed. Philadelphia, WB Saunders, 1989.

Cunningham FG, MacDonald PC, Grand NF (eds): *Williams Obstetrics,* 18th ed. Norwalk, Appleton & Lange, 1990.

Fox H: *Pathology of the Placenta.* Philadelphia, WB Saunders, 1978.

Hamilton WJ, Boyd JD: Development of the human placenta. *In* Philipp EE, Barnes J, Newton M (eds): *Scientific Foundations of Obstetrics and Gynecology.* London, William Heinemann, 1970.

Hay WW: In vivo measurements of placental transport and metabolism. *Proc Nutr Soc 50*:355, 1991.

Jauniaux E, Campbell S: Ultrasonographic assessment of placental abnormalities. *Am J Obstet Gynecol 163*:1650, 1990.

Jauniaux E, Jurkovic D, Henriet Y, Rodesch F, Hustin J: Development of the secondary human yolk sac — correlation of sonographic and anatomical features. *Hum Reprod 6*:1160, 1991.

Lindsay DJ, Lovett IS, Lyons EA, Levi CS, Zheng X-H, Holt SC, Daschefsky SM: Endovaginal sonography: yolk sac diameter and shape as a predictor of pregnancy outcome in the first trimester. *Radiology 183*:115, 1992.

Lyons EA, Levi CS: *Ultrasound of the normal first trimester of pregnancy.* Syllabus. Special Course. Ultrasound, Radiological Society of North America, 1991.

Moore KL, Persaud TVN: *The Developing Human. Clinically Oriented Embryology,* 5th ed. Philadelphia, WB Saunders, 1993.

Mossman HW: Classics revisited: comparative morphogenesis of fetal membranes and accessory uterine structures. *Placenta 12*:1, 1991.

Naeye RL: *Disorders of the Placenta, Fetus, and Neonate.* St. Louis, Mosby Year Book, 1992.

Nyberg DA, Callen PW: Ultrasound evaluation of the placenta. *In* Callen PW (ed): *Ultrasonography in Obstetrics and Gynecology,* 2nd ed. Philadelphia, WB Saunders, 1988.

Oxorn H: *Human Labor and Birth,* 5th ed. Norwalk, Appleton-Century-Crofts, 1989.

Peipert JF, Dennerfeld AE: Oligohydramnios: a review. *Obstet Gynecol 46*:325, 1991.

Petraglia F, Angioni S, Coukos G, Uccelli E, Didomenica P, Deramundo BM, Genazzani AD, Garuti GC, Segre A: Neuroendocrine mechanisms regulating placental hormone production. *Contr Gynecol Obstet 18*:147, 1991.

Schneider H: Placental transport function. *Reprod Fert Develop 3*:345, 1991.

Scott JR, DiSaia PJ, Hammond CB, Spellacy WN (eds): *Danforth's Obstetrics and Gynecology,* 6th ed. Philadelphia, JB Lippincott, 1990.

Thompson MW, McInnes RR, Willard HF: *Thompson & Thompson Genetics in Medicine,* 5th ed. Philadelphia, WB Saunders, 1991.

Yen SSC, Jaffe RB: *Reproductive Endocrinology, Physiology, Pathophysiology and Clinical Management,* 3rd ed. Philadelphia, WB Saunders, 1991.

9

HUMAN BIRTH DEFECTS AND THEIR CAUSES

Birth defects, congenital malformations, deformities, and congenital anomalies are all-encompassing terms currently used to describe developmental defects present at birth (L. *congenitus*, born with)[1]. Birth defects or congenital anomalies may be structural, functional, metabolic, behavioral, or hereditary. According to data from the U.S. Centers for Disease Control, the leading cause of death in 1989 for white infants was birth defects. *More than 20 per cent of infant deaths in North America are attributed to birth defects.* Major structural anomalies (e.g., cleft lip) are observed in about three per cent of newborn infants, and congenital abnormalities are detected in an additional three percent during infancy. Thus, the incidence reaches about six per cent in 2-year-olds and eight per cent in 5-year-olds.

Teratology is the study of all aspects of abnormal embryonic development including the *causes and pathogenesis of congenital anomalies or defects.* A fundamental concept in teratology is that certain stages of embryonic development are more vulnerable to *teratogens* (e.g., drugs and viruses) *than others.*

It is customary to divide the causes of congenital anomalies into: (1) *genetic factors* (e.g., chromosome abnormalities), and (2) *environmental factors* such as drugs. Many common anomalies, however, are caused by genetic and environmental factors acting together. This is called *multifactorial inheritance* (p. 139), which affects about 20 to 25 per cent of individuals. For 50 to 60 per cent of congenital anomalies, the causes of the birth defects are unknown (Table 9–1).

Anomalies (structural abnormalities of any type) may be single or multiple and of major or minor clinical significance. Single *minor anomalies* are present in about 14 per cent of newborns. These anomalies (e.g., of the external ear [see Fig. 18–12] or a simian crease in the hand [see Fig. 9–4B]) are of no serious medical or cosmetic significance, but they alert the clinician to the possible presence of associated major anomalies; for example, a single umbilical artery (see Fig. 8–12B) alerts the clinician to the pos-

Table 9–1. ESTIMATED INCIDENCE OF CAUSES OF MAJOR CONGENITAL ANOMALIES[1]

Causes	Incidence (%)
Chromosome abnormalities	6–7
Mutant genes	7–8
Environmental factors	7–10
Multifactorial inheritance	20–25
Unknown etiology[2]	50–60

[1] Based on data, combined with reasoning, from Connor and Ferguson-Smith (1987), Persaud (1990), and Thompson et al. (1991).
[2] It is likely that the majority of infants with birth defects or congenital anomalies of unknown cause has a genetic disorder. Molecular biological techniques are likely to reduce the number of anomalies of unknown etiology.

[1] Persons desiring explanations of the various terms used to describe birth defects should consult the glossary in Moore and Persaud (1993).

118

sible presence of cardiovascular and renal anomalies.

Ninety per cent of infants with multiple minor anomalies have an associated major anomaly. Of the three per cent of infants born with congenital anomalies, 0.7 per cent have multiple major anomalies. Most of these infants die during infancy (e.g., those with trisomy 13 [see Fig. 9–6]). Major developmental defects are much more common in early embryos (10 to 15 per cent), but most of them abort spontaneously. Chromosome abnormalities are present in 50 to 60 per cent of spontaneously aborted embryos (Shepard et al., 1989).

ANOMALIES CAUSED BY GENETIC FACTORS[2]

Genetic factors are the most common causes of congenital anomalies. They cause about a third of all birth defects (Table 9–1) and nearly 85 per cent of all those with known causes. Any mechanism as complex as mitosis or meiosis may occasionally malfunction; thus, *chromosomal aberrations are common* and are thought to be present in about six per cent of zygotes. Many of these primordial cells never undergo normal cleavage (mitosis) and become blastocysts. *In vitro studies* of cleaving human pre-embryos less than five days old have revealed a high incidence of abnormalities. More than 60 per cent of day two zygotes were found to be abnormal. Many defective zygotes, blastocysts, and pre-embryos abort spontaneously during the first two weeks (p. 43).

Chromosome complements are subject to two kinds of change: numerical and structural, and these abnormalities may affect the sex chromosomes and/or the autosomes[3]. In some cases, both kinds of chromosome are affected. Persons with chromosome abnormalities usually have characteristic *phenotypes* (e.g., the physical characteristics of infants with Down syndrome

[see Fig. 9–4]). They often look more like other persons with the same chromosome abnormality than like their own siblings (brothers or sisters). This characteristic appearance results from the genetic imbalance that disrupts normal development.

Genetic factors initiate anomalies by biochemical or other means at the subcellular, cellular, or tissue level. The abnormal mechanism initiated by the genetic factor may be identical or similar to the causal mechanism initiated by a teratogen (e.g., a drug). **A teratogen** is any agent that can produce a congenital anomaly or raise the incidence of the anomaly in the population (p. 128).

Numerical Chromosome Abnormalities

Numerical aberrations of chromosomes usually result from *nondisjunction,* an error in cell division in which there is failure of a chromosome pair or two chromatids to separate (disjoin) during mitosis or meiosis (Chapter 2). This error may occur during a mitotic division or the first or second meiotic division (Fig. 9–1). Nondisjunction may occur during maternal or paternal gametogenesis (p. 14). Chromosomes normally exist in pairs (Fig. 9–2); the two chromosomes making up a pair are called *homologs.* Normal human females have 22 pairs of autosomes plus two X chromosomes; whereas, normal males have 22 pairs of autosomes plus one X and one Y chromosome.

During embryogenesis, one of the two X chromosomes in somatic cells of female somatic cells is randomly inactivated and appears as a mass of *sex chromatin* (see Fig. 9–8B). This chromatin mass is not present in cells of normal males or in females lacking a sex chromosome (see Fig. 9–8A). Although sex chromatin studies are useful in diagnosing errors of sex development (see Fig. 9–14), they provide no information about the presence or absence of the Y chromosome. The Y chromosome can be detected in interphase cells by means of quinacrine fluorescence staining (see Fig. 7–12C).

Inactivation of genes on one X chromosome is important clinically because it means that each cell from a carrier of an X-linked disease has the mutant gene causing the disease, either on the active X chromosome or on the inactivated X chromosome that is represented by sex chromatin. For more information about X inactivation

[2] We are grateful to Dr. A.E. Chudley, M.D., F.R.C.P.C., F.C.C.M.G., Professor of Pediatrics and Child Health; Director of Clinical Genetics, Health Sciences Centre, University of Manitoba, Winnipeg, Manitoba, for assistance with the preparation of this section. We also relied heavily on the commendable work of Thompson et al., 1991.
[3] Autosomes are any chromosomes other than the sex chromosomes. There are 22 pairs in the human karyotype (the chromosome constitution of an individual). For information about them and gene mapping, see Thompson et al., 1991.

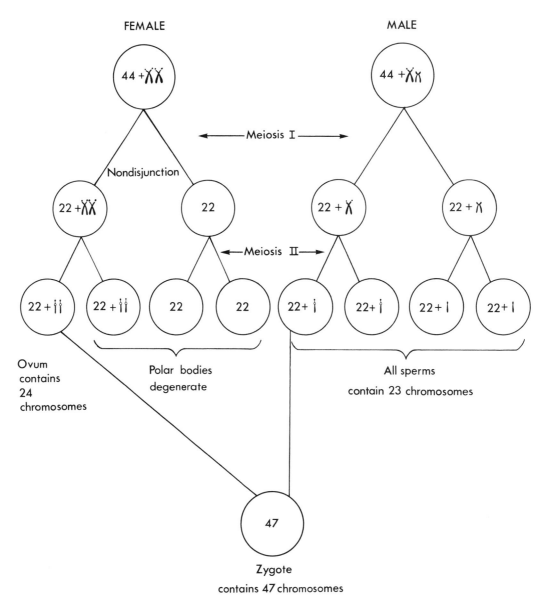

Figure 9–1. Diagram showing nondisjunction of chromosomes during the first meiotic division of a primary oocyte during oogenesis, resulting in an abnormal oocyte (ovum) with 24 chromosomes. Subsequent fertilization by a normal sperm produces a zygote with 47 chromosomes, a condition called aneuploidy.

and its clinical implications see Thompson et al. (1991).

Changes in chromosome number represent either aneuploidy or polyploidy.

ANEUPLOIDY. Any deviation from the human diploid number of 46 chromosomes is called aneuploidy. An *aneuploid* is an individual or a cell that has a chromosome number that is not an exact multiple of the haploid number of 23 (e.g., 45 or 47). The principal cause of aneuploidy is nondisjunction during cell division

(Fig. 9–1). This results in an unequal distribution of one pair of homologous chromosomes to the daughter cells. One cell has two chromosomes, and the other has neither chromosome of the pair. As a result, the embryo's cells may be *hypodiploid* (45,X as in *Turner syndrome* [Fig. 9–3]), or *hyperdiploid* (usually 47, as in *Down syndrome* [Fig. 9–4]).

Monosomy. Embryos missing a chromosome usually die and are spontaneously aborted. Monosomy of an autosome is extremely uncommon

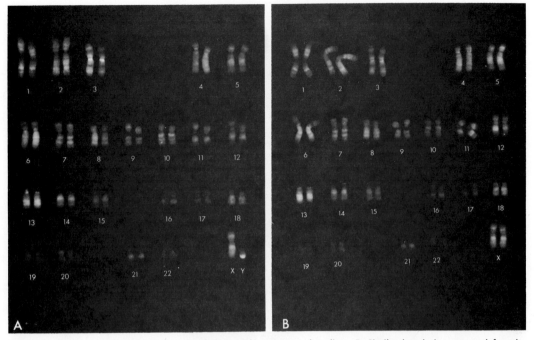

Figure 9–2. *A*, Normal male karyotype showing chromosome banding. *B*, Similar bands in a normal female karyotype. When chromosomes are stained with quinacrine mustard or related compounds and examined by fluorescent microscopy, each pair of chromosomes stains in a distinctive pattern of bright and dim bands. They form the basis of the classification of chromosomes.

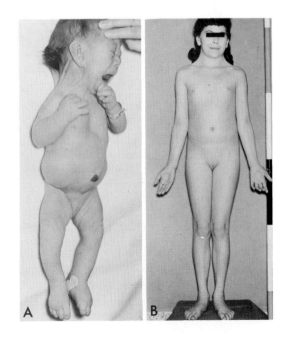

Figure 9–3. Females with 45,X Turner syndrome. *A*, Newborn infant. Note the webbed neck and lymphedema of the hands and feet. *B*, 13-year-old girl, showing the classic features: short stature, webbed neck, absence of sexual maturation, and broad, shieldlike chest with widely spaced nipples. (From Medovy H: In Moore KL: *The Sex Chromatin.* Philadelphia, WB Saunders, 1966).

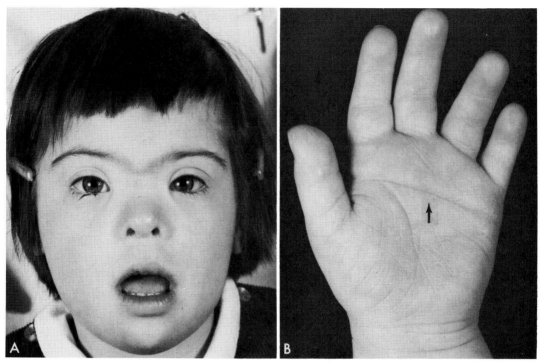

Figure 9–4. *A,* Photograph of a 3½-year-old girl, showing the typical facial appearance associated with Down syndrome (trisomy 21). Note the flat, broad face, oblique palpebral fissures, epicanthus, speckling of the iris, and furrowed lower lip. *B,* The typical short, broad hand of this child shows the characteristic single, transverse, flexion (simian) crease *(arrow).* About half the palms of patients with Down syndrome have a simian crease, and about 1 per cent of normal persons have this unusual palm pattern. (From Bartalos M, Baramki TA: *Medical Cytogenetics.* Baltimore, Williams & Wilkins, © 1967.)

in living persons; furthermore, about 99 per cent of embryos lacking a sex chromosome also die, but some survive and develop characteristics of *Turner syndrome* (Fig. 9–3). The incidence of *monosomy X* (45,X), or Turner syndrome, in newborn females is approximately one in 5000 live female births (Thompson et al., 1991).

The phenotype of Turner syndrome *(observable characteristics)* is illustrated in Figure 9–3. The *XO chromosome abnormality* is the most common cytogenetic abnormality observed in fetuses that abort spontaneously, and it accounts for about 18 per cent of all abortions caused by chromosome abnormalities. The error in gametogenesis (nondisjunction) that causes Turner syndrome, when it can be traced, is usually (about 75 per cent) in the paternal gamete (i.e., it is the paternal X chromosome that is missing). Maternal age is not advanced.

Trisomy. If three chromosomes are present instead of the usual pair, the disorder is called trisomy. The usual cause of this error is *nondisjunction* (Fig. 9–1), resulting in a germ cell with 24 instead of 23 chromosomes and, subsequently, in a zygote with 47 chromosomes.

Trisomy of the autosomes is associated primarily with three syndromes (see Table 9–2). The most common condition is *trisomy 21* or *Down syndrome* (Fig. 9–4) in which three number 21 chromosomes are present. *Trisomy 18* (Fig. 9–5) and *trisomy 13* (Fig. 9–6) are much less common (Table 9–2); infants with these chromosome abnormalities are severely malformed and mentally retarded, and they usually die early in infancy.

Autosomal trisomies occur with increasing frequency as maternal age increases, particularly trisomy 21 (Down syndrome), which is present once in about 1400 births in mothers aged 20 to 24 years (Table 9–3), but once in about 25 births in mothers 45 years and older.

Trisomy of the sex chromosomes is a common condition (Table 9–4); however, because there are no characteristic physical findings in infants

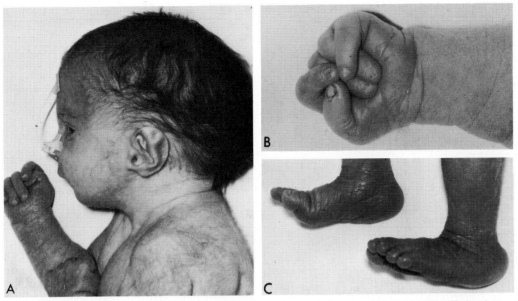

Figure 9–5. Photographs of an infant with trisomy 18 syndrome. *A,* Prominent occiput and malformed ears. *B,* Typical flexed fingers. *C,* Rocker-bottom feet showing posterior prominences of the heels. About 95 per cent of trisomy 18 conceptuses are aborted spontaneously. (Courtesy of Dr. Harry Medovy, Children's Centre, Winnipeg.)

Figure 9–6. Female infants with trisomy 13 syndrome. Trisomy 13 results in a clinically severe condition, lethal in almost all cases by the age of six months. Note bilateral cleft lip, sloping forehead, and rocker-bottom feet. (From Smith DW: *Am J Obstet Gynecol 90:*1055, 1964.)

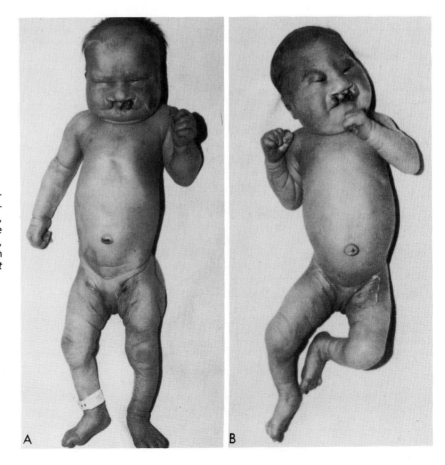

Table 9-2. TRISOMY OF THE AUTOSOMES

Disorder	Incidence	Usual Characteristics
Trisomy 21 or Down syndrome*	1:800	Mental deficiency; hypotonia; flat nasal bridge; upward slant to palpebral fissures; protruding tongue; simian crease; congenital heart defects
Trisomy 18†	1:8000	Mental deficiency; growth retardation; prominent occiput; short sternum; ventricular septal defect; micrognathia; low-set malformed ears; flexed fingers
Trisomy 13†	1:25000	Mental deficiency; sloping forehead; malformed ears; microphthalmos; bilateral cleft lip and/or palate; polydactyly; posterior prominence of the heels

*The importance of this disorder in the overall problem of mental retardation is indicated by the fact that persons with Down syndrome represent 10 to 15 per cent of institutionalized mental defectives. Down syndrome is by far the most common and best known of the chromosomal disorders. The old name "mongolism" should not be used; it refers to the somewhat oriental appearance of the face caused by the apparent slanting of the eyes.

†Infants with this syndrome rarely survive beyond a few months.

Table 9-3. INCIDENCE OF DOWN SYNDROME IN NEWBORN INFANTS

Maternal Age (Years)	Incidence
20–24	1:1400
25–29	1:1100
30–34	1:700
35	1:350
37	1:225
39	1:140
41	1:85
43	1:50
45+	1:25

or children, this disorder is not usually detected until adolescence (Fig. 9–7). *Sex chromatin studies* are useful in detecting some types of trisomy of the sex chromosomes because two masses of sex chromatin are present in XXX females (Fig. 9–8C), and nuclei of cells of XXY males are chromatin positive (i.e., contain sex chromatin).

TETRASOMY AND PENTASOMY OF THE SEX CHROMOSOMES. Some persons, usually mentally retarded, have four or five sex chromosomes. The following chromosome complexes have been reported: *in females*, 48,XXXX and 49,XXXXX; and *in males*, 48,XXXY, 48,XXYY, 49,XXXYY, and 49,XXXXY. The extra sex chromosomes do not accentuate sexual characteristics; however, usually the greater the number of sex chromosomes present, the greater the severity of the mental retardation and physical impairment.

MOSAICISM. A mosaic is a person derived from one zygote that has cells with *two or more different genotypes* (genetic constitutions). The anomalies are usually less serious than in persons with monosomy or trisomy, e.g., the features of Turner syndrome are not as evident in 45,X/46,XX mosaic females as in the usual 45,X females shown in Figure 9–3. Mosaicism usually results from nondisjunction during early cleavage of the zygote (see Fig. 3–3). Mosaicism due to loss of a chromosome by so-called *anaphase lagging* is also known to occur. The chromosomes separate normally, but one chromosome is delayed in its migration and is eventually lost.

POLYPLOIDY. Polyploid cells contain multiples of the haploid number of chromosomes (e.g., 69 and 92). Polyploidy is a significant cause of spontaneous abortion. The most common type of polyploidy in human embryos is **triploidy** (69 chromosomes). This can result from the second polar body failing to separate from the oocyte during the second meiotic division (see Chapter 2) or by an ovum being fertilized by two sperms

Table 9-4. TRISOMY OF THE SEX CHROMOSOMES

Chromosome Complement*	Sex	Incidence	Usual Characteristics
47,XXX	Female	1:960	Normal in appearance; fertile; 15 to 25 per cent are mentally retarded
47,XXY	Male	1:1080	Klinefelter syndrome; small testes and hyalinization of seminiferous tubules; aspermatogenesis; may be mentally retarded; often tall with long lower limbs
47,XYY	Male	1:1080	Normal in appearance, often tall; may have personality disorder

*The number designates the total number of chromosomes, including the sex chromosomes shown after the comma.

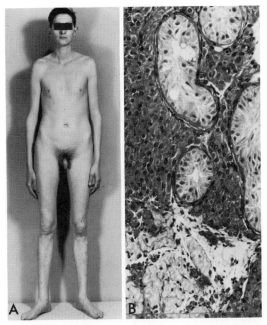

Figure 9–7. *A*, Adult male with Klinefelter syndrome (XXY trisomy). Note the long limbs and normal trunk length. *B*, Section of a testicular biopsy showing some seminiferous tubules without germ cells and others that have degenerated. (From Ferguson-Smith MA: Sex chromatin, Klinefelter's syndrome and mental deficiency. *In* Moore KL [ed]: *The Sex Chromatin.* Philadelphia, WB Saunders, 1966.)

almost simultaneously. It has been estimated that 66 per cent of **triploid embryos** result from double fertilization *(dispermy)*. Triploidy occurs in about two per cent of embryos, but most of them abort spontaneously. Although *triploid fetuses* have been born alive, this occurrence is exceptional. They all died within a few days because of multiple anomalies and low birth weight (Connor and Ferguson-Smith, 1987).

Doubling of the diploid chromosome number to 92 *(tetraploidy)* probably occurs during the first cleavage division (see Fig. 3–3*A*). Division of this abnormal zygote would subsequently result in an embryo with cells containing 92 chromosomes. *Tetraploid embryos* abort very early; and often, all that is recovered is an empty chorionic sac. This is often referred to clinically as a "blighted embryo."

Structural Chromosome Abnormalities

Most abnormalities of chromosome structure result from chromosome breakage that is induced by various environmental factors, e.g., radiation, drugs, chemicals, and viruses. The type

of abnormality that results depends upon what happens to the broken pieces of the chromosomes (Fig. 9–9). The only aberrations of chromosome structure that are likely to be transmitted from parent to child are structural rearrangements, such as inversion and translocation (Thompson et al., 1991).

TRANSLOCATION. This is the transfer of a piece of one chromosome to a nonhomologous chromosome. If two nonhomologous chromosomes exchange pieces, it is called a *reciprocal translocation* (Fig. 9–9*A* and *G*). Translocation does not necessarily lead to abnormal development. A person with a translocation, for example, between a number 21 chromosome and a number 14 (Fig. 9–9*G*), is phenotypically normal. Such persons are called *balanced translocation carriers.* They have a tendency, independent of age, to produce germ cells with an abnormal translocation chromosome. Three to four per cent of persons with Down syndrome have translocation trisomies, i.e., the extra 21 chromosome is attached to another chromosome.

DELETION. When a chromosome breaks, a portion of the chromosome may be lost (Fig. 9–9*B*). A partial terminal deletion from the short arm of chromosome number 5 causes the **cri du chat syndrome** (Fig. 9–10*A*). Affected infants have a weak, catlike cry, microcephaly, severe mental retardation, and congenital heart disease. The only invariable feature is mental retardation. A *ring chromosome* is a type of deletion chromosome from which both ends have been lost, and the broken ends have rejoined to form a ring-shaped chromosome (Fig. 9–9*C*). These abnormal chromosomes have been described in persons with Turner syndrome, trisomy 18, and other abnormalities (Hirschhorn, 1992).

Microdeletions. High-resolution banding techniques have allowed detection of very small

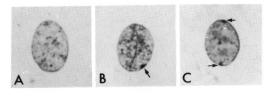

Figure 9–8. Oral epithelial nuclei stained with cresylecht violet (× 2000). *A*, From normal chromatin-negative male. No sex chromatin is visible. *B*, From normal chromatin-positive female. The arrow indicates a typical mass of sex chromatin. *C*, Female with 47,XXX trisomy. The arrows indicate two masses of sex chromatin. (*A* and *B* from Moore KL, Barr ML: *Lancet* 2:57, 1955.)

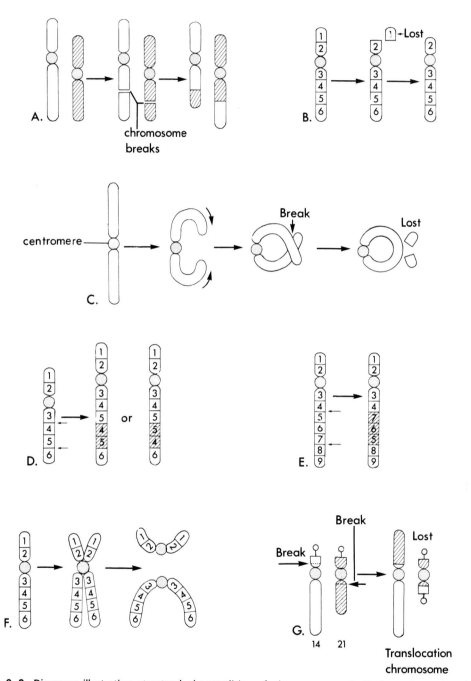

Figure 9–9. Diagrams illustrating structural abnormalities of chromosomes. *A*, Reciprocal translocation. *B*, Terminal deletion. *C*, Ring. *D*, Duplication. *E*, Paracentric inversion. *F*, Isochromosome. *G*, Robertsonian translocation.

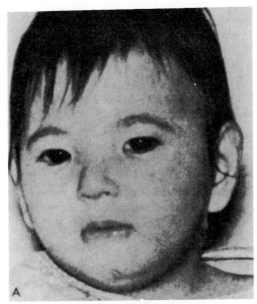
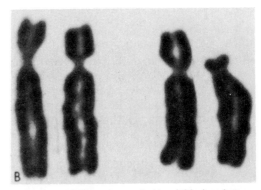

Figure 9–10. *A*, Male infant with cri du chat syndrome. *B*, A partial karyotype of this child showing a terminal deletion of the short arm end of the chromosome number 5 on the right. The arrow indicates the abnormal short arm. (Courtesy of Dr. J. de Grouchy, Paris).

interstitial and terminal deletions in a number of disorders. Normal resolution chromosome banding reveals 350 bands per haploid set; whereas, *high-resolution chromosome banding* reveals up to 1300 bands per haploid set. Because the deletions span several contiguous genes, these disorders have been referred to as *contiguous gene syndromes.* Two examples are: the *Prader-Willi syndrome,* a sporadically occurring disorder associated with short stature, mild mental retardation, obesity, hyperphagia (overeating) and hypogonadism; and the *Angelman syndrome,* characterized by severe mental retardation, microcephaly, brachycephaly, seizures and ataxic (jerky) movements of limbs and trunk. Both disorders are often associated with a visible deletion of band q12 on chromosome 15. The clinical phenotype is determined by the parental origin of the deleted chromosome 15. If the deletion arises in the mother, Angelman syndrome will occur. If passed on by the father, the child will exhibit the Prader-Willi phenotype. This suggests the phenomenon of genetic imprinting whereby differential expression of genetic material is dependent on the sex of the transmitting parent.

Molecular Cytogenetics. Several new methods involve the merging of classical cytogenetics with DNA technology and have facilitated a more precise definition of chromosome abnormalities, location or origins, including unbalanced translocations, accessory or marker chromosomes, as well as gene mapping. One new approach to chromosome identification is based on *fluorescent in situ hybridization* (FISH), whereby chromosome-specific DNA probes can adhere to complementary regions located on specific chromosomes. This allows improved identification of chromosome location and number in metaphase spreads or even in interphase cells. FISH techniques using interphase cells may soon obviate the need to culture cells for specific chromosome analysis, such as in the case of prenatal diagnosis of fetal trisomies.

DUPLICATION. This abnormality may be represented as a duplicated portion of a chromosome: (1) within a chromosome (Fig. 9–9*D*), (2) attached to a chromosome, or (3) as a separate fragment. *Duplications are more common than deletions, and they are less harmful* because there is no loss of genetic material. Duplication may involve part of a gene, a whole gene, or a series of genes.

INVERSION. This is a chromosomal aberration in which a segment of a chromosome is reversed. Paracentric inversion (Fig. 9–9*E*) is confined to a single arm of the chromosome; whereas, pericentric inversion involves both arms and includes the centromere. Carriers of pericentric inversions are at risk of having offspring with abnormalities as a result of unequal crossing over and malsegregation at meiosis (Thompson et al., 1991).

ISOCHROMOSOME. This abnormality results when the centromere divides transversely instead of longitudinally (Fig. 9–9*F*). It appears to be *the most common structural abnormality of the X chromosome*. Patients with this chromosomal abnormality are often short in stature and have other stigmata of Turner syndrome. These characteristics are related to the loss of a short arm of one X chromosome.

Anomalies Caused by Mutant Genes

Seven to eight per cent of congenital anomalies or birth defects are caused by mutant genes (Table 9–1). A *mutation* usually involves a loss or a change in the function of a gene. Because a random change is unlikely to lead to an improvement in development, most mutations are deleterious and some are lethal. The mutation rate can be increased by a number of environmental agents, e.g., large doses of radiation and many chemicals, especially carcinogenic (cancer-inducing) ones (Table 9–5). Anomalies resulting from gene mutation are inherited according to mendelian laws; consequently, predictions can be made about the probability of their occurrence in the affected person's children and in other relatives.

Examples of dominantly inherited congenital anomalies are **achondroplasia** (Fig. 9–11) and **polydactyly** (extra digits [see Chapter 16]). Other anomalies are attributed to *autosomal recessive inheritance*, e.g., congenital adrenal hyperplasia (see Fig. 14–16) and microcephaly (see Fig. 17–24). Autosomal recessive genes manifest themselves only when homozygous; as a consequence, many carriers of these genes (heterozygous persons) remain undetected.

The fragile X syndrome is the most common inherited cause of moderate mental retardation. The diagnosis can be confirmed by chromosome analysis demonstrating the fragile X chromosome[4] or by DNA studies of the fragile X gene. X-linked recessive genes are usually manifest in affected (hemizygous) males and occasionally in carrier (heterozygous) females, e.g., fragile X syndrome (Chudley and Hagerman, 1987; Heitz et al., 1991).

The human genome contains an estimated 50,000 to 100,000 structural genes per haploid set. The fact that, up to 1992, less than 5000 gene mutations have been identified suggests that the majority of gene mutations have yet to be discovered. It is plausible that the majority

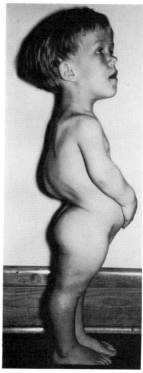

Figure 9–11. A child with achondroplasia, showing short limbs, large head, thoracic kyphosis (humpback), sharply angled upper lumbar lordosis (hollow back), and protrusion of the abdomen. (Courtesy of Dr. Harry Medovy, Children's Centre, Winnipeg.)

of children with congenital anomalies of unknown cause likely have a genetic disorder. Molecular biological techniques will accelerate gene discoveries over the next few decades.

ANOMALIES CAUSED BY ENVIRONMENTAL FACTORS

Although the human embryo is well protected in the uterus, certain environmental agents called **teratogens** may induce developmental disruptions following maternal exposure when the embryo's organs are forming. The organs and parts of an embryo are most sensitive to teratogenic agents during periods of rapid differentiation. Environmental factors called teratogenic agents cause about seven to ten per cent of congenital anomalies (Tables 9–1 and 9–5). Because biochemical differentiation precedes morphological differentiation, the period during which structures are sensitive to interference often precedes the stage of their visible development by a few days (Fig. 9–12). Teratogens

---

[4] An area at the end of the long arm of the chromosome looks like it is breaking off from the chromosome.

Table 9–5. TERATOGENS KNOWN TO CAUSE HUMAN BIRTH DEFECTS*

Agents	Most Common Congenital Anomalies
Drugs	
Alcohol	*Fetal alcohol syndrome (FAS):* intrauterine growth retardation (IUGR); mental retardation, microcephaly; ocular anomalies; joint abnormalities; short palpebral fissures (Fig. 9–13).
Androgens and high doses of progestogens	Varying degrees of masculinization of female fetuses: ambiguous external genitalia resulting in labial fusion and clitoral hypertrophy.
Aminopterin	IUGR; skeletal defects (Fig. 9–15); malformations of the central nervous system, notably meroanencephaly (most of the brain is absent).
Busulfan	Stunted growth; skeletal abnormalities; corneal opacities; cleft palate; hypoplasia of various organs.
Cocaine	IGUR; microcephaly; cerebral infarction; urogenital anomalies; neurobehavioral disturbances.
Diethylstilbestrol	Abnormalities of the uterus and vagina: cervical erosion and ridges.
Isotretinoin (13-*cis*-retinoic acid)	Craniofacial abnormalities; neural tube defects (NTDs), such as spina bifida cystica; cardiovascular defects.
Lithium carbonate	Various anomalies, usually involving the heart and great vessels.
Methotrexate	Multiple malformations, especially skeletal, involving the face, skull, limbs, and vertebral column.
Phenytoin (Dilantin)	*Fetal hydantoin syndrome (FHS):* IUGR; microcephaly; mental retardation; ridged metopic suture; inner epicanthal folds; eyelid ptosis; broad depressed nasal bridge; phalangeal hypoplasia.
Tetracycline	Stained teeth; hypoplasia of enamel.
Thalidomide	Abnormal development of the limbs (Fig. 9–16), e.g., meromelia (partial absence) and amelia (complete absence); facial anomalies; systemic anomalies, e.g., cardiac and kidney defects.
Trimethadione	Development delay; V-shaped eyebrows; low-set ears; cleft lip and/or palate.
Valproic acid	Craniofacial anomalies; NTDs; often hydrocephalus; heart and skeletal defects.
Warfarin	Nasal hypoplasia; stippled epiphyses; hypoplastic phalanges; eye anomalies; mental retardation.
Chemicals	
Methyl mercury	Cerebral atrophy; spasticity; seizures; mental retardation.
PCBs	IGUR; skin discolorization.
Infections	
Cytomegalovirus	Microcephaly; chorioretinitis; sensorineural loss; delayed psychomotor/mental development; hepatosplenomegaly; hydrocephaly; cerebral palsy; brain (periventricular) calcification.
Herpes simplex virus	Skin vesicles and scarring; chorioretinitis; hepatomegaly; thrombocytopenia; petechiae; hemolytic anemia; hydranencephaly.
Human immunodeficiency virus (HIV)	Growth failure; microcephaly; prominent boxlike forehead; flattened nasal bridge; hypertelorism; triangular philtrum and patulous lips.
Human parvovirus B19	Eye defects; degenerative changes in fetal tissues.
Rubella virus	IUGR; postnatal growth retardation; cardiac and great vessel malformations; microcephaly; sensorineural deafness; cataract; microphthalmos; glaucoma (Fig. 9–17); pigmented retinopathy; mental retardation; newborn bleeding; hepatosplenomegaly; osteopathy.
Toxoplasma gondii	Microcephaly; mental retardation; microphthalmia; hydrocephaly; chorioretinitis; cerebral calcifications.
Treponema pallidum	Hydrocephalus; congenital deafness; mental retardation; abnormal teeth and bones.
Venezuelan equine encephalitis virus	Microcephaly; microphthalmia; cerebral agenesis; CNS necrosis; hydrocephalus.
Varicella virus	Cutaneous scars (dermatome distribution); neurological anomalies (limb paresis, hydrocephaly, seizures, etc.); cataracts; microphthalmia; Horner syndrome; optic atrophy; nystagmus; chorioretinitis; microcephaly; mental retardation; skeletal anomalies (hypoplasia of limbs, fingers, and toes, etc.); urogenital anomalies.
High Levels of Ionizing Radiation	Microcephaly; mental retardation; skeletal anomalies.

*The spectrum and severity of congenital anomalies may vary from one case to another. For more information see Shephard, 1992; Gibbs and Sweet, 1989; Persaud, 1990; Remington and Klein, 1990; Holmes, 1992.

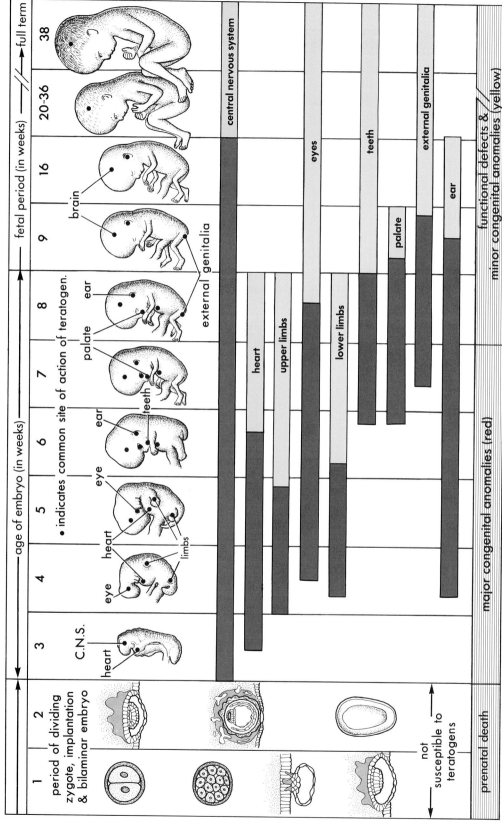

Figure 9–12. Schematic illustration of the critical periods in human development. During the first two weeks of development, the embryo is not usually susceptible to teratogens. During these pre-embryonic stages, a substance either damages all or most of the cells of the embryo resulting in death, or damages only a few cells, allowing the conceptus to recover and the embryo to develop without birth defects. *Red denotes highly sensitive periods when major defects may be produced* (e.g., limb deficiencies). Yellow indicates stages that are less sensitive to teratogens when minor defects may be induced (e.g., hypoplastic thumbs).

do not appear to be effective in causing anomalies until cellular differentiation has begun; however, their early actions may cause the death of an embryo before anomalies are established (Fig. 9–12).

The exact *mechanisms* by which drugs, chemicals, and other environmental factors interfere with embryonic development and induce abnormalities still remain obscure. Even the mechanisms of action of thalidomide[5] on the embryo are a mystery, and more than 20 different hypotheses have been postulated to explain how it affects the embryo. Many studies have shown that certain hereditary and environmental influences may adversely affect embryonic development by altering such fundamental processes as the intracellular compartment, the surface of the cell, extracellular matrix, and the fetal environment; but, as yet, there is no fundamental hypothesis to explain the underlying mechanisms (Persaud et al., 1985).

Critical Periods in Human Development

The stage of development of the embryo determines its susceptibility to teratogens. The most critical period in the development of an embryo or in the growth of a particular tissue or organ is during the time of most rapid cell division (Fig. 9–12). The critical period varies in accordance with the timing and duration of the period of increasing cell numbers for the tissue or organ concerned. Table 9–6 indicates the relative frequencies of anomalies for certain organs.

The most critical period for brain development is from three to 16 weeks (Fig. 9–12). Major anomalies develop during the third and fourth weeks (e.g., neural tube defects [NTDs]; see Chapter 17). Teratogens (e.g., alcohol) may also produce *mental retardation* during the fetal period (Fig. 9–12). The brain is growing rapidly at birth and continues to do so throughout the first two years after birth; hence, mental retardation can also result from injury during infancy.

Tooth development also continues long after birth (see Chapter 19); hence, the development of the permanent teeth may be affected by *tetracyclines* (p. 134) from 18 weeks (prenatal) to 16 years. The *skeletal system* has a prolonged

---

[5] One of the best known and most studied teratogens (Table 9–5).

Table 9–6. INCIDENCE OF MAJOR MALFORMATIONS IN HUMAN ORGANS AT BIRTH*

Organ	Incidence of Malformations
Brain	10:1000
Heart	8:1000
Kidneys	4:1000
Limbs	2:1000
All other	6:1000
Total	30:1000

* Data from Connor and Ferguson-Smith (1987).

critical period of development extending into childhood; hence, the growth of skeletal tissues provides a good gauge of general growth.

Environmental disturbances during the first two weeks after fertilization may interfere with cleavage of the zygote and implantation of the blastocyst and/or cause early death and spontaneous abortion of the embryo, but they are not known to cause congenital anomalies in human embryos (Fig. 9–12).

Development of the embryo is most easily disturbed during the organogenetic period (i.e., when the organs are forming [Chapters 5 and 6]). During this period teratogenic agents may produce major congenital anomalies. Physiological defects, minor morphological abnormalities, and functional disturbances (e.g., *mental retardation*) are likely to result from disturbances during the fetal period. Certain microorganisms, however, are known to cause serious congenital anomalies, particularly of the brain and eyes (e.g., *Toxoplasma gondii* [p. 138]), when they infect the fetus (see Table 9–5).

Each part and organ of an embryo has a critical period during which its development may be disrupted (Fig. 9–12). The type of congenital anomalies produced depends upon which organ is most susceptible at the time the teratogen is active. The following examples illustrate that teratogens may affect different organ systems that are developing at the same time:

1. High levels of radiation produce abnormalities of the central nervous system and eyes, as well as mental retardation (p. 139). The period of greatest sensitivity for *radiation damage to the brain* leading to severe mental retardation is from eight to 16 weeks after fertilization.

2. The *rubella virus* causes eye defects (glaucoma and cataracts), deafness, and cardiac anomalies (p. 137).

3. *Thalidomide* is a potent teratogen that induces limb defects and several other anomalies (Table 9–5).

> *Embryological timetables* (e.g., Fig. 9–12) are helpful in studying the causes of human abnormalities, but it is wrong to assume that anomalies always result from a single event occurring during the critical period or that one can determine from these tables the day on which the anomaly was produced. All one can reliably state is that the teratogen would have had to disrupt development before the end of the organogenetic period of the structure or organ concerned (indicated by *red* in Fig. 9–12). The critical period for limb development, for example, is 24 to 36 days after fertilization (38 to 50 days after LNMP).

Human Teratogens and Congenital Anomalies

A teratogen is any agent that can induce or increase the incidence of a congenital anomaly. Recognition of human teratogens offers the opportunity for the prevention of some congenital anomalies (Table 9–5); for example, if women are made aware of the harmful effects of alcohol and certain drugs and viruses, most of them will not expose their embryos to these teratogenic agents. The general objective of teratogenicity testing of drugs, food additives, and pesticides is to identify agents that may be teratogenic during human development and to alert pregnant women of this possible danger to the embryo/fetus (Shepard, 1992).

> To prove that an agent is a teratogen, one must show either that the frequency of anomalies is increased above the spontaneous rate in pregnancies in which the mother is exposed to the agent *(the prospective approach)* or that malformed infants have a history of maternal exposure to the agent more often than normal children *(the retrospective approach)*. Both types of data are difficult to obtain in an unbiased form. Individual *case reports are not convincing* unless both the agent and type of anomaly are so rare that their association in several cases can be judged not coincidental (e.g., thalidomide).
>
> **DRUG TESTING IN PREGNANT ANIMALS.** Although the testing of drugs in animals is important, it should be emphasized that the results are of limited value for predicting drug effects on human embryos. *Animal experiments can only suggest that similar effects may occur in humans.* If two or three species respond to a specific compound, however, even if the anomalies

differ among species, the probability of potential human hazard must be considered high.

The fact that a drug is teratogenic in two or more animal species is only one of many criteria that are used for deciding whether a drug should be used by women during pregnancy. Many drugs produce anomalies in animals when administered at many times the usual therapeutic dose; consequently, the dose, species, and anomaly produced are all important when considering a particular drug's teratogenic potential in human pregnancy.

Drugs as Teratogens

Drugs vary considerably in their teratogenicity. Some cause severe anomalies if administered during the organogenetic period (e.g., thalidomide). Other socially used drugs produce mental and growth retardation if used excessively throughout development (e.g., alcohol). The use of prescription and nonprescription drugs during pregnancy is surprisingly high. From 40 to 90 per cent of pregnant women consume at least one drug. Several studies have indicated that pregnant women take an average of four drugs, excluding nutritional supplements, and about half of these women take them during the first trimester of pregnancy, the most vulnerable period.

Drug consumption also tends to be higher during this critical period of development among heavy smokers and heavy drinkers (Persaud, 1990). Despite this, less than two per cent of congenital anomalies are caused by drugs and chemicals. Only a few drugs have been positively implicated as human teratogenic agents (Table 9–5). Their use should be avoided by pregnant women and those likely to conceive.

> It is best for women to avoid using all medication during the first eight weeks after conception (ten weeks after LNMP) unless there is a strong medical reason for its use, and then only if it is recognized as reasonably safe for the human embryo. The reason for this caution is that even though well-controlled studies of certain drugs (e.g., *marijuana*) have failed to demonstrate a teratogenic risk to human embryos (p. 137), they harm the embryo (i.e., they decrease birth weight [Holmes, 1992]).

CIGARETTE SMOKING. Maternal smoking is a well-established cause of *intrauterine growth retardation* (IUGR). Epidemiological studies have not indicated a strong association between maternal smoking and the overall occurrence of

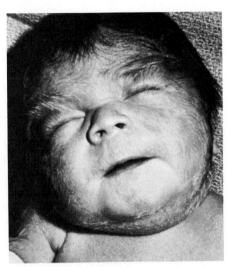 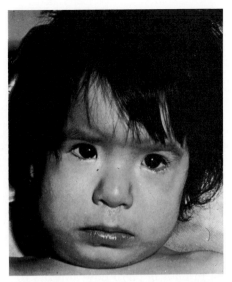

Figure 9–13. Photographs showing the facial appearance of an infant with the fetal alcohol syndrome (FAS). The characteristic triad of abnormalities includes growth deficiency, mental retardation, and abnormal facial features. Note the widely spaced eyes, long philtrum and thin upper lip. *A*, At birth. *B*, At one year. (*A* is from Jones KL, Smith DW: *Lancet 2:*999, 1973; *B*, is from Jones K, et al.: *Lancet 1:*1267, 1973.)

congenital anomalies. There is, however, some evidence that maternal smoking may cause *behavioral problems and decreased physical growth.* Infants of mothers who stop smoking during pregnancy show an improvement in their birth weights. The benefit is greatest in those mothers who quit smoking before 16 weeks of gestation.

CAFFEINE. Caffeine is not known to be a human teratogen when taken in moderation, but there is no assurance that excessive maternal consumption of it is safe for the embryo. For this reason, excessive drinking of coffee, tea, and colas containing caffeine should be avoided.

ALCOHOL. Infants born to chronic alcoholic mothers exhibit a specific pattern of defects known as the *fetal alcohol syndrome* (FAS). This includes prenatal and postnatal growth deficiency, mental retardation, and other anomalies (Fig. 9–13). *Maternal alcohol abuse* is considered to be the most common cause of mental retardation. The incidence of FAS, estimated to be about 2 per 1000 live births, is related to the population studied (Persaud, 1988). Even moderate maternal alcohol consumption (e.g., two to three ounces per day) may produce *fetal alcohol effects* (FAE); (i.e., behavioral and learning difficulties). *Binge drinking* (heavy consumption of alcohol for one to three days) during pregnancy is very likely to produce **FAE**. The susceptible period of brain development spans the major

part of gestation (Fig. 9–12); therefore, the best advice is total abstinence from alcohol during pregnancy.

ANDROGENS AND PROGESTOGENS[6]. Any hormone that has androgenic masculinizing activities may affect the fetus, producing masculinization of the female external genitalia (Fig. 9–14). The incidence of anomalies varies with the drug and the dosage. The preparations most frequently involved were the *progestins,* ethisterone and norethisterone. From a practical standpoint the teratogenic risk of these hormones is low (Persaud, 1990). Progestin exposure during the critical period of development is also associated with an increased prevalence of cardiovascular abnormalities. Obviously, the administration of *testosterone* to pregnant women is very likely to produce masculinizing effects in female fetuses.

Oral contraceptives containing progestogens and estrogens taken during the early stages of an unrecognized pregnancy are suspected of being teratogenic agents. The infants of mothers

---

[6] The terms "progestogens" and "progestins" are used for substances, natural or synthetic, that produce some or all the biological changes produced by progesterone, a hormone produced by the corpus luteum that promotes and maintains a gravid endometrium or decidua (p. 20). Some of these substances have androgenic or masculinizing properties.

who have taken *birth control pills* during the critical period of development exhibited the Vacterl syndrome. The acronym *VACTERL* stands for vertebral, anal, cardiac, tracheoesophageal, renal, and limb anomalies. As a precaution, use of oral contraceptives should be stopped as soon as pregnancy is detected.

Diethylstilbestrol (stilbestrol) is recognized as a human teratogen. Both gross and microscopic congenital abnormalities of the uterus and vagina have been detected in women who were exposed to diethylstilbestrol (DES) *in utero.* A number of young women aged 16 to 22 years have developed *adenocarcinoma of the vagina* after a common history of exposure to this synthetic estrogen *in utero;* however, the probability of cancers developing at this early age in females exposed to DES *in utero* now appears to be low (Noller, 1990).

ANTIBIOTICS. *Tetracyclines* cross the placental membrane (see Fig. 8–7) and are deposited in the embryo's bones and teeth at sites of active calcification. As little as 1 gm per day of tetracycline during the third trimester of pregnancy can produce *yellow staining of the primary or deciduous teeth;* hence, tetracycline therapy during the second and third trimesters of pregnancy may also cause tooth defects (e.g., hypoplasia of

enamel), and diminished growth of long bones (Cohlan, 1986).

Deafness has been reported in infants of mothers who have been treated with high doses of streptomycin and dihydrostreptomycin as *antituberculosis agents.* More than 30 cases of hearing deficit and eighth cranial nerve damage have been reported in infants exposed to streptomycin derivatives *in utero.* **Penicillin** has been used extensively during pregnancy and *appears to be harmless* to the human embryo and fetus.

ANTICOAGULANTS. With the exception of heparin, all anticoagulants cross the placental membrane (see Fig. 8–7) and may cause hemorrhage in the fetus. *Warfarin* and other coumarin derivatives are antagonists of vitamin K. Warfarin is used for the treatment of thromboembolitic disease and for patients with artificial heart valves.

Warfarin is definitely a teratogen. There are reports of infants with hypoplasia of the nasal cartilage, stippled epiphyses, and various central nervous system defects whose mothers took this anticoagulant during the critical period of their embryo's development. The period of greatest sensitivity is between six and 12 weeks after fertilization (eight to 14 weeks after LNMP). Second- and third-trimester exposure may result in mental retardation, optic atrophy, and microcephaly.

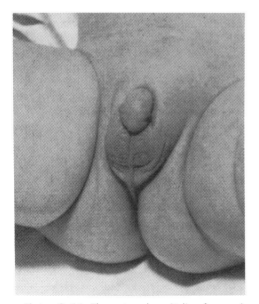 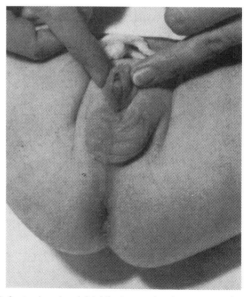

Figure 9–14. The external genitalia of a newborn female infant, showing labial fusion and enlargement of the clitoris. The masculinization was caused by an androgenic agent given to the infant's mother during the first trimester. (From Jones HW, Scott WW: *Hermaphroditism, Genital Anomalies and Related Endocrine Disorders.* Baltimore, Williams & Wilkins, © 1958.)

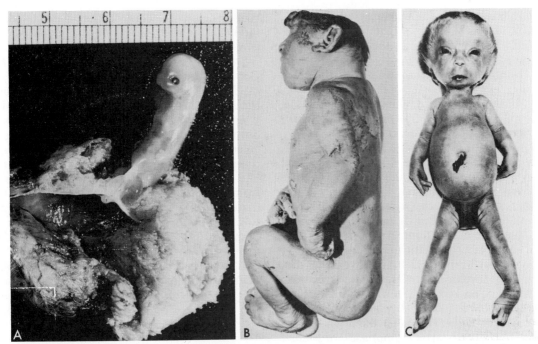

Figure 9–15. Aminopterin-induced congenital anomalies. *A,* Grossly malformed embryo and its membranes. (Courtesy of Dr. J.B. Thiersch, Seattle, Washington.) *B,* Newborn infant with meroanencephaly or partial absence of the brain. (From Thiersch JB: *In* Wolstenholme GEW, O'Connor CM [eds]: Ciba Foundation Symposium on Congenital Malformations. London, J. & A. Churchill, 1960). *C,* Newborn infant showing marked intrauterine growth retardation, a large head, a small mandible, deformed ears, clubhands, and clubfeet. (From Warkany J, Beaudry PH, Hornstein S: *Am J Dis Child 97:*274–281, 1960.)

As it does not cross the placental membrane, *heparin is not a teratogen* and so is the drug of choice for pregnant women requiring anticoagulant therapy.

ANTICONVULSANTS. Approximately one of 200 pregnant women is epileptic and requires treatment with an anticonvulsant. Of the anticonvulsant drugs available, there is strong evidence that *trimethadione* (Tridione) is teratogenic. **Phenytoin** (Dilantin, Novophenytoin) is definitely a teratogen. The *fetal hydantoin syndrome* consists of the following abnormalities: intrauterine growth retardation (IUGR), microcephaly, mental retardation, inner epicanthal folds, eyelid ptosis, a broad depressed nasal bridge, nail and/or distal phalangeal hypoplasia, and hernias (Persaud, 1990).

Valproic acid had been the drug of choice for the management of different types of epilepsy; however, its use by pregnant women has led to a pattern of anomalies comprised of craniofacial, heart and limb defects. There is also an increased risk of neural tube defects. *Phenobarbital* appears to be a safe antiepileptic drug for use during pregnancy (Persaud, 1990).

ANTINEOPLASTIC AGENTS. Tumor-inhibiting chemicals are highly teratogenic. This is not surprising because these agents inhibit mitosis in rapidly dividing cells. *Busulfan and 6-mercaptopurine* administered in alternating courses throughout pregnancy have produced multiple severe abnormalities, but neither drug alone appears to cause major anomalies. *Aminopterin is a potent teratogen* that produces major congenital anomalies (Fig. 9–15), especially of the skeletal and central nervous systems.

CORTICOSTEROIDS. Cortisone causes cleft palate and cardiac defects in susceptible strains of mice and rabbits, but cortisone is not a human teratogen (Shepard, 1992).

ANGIOTENSIN-CONVERTING ENZYME (ACE) INHIBITORS. ACE inhibitors are used as antihypertensive agents. Fetal exposure to this drug results in oligohydramnios (p. 109), fetal death, longlasting hypoplasia, and renal dysfunction. During *early* pregnancy the risk to the embryo is apparently less, and there is no indication in such a case to terminate a wanted pregnancy.

INSULIN AND HYPOGLYCEMIC DRUGS. Insulin is not teratogenic in human embryos except possibly in maternal insulin coma therapy. Hypoglycemic drugs (e.g., tolbutamide) have been implicated, but evidence for their teratogenicity is very weak; consequently, despite their marked teratogenicity in rodents, there is no convincing evidence that oral hypoglycemic agents (particularly sulfonylureas) are teratogenic in human embryos. The incidence of congenital anomalies (e.g., *sacral agenesis*) is increased two to three times in the offspring of diabetic mothers, and about 40 per cent of all perinatal deaths among diabetic infants are the result of congenital anomalies.

RETINOIC ACID (VITAMIN A). *Isotretinoin* (13-*cis*-retinoic acid), used for the oral treatment of severe cystic acne, *is teratogenic at very low doses in humans.* The critical period for exposure appears to be from the third week to the fifth week of development (five to seven weeks after LNMP). The risk of spontaneous abortion and birth defects following *in utero* exposure to retinoic acid is high. The most common major anomalies observed are *craniofacial dysmorphism* (microtia [small ears], micrognathia [smallness of the jaws]), cleft palate and/or thymic aplasia defects, cardiovascular anomalies, and neural tube defects (see Chapter 17).

SALICYLATES. There is some evidence that *aspirin* (salicylates), the most commonly ingested drug during pregnancy, is potentially harmful to the embryo or fetus when administered to the mother in *large doses.* The fact that the labeling for acetylsalicylic acid bears no restriction for use in pregnancy indicates that the possibility of embryonic/fetal harm is remote. From the results of recent epidemiological studies, *there is no reason to believe aspirin is teratogenic if taken in the usual therapeutic doses.*

THYROID DRUGS. *Potassium iodide* in cough mixtures and large doses of *radioactive iodine* may cause congenital goiter. Iodides readily cross the placental membrane and interfere with thyroxin production, and they may cause thyroid enlargement and *cretinism* (arrested physical and mental development and dystrophy of bones and soft parts). Pregnant women have been advised to avoid using douches or creams containing povidone-iodine because it is absorbed by the vagina.

Propylthiouracil interferes with thyroxin formation in the fetus and may cause goiter. The administration of *antithyroid substances* for the treatment of maternal disorders of the thyroid gland may cause congenital goiter in an infant if the mother is given the substance in excess of requirements to control the disease. Maternal iodine deficiency may cause congenital cretinism.

TRANQUILIZERS. *Thalidomide is a potent teratogen.* This hypnotic agent was once widely used in Europe as a tranquilizer and sedative. The *thalidomide epidemic* started in 1959. It has been estimated that nearly 12,000 infants were born with defects caused by this drug. The characteristic feature of the *thalidomide syndrome* is **meromelia** (e.g., phocomelia or seal-like limbs [Fig. 9–16]), but the anomalies ranged from **amelia** (absence of limbs) through intermediate stages of development (rudimentary limbs) to **micromelia** (abnormally small and/or short limbs). *Thalidomide also caused anomalies of other organs* (e.g., heart defects).

LITHIUM is the drug of choice for the long-term maintenance of patients with manic-depressive

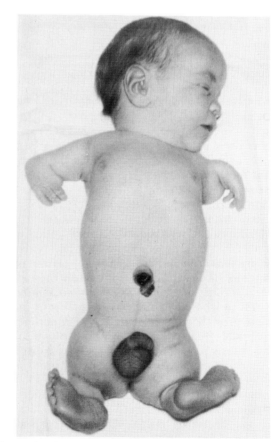

Figure 9–16. Newborn male infant showing typically malformed limbs (meromelia [limb reduction]) caused by thalidomide ingested by his mother during the critical period of limb development (Fig. 9–12). (From Moore KL: *Manitoba Med Rev 43:*306, 1963.)

psychosis; however, it has caused congenital anomalies, mainly of the heart and great vessels, in infants born to mothers given the drug early in pregnancy (Table 9–5).

Benzodiazepine derivatives (psychoactive drugs), including *diazepam* and *oxazepam* readily cross the placental membrane (see Fig. 8–7). The use of these drugs during the first trimester of pregnancy is associated with transient withdrawal symptoms and craniofacial deformities in the newborn.

ILLICIT (STREET) DRUGS. *Lysergic acid diethylamide* (LSD), an hallucinogen, is not currently thought to be a teratogen. Neither is there strong evidence to indicate that *marijuana* is a human teratogen. There is some indication that its use during the first two months of pregnancy affects fetal length, but not birth weight. In addition, sleep and EEG patterns in newborns exposed prenatally to marijuana were altered. For these reasons, pregnant women should not use marijuana.

Phencyclidine (PCP, "Angel Dust") is not known to be teratogenic. A case of an infant with several birth defects and behavioral disturbances whose mother used PCP throughout her pregnancy has been reported. This suggests, but does not prove, a causal association.

COCAINE is now one of the most commonly abused illicit drugs in North America, and of concern is its increasing use by women of childbearing age. There have been many reports dealing with the prenatal effects of cocaine. These include spontaneous abortion, prematurity, intrauterine growth retardation, microcephaly, cerebral infarction, urogenital anomalies, and neurobehavioral disturbances. The use of cocaine during pregnancy should be avoided because of its teratogenic effects.

METHADONE has proven valuable for the treatment of heroin addiction; however, infants born to narcotic-dependent women maintained on methadone therapy were found to have smaller birth weights and head circumferences than nonexposed infants. There is also concern about the long-term postnatal developmental effects of methadone.

Environmental Chemicals as Teratogens

ORGANIC MERCURY. Infants of mothers whose main diet during pregnancy consisted of fish containing abnormally high levels of organic mercury acquire fetal *Minamata disease* and exhibit neurological and behavioral disturbances resembling cerebral palsy. In some cases, severe *brain damage*, mental retardation, and blindness have been present in the infants of mothers who received *methylmercury* in their food. Methylmercury is considered to be a teratogen that causes cerebral atrophy, spasticity, seizures, and *mental retardation.*

LEAD. Lead is abundantly present in the workplace and environment. It is transferred across the placental membrane and accumulates in fetal tissues. *In utero* exposure to lead has been associated with increased abortions, fetal anomalies, intrauterine growth retardation, and functional deficits. Children born to mothers who were exposed to subclinical levels of lead revealed neurobehavioral and psychomotor disturbances (Persaud, 1990).

POLYCHLORINATED BIPHENYLS (PCBs). These teratogenic chemicals produce *intrauterine growth retardation* (IUGR) and skin discoloration. The main dietary source of PCBs in North America is probably sport fish caught in contaminated waters.

Infectious Agents as Teratogens

Throughout prenatal life the embryo and fetus are endangered by a variety of microorganisms. In most cases the assault is resisted; in some cases, an abortion or stillbirth occurs, and in others the infants are born with growth retardation, congenital anomalies or neonatal diseases (Table 9–5).

RUBELLA (GERMAN OR THREE-DAY MEASLES). This virus is the prime example of an *infective teratogen*. In cases of primary maternal infection during the first trimester of pregnancy, the overall risk of **congenital rubella syndrome** (CRS) is about 20 per cent. The usual features of congenital rubella syndrome are *cataract, cardiac defects*, and *deafness*, but the following abnormalities are occasionally observed: chorioretinitis, glaucoma (Fig. 9–17), microphthalmia, and tooth defects.

CYTOMEGALOVIRUS (CMV). Infection with CMV is the most common viral infection of the human fetus. Because the disease seems to be fatal when it affects the embryo, it is believed that most pregnancies end in spontaneous abortion when the infection occurs during the first trimester. At birth, the infected infants usually show no clinical signs and are identified through screening programs. Later in pregnancy, infection may result in intrauterine growth retardation,

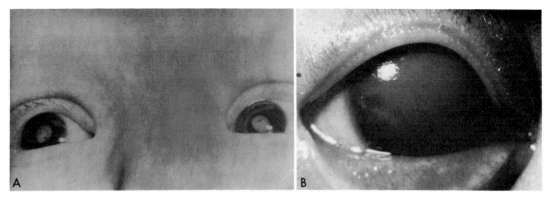

Figure 9–17. Congenital anomalies of the eye caused by the rubella virus. *A*, Cataracts. (Courtesy of Dr. Richard Baragry, Department of Ophthalmology, Cornell-New York Hospital). *B*, Glaucoma. (Courtesy of Dr. Daniel I. Weiss, Department of Ophthalmology, New York University School of Medicine). (Photos from Cooper LA et al.: *Am J Dis Child 110:*416–427, 1965. Copyright 1965, American Medical Association.)

microphthalmia, chorioretinitis, blindness, microcephaly, cerebral calcification, mental retardation, deafness, cerebral palsy, and hepatosplenomegaly (Persaud, 1990).

HERPES SIMPLEX VIRUS (HSV). Maternal infection with HSV in early pregnancy increases the abortion rate, and infection after the twentieth week is associated with a higher rate of prematurity. Infection of the fetus with HSV usually occurs very late in pregnancy, probably most often during delivery. Congenital abnormalities that have been observed in the offspring included: cutaneous lesions and, in some cases, microcephaly, microphthalmia, spasticity, retinal dysplasia, and mental retardation (Persaud, 1990).

VARICELLA (CHICKENPOX). Varicella and herpes zoster (shingles) are caused by the same virus, *varicella-zoster virus.* There is convincing evidence that maternal varicella infection during the first four months of pregnancy causes congenital anomalies (skin scarring, muscle atrophy, hypoplasia of the limb, rudimentary digits, and mental retardation). There is about a 20 per cent chance of these or other abnormalities when the infection occurs during the critical periods of development (Fig. 9–12).

HUMAN IMMUNODEFICIENCY VIRUS (HIV). This retrovirus causes acquired immunodeficiency syndrome (AIDS), a major public health problem worldwide. As yet, there is no treatment for this disease, which is increasing in prevalence among women of childbearing age. There is conflicting information on the fetal effects of *in utero* infection with HIV; some of the congenital anomalies reported included growth failure and specific craniofacial features. Preventing the transmission of the virus to women and their infants is of obvious importance because of any potential embryopathic effects.

TOXOPLASMA GONDII. Maternal infection with *Toxoplasma gondii (an intracellular parasite)* can be contracted from eating raw or poorly cooked meat (usually pork or lamb) containing *Toxoplasma cysts*, through close contact with infected domestic animals (usually cats), or from the soil. It is thought that the soil or garden vegetables may become contaminated with infected cat feces carrying oocysts. The *Toxoplasma gondii organism* crosses the placental membrane and infects the fetus, causing destructive changes in the brain and eyes that result in microcephaly, microphthalmia, and hydrocephaly. Because animals (cats, dogs, rabbits, and other domestic and wild animals) may be infected with this parasite, pregnant women should avoid them and the eating of raw meat from them (e.g., rabbits).

SYPHILIS. *Treponema pallidum,* the small, spiral microorganism that causes syphilis, rapidly crosses the placental membrane after the twentieth week of gestation. The fetus can become infected at any stage of the disease or at any stage of pregnancy. Untreated *primary maternal infections* (acquired during pregnancy) nearly always cause serious fetal infection and congenital anomalies. *Secondary maternal infections* (acquired before pregnancy) seldom result in fetal disease and anomalies. If the mother is untreated, stillbirths occur in about one fourth of the cases.

Two clinically distinct forms of congenital syphilis, early (under two years of age) and late (over two years of age), have been described. It is well established that *Treponema pallidum* may produce congenital deafness, abnormal teeth and bones, hydrocephalus, and mental retardation. Late manifestations of untreated congenital syphilis are destructive lesions of the palate and nasal septum, dental abnormalities (centrally notched, widely spaced, peg-shaped upper central incisors called *Hutchinson's teeth*), and abnormal facies (frontal bossing, saddlenose, and poorly developed maxilla).

Radiation as a Teratogen

Exposure to *ionizing radiation* may injure embryonic cells, resulting in cell death, chromosome injury, and retardation of mental development and physical growth. The severity of the embryonic damage is related to the absorbed dose, the dose rate, and the stage of embryonic or fetal development during which the exposure occurs (Brent, 1986). Growth retardation, microcephaly, spina bifida cystica, pigment changes in the retina, cataracts, cleft palate, skeletal and visceral abnormalities, and mental retardation were observed in the infants who survived after receiving high levels of ionizing radiation. Development of the central nervous system was nearly always affected.

There is no proof that human congenital anomalies have been caused by diagnostic levels of radiation. Scattered radiation from an x-ray examination of a part of the body that is not near the uterus (e.g., the chest, sinuses, teeth) produces a dose of only a few millirads, which is not teratogenic to the embryo. For example, a radiograph of the chest of a pregnant woman in the first trimester results in a whole-body dose to her embryo or fetus of approximately 1 millirad. If the embryonic radiation exposure is 5 rads or less, the radiation risks to the embryo are minuscule (Brent, 1986).

Maternal Factors as Teratogens

Maternal diseases can sometimes lead to a higher risk of abnormalities in the offspring. Poorly controlled *diabetes mellitus* in the mother with persisting hyperglycemia and ketosis, particularly during embryogenesis, is associated with a two- to threefold higher incidence of birth defects. No specific diabetic embryopathic syndrome exists, but common abnormalities include holoprosencephaly, meroencephaly, sacral agenesis, vertebral anomalies, congenital heart defects and limb abnormalities.

If untreated, women who are homozygous for phenylalanine hydroxylase deficiency (*phenylketonuria* [PKU]) and those with hyperphenylalaninemia are at a high risk of having an offspring with microcephaly, septal cardiac defects, and mental retardation. The congenital anomalies can be prevented if the PKU mother is placed on a phenylalanine-restricted diet prior to and during the pregnancy (Lenke and Levy, 1980).

Mechanical Factors as Teratogens

The significance of mechanical influences in the uterus on congenital postural deformities is still an open question. The amniotic fluid absorbs mechanical pressures, thereby protecting the embryo from most external trauma. *Congenital dislocation of the hip and clubfoot* may be caused by mechanical forces, particularly in a malformed uterus. Such deformations may be caused by any factor that restricts the mobility of the fetus, thereby causing prolonged compression in an abnormal posture. A significantly reduced quantity of amniotic fluid (*oligohydramnios* [p. 109]) may result in mechanically induced deformation of the limbs, e.g., hyperextension of the knee. Intrauterine amputations or other anomalies caused by local constriction during fetal growth may result from *amniotic bands,* presumably formed as a result of rupture of the fetal membranes (amnion) during early pregnancy (Moore and Persaud, 1993).

ANOMALIES CAUSED BY MULTIFACTORIAL INHERITANCE

Most common congenital anomalies have familial distributions consistent with multifactorial inheritance (MFI). This may be represented by a model in which "liability" to a disorder is a continuous variable determined by a combination of genetic and environmental factors, with a developmental threshold dividing individuals with the anomaly from those without it. *Multifactorial traits are often single major anomalies,* such as cleft lip, isolated cleft palate, neural tube defects (meroanencephaly and spina bifida cystica), pyloric stenosis, and congenital dislocation of the hip. Some of these anomalies may also occur as part of the phenotype in syndromes determined by single-gene inheritance, chromosome abnormality, or an environmental teratogen, or their etiology may be unknown.

The *recurrence risks* used for genetic counseling of families having congenital anomalies determined by MFI are *empirical risks* based on the frequency of the anomaly in the general population and in different categories of relatives. In individual families, such estimates may be inaccurate because they are usually averages for the population rather than precise probabilities for the individual family (Thompson et al. [1991]).

SUMMARY

A congenital anomaly is a structural abnormality present at birth. Much progress has been made in recent years in the search for causes of anomalies, but satisfactory explanations are still lacking for most of them. Developmental abnormalities may be macroscopic or microscopic, on the surface or within the body.

Some congenital anomalies are caused by *genetic factors* (chromosomal abnormalities and mutant genes) and a few are caused by *environmental factors* (infectious agents and teratogenic drugs), but most common anomalies result from complex interaction of genetic and environmental factors (*multifactorial inheritance*).

During the first two weeks of development, teratogenic agents may kill the embryo, but they do not cause congenital anomalies. During the *organogenetic period* teratogenic agents may cause major congenital anomalies. During the *fetal period* teratogens may produce minor morphological and functional abnormalities, particularly of the brain and the eyes. *Mental retardation* may result from the teratogenic actions of infectious agents, high levels of radiation, and alcohol abuse.

Commonly Asked Questions

1. If a pregnant woman takes *aspirin* in normal doses, will it cause congenital anomalies?
2. If a woman is a drug addict, will her child show signs of drug addiction?
3. Are all drugs tested for teratogenicity (the ability to produce congenital anomalies) before they are marketed? If the answer is "yes," why are these teratogens still sold?
4. Is cigarette smoking during pregnancy harmful to the embryo or fetus? If the answer is "yes," would refraining from inhaling the smoke be safer?
5. Are there any drugs that are safe to take during pregnancy? If so, what are they?

The answers to these questions are given on page 330.

REFERENCES[7]

Beckman DA, Brent RL: Mechanisms of teratogenesis. *Annual Rev Pharmacol Toxicol* 24:483, 1984.

Brent RL: Radiation teratogenesis. *In* Sever JL, Brent RL (eds): *Teratogen Update: Environmentally Induced Birth Defect Risks.* New York, Alan R. Liss, 1986.

Briggs GG, Freeman RK, Yaffe SJ: *Drugs in Pregnancy and Lactation,* 3rd ed. Baltimore, Williams & Wilkins, 1990.

Brown RT, Coles CD, Smith IE, Platzman KA, Silverstein J, Erickson S, Falek A: Effects of prenatal alcohol exposure at school age. II. Attention and behavior. *Neurotoxicol Teratol* 13:369, 1991.

Buitendijk S, Bracken MB: Medication in early pregnancy—prevalence of use and relationship to maternal characteristics. *Am J Obstet Gynecol* 165:33, 1991.

Burbacher TM, Rodier PM, Weiss B: Methylmercury developmental neurotoxicity: a comparison of effects in humans and animals. *Neurotoxicol Teratol* 12:191, 1990.

Chodirker BN, Chudley AE, Reed MH, Persaud TVN: Possible prenatal hydantoin effect in a child born to a nonepileptic mother. *Am J Med Genet* 27:373, 1987.

Chudley AE, Hagerman RJ: The fragile X syndrome. *J Pediatr* 110:821, 1987.

Cohen Jr, MM: *The Child with Multiple Birth Defects.* New York, Raven Press, 1982.

Cohlan SQ: Tetracycline staining of teeth. *In* Sever JL, Brent RL (eds): *Teratogen Update: Environmentally Induced Birth Defect Risks.* New York, Alan R. Liss, 1986.

Connor JM, Ferguson-Smith MA: *Essential Medical Genet-*

---

[7]Persons wishing more information and references on human birth defects should consult Moore and Persaud (1993).

ics, 2nd ed. Oxford, Blackwell Scientific Publications, 1987.

Corby DG: Aspirin in pregnancy: Maternal and fetal effects. Pediatrics 62:930, 1978.

Dansky LV, Finnell RH: Parental epilepsy, anticonvulsant drugs, and reproductive outcome—epidemiologic and experimental findings spanning 3 decades. 2. Human studies. Reprod Toxicol 5:301, 1991.

Davis JM, Otto DA, Weil DE, Grant LD: The comparative developmental neurotoxicity of lead in humans and animals. Neurotoxicol Teratol 12:215, 1990.

Day N, Sambamoorthi V, Taylor P, Richardson G, Robles N, Jhon Y, Scher M, Stoffer D, Cornelius M, Jasperse D: Prenatal marijuana use and neonatal outcome. Neurotoxicol Teratol 13:329, 1991.

Embree JE, Braddick M, Datta P, et al: Lack of correlation of maternal human immunodeficiency virus infection with neonatal malformations. Pediatr Infect Dis J 8:700, 1989.

Fantel AG, Shepard TH: Prenatal cocaine exposure. Reprod Toxicol 4:83, 1990.

Ferguson-Smith MA: Sex chromatin, Klinefelter's syndrome and mental deficiency. In Moore KL (ed): The Sex Chromatin. Philadelphia, WB Saunders, 1966.

Forrest DD, Fordyce RR: Fam Plan Perspect 20:112, 1988. (Cited in Djerassi C: The bitter pill. Science 245:356, 1989.)

Fraser FC: Of mice and children: reminiscences of a teratogeneticist. In Kalter H (ed): Issues and Reviews in Teratology. Vol 5. New York, Plenum Press, 1990.

Fuccillo D: Congenital varicella. In Sever JL, Brent RL (eds): Teratogen Update: Environmentally Induced Birth Defect Risks. New York, Alan R. Liss, 1986.

Ganguin G, Rempt E: Streptomycinbehandlung in der Schwangerschaft und ihre Auswirkung auf das Gehör des Kindes. Z Laryngol Rhinol Otol 49:496, 1970.

Garber JE: Long-term follow-up of children exposed in utero to antineoplastic agents. Seminar in Oncology 16:437, 1989.

Gardner EJ, Simons MJ, Snustad DP: Principles of Genetics, 8th ed. New York, John Wiley & Sons, 1991.

Garza A, Cordero JF, Mulinare J: Epidemiology of the early amnion rupture spectrum of defects. Am J Dis Chld 142:541, 1988.

Gibbs RS, Sweet RL: Maternal and fetal infections—clinical disorders. In Creasy RK, Resnik R (eds): Maternal-Fetal Medicine: Principles and Practice, 2nd ed. Philadelphia, WB Saunders, 1989.

Ginsberg JS, Hirsh J: Optimum use of anticoagulants in pregnancy. Drugs 36:505, 1988.

Ginsburg KA, Blacker CM, Abel EL, Sokol RJ: Fetal alcohol exposure and adverse pregnancy outcome. Contr Gynecol Obstet 18:115, 1991.

Gregg NM: Congenital cataract following German measles in the mother. Trans Ophthalmol Soc Aust 3:35, 1941.

Hansen N, Coury DL: Congenital anomalies of the neonate. In Quilligan EJ, Zuspan FP (eds): Current Therapy in Obstetrics and Gynecology, Vol 3. Philadelphia, WB Saunders, 1990.

Hanssens M, Keirse MJNC, Vankelecom F, Van Assche FA: Fetal and neonatal effects of treatment with angiotensin-converting enzyme inhibitors in pregnancy. Obstet Gynecol 78:128, 1991.

Heitz D, Rousseau F, Devys D, et al: Isolation of sequences that span the fragile X and identification of a fragile X-related CpG island. Science 251:1236, 1991.

Hirschhorn K: Chromosomes and their abnormalities. In Behrman RE: Nelson Textbook of Pediatrics, 14th ed. Philadelphia, WB Saunders, 1992.

Holmes KK: Syphilis. In Thor GW, Adams RD, Braunwald E, et al (eds): Harrison's Principles of Internal Medicine, 8th ed. New York, McGraw-Hill, 1992.

Holmes LB: Teratogens. In Behrman RE (ed): Nelson Textbook of Pediatrics, 14th ed. Philadelphia, WB Saunders, 1992.

Isada N, Sever J, Larsen J: Rubella. In Quilligan EJ, Zuspan FP (eds): Current Therapy in Obstetrics and Gynecology, vol 3. Philadelphia, WB Saunders, 1990.

Jones KL: Smith's Recognizable Patterns of Human Malformation, 4th ed. Philadelphia, WB Saunders, 1988.

Kirkilionis AJ, Chudley AE, Gregory CA, Hamerton JL: Molecular and clinical overlap of Angelman and Prader-Willi syndrome phenotypes. Am J Med Genet 40:454, 1991.

Koren G (ed): Maternal-Fetal Toxicology: A Clinicians Guide. New York, Marcel Dekker, 1990.

Kriegel H, Schmahl W, Kistner G, Stieve FE (eds): Developmental Effects of Prenatal Irradiation. Stuttgart, Gustav Fischer, 1982.

Laegreid L, Olegard R, Walstrom J, Conradi N: Teratogenic effects of benzodiazepine use during pregnancy. J Pediatr 114:126, 1989.

Lenke RR, Levy HL: Maternal phenylketonuria and hyperphenyl-alanimemia. An international survey of untreated and treated pregnancies. N Engl J Med 303:1202, 1980.

Melkonian R, Baker D: Risks of industrial mercury exposure in pregnancy. Obstet Gynecol Surv 43:637, 1988.

Moore KL (ed): The Sex Chromatin. Philadelphia, WB Saunders, 1966.

Moore KL, Persaud TVN: The Developing Human. Clinically Oriented Embryology, 5th ed. Philadelphia, WB Saunders, 1993.

Noller KL: In utero DES exposure. In Quilligan EJ, Zuspan FP (eds): Current Therapy in Obstetrics and Gynecology, Vol 3. Philadelphia, WB Saunders, 1990.

Persaud TVN: Problems of Birth Defects. From Hippocrates to Thalidomide and After. Baltimore, University Park Press, 1977.

Persaud TVN: Teratogenesis. Experimental Aspects and Clinical Implications. Jena, Gustav Fischer Verlag, 1979.

Persaud TVN: Fetal alcohol syndrome. Critical Rev Anat Cell Biol 1:277, 1988.

Persaud TVN: Environmental Causes of Human Birth Defects. Springfield, Charles C Thomas, 1990.

Persaud TVN, Chudley AE, Skalko RG: Basic Concepts in Teratology. New York, Alan R. Liss, 1985.

Persaud TVN, Ellington AC: Teratogenic activity of cannabis resin. Lancet 2:406, 1968.

Persaud TVN, Moore KL: Causes and prenatal diagnosis of congenital abnormalities. J Obstet Gynecol Nursing 3:40, 1974.

Reece EA, Hobbins JC: Diabetic embryopathy: pathogenesis, prenatal diagnosis and prevention. Obstet Gynecol Surv 41:325, 1986.

Remington JS, Klein JO (eds): Infectious Diseases of the Fetus and Newborn Infant, 3rd ed. Philadelphia, WB Saunders, 1990.

Sever JL, Brent RL (eds): Teratogen Update: Environmentally Induced Birth Defect Risks. New York, Alan R. Liss, 1986.

Shepard TH: Catalog of Teratogenic Agents, 7th ed. Baltimore, The Johns Hopkins University Press, 1992.

Shepard TH, Fantel AG, Fitzsimmons J: Congenital defect rates among spontaneous abortuses. Twenty years of monitoring. Teratology 39:325, 1989.

Thompson MW, McInnes RR, Willard HF: Thompson and Thompson Genetics in Medicine, 5th ed. Philadelphia, WB Saunders, 1991.

10

BODY CAVITIES, PRIMITIVE MESENTERIES, AND THE DIAPHRAGM

Early development of the **intraembryonic coelom** (primordium of the embryonic body cavities) during the third week is described in Chapter 5 (p. 53). By the fourth week, the coelom appears as a horseshoe-shaped cavity in the cardiogenic and lateral mesoderm (see Figs. 5–5 and 10–1A). The curve or bend of this cavity represents the future *pericardial cavity,* and its limbs (lateral parts) indicate the future *pleural and peritoneal cavities.*

The intraembryonic coelom provides room for organ development and movement[1]. For about seven weeks the distal part of each limb of the intraembryonic coelom communicates with the extraembryonic coelom at the lateral edges of the embryonic disc (Fig. 10–1A and B). This communication is greatly reduced during folding of the embryonic disc into a cylindrical embryo but persists for awhile around the stalk of the yolk sac (Fig. 10–2E). This communication is important because most of the midgut herniates through this communication into the umbilical cord where it develops into most of the small intestine and part of the large intestine (see Figs. 7–3 and 13–6).

During horizontal folding of the embryo, the limbs of the intraembryonic coelom are brought together on the ventral aspect of the embryo (Fig. 10–2C and F). The ventral mesentery degenerates in the region of the future peritoneal cavity, forming a large peritoneal cavity extending from the heart to the pelvic region (Figs. 10–2F and 10–3).

THE EMBRYONIC BODY CAVITY

The intraembryonic coelom gives rise to three primitive embryonic body cavities during the fourth week: (1) a large *pericardial cavity* around the heart (Figs. 10–2B and 10–4), (2) two *pericardioperitoneal canals* connecting the pericardial and peritoneal cavities (Fig. 10–3), and (3) a large *peritoneal cavity* containing the primordium of the abdominal and pelvic viscera (see Figs. 10–2F and 13–6). The peritoneal cavity has a parietal wall lined by mesothelium (future peritoneum) derived from somatic mesoderm and a visceral wall covered by mesothelium derived from the splanchnic mesoderm (Fig. 10–2F).

During formation of the *head fold,* the heart and pericardial cavity move ventrocaudally, anterior to the foregut (see Figs. 6–1 and 10–2B and E). As a result, the pericardial cavity opens dorsally into the pericardioperitoneal canals, which pass dorsal to the septum transversum on each side of the foregut and enter the peritoneal cavity (Fig. 10–3). The *septum transversum* is a transverse sheet of mesoderm that separates the pericardial cavity from the peritoneal cavity,

---

[1] In embryos of lower animal forms, the intraembryonic coelom provides short-term storage for excretory products.

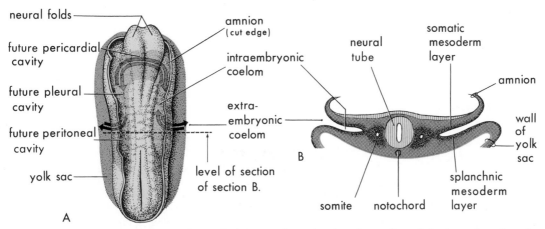

Figure 10–1. *A,* Drawing of an embryo of about 22 days, showing the outline of the horseshoe-shaped intraembryonic coelom. The amnion has been removed, and the coelom is shown as if the embryo were translucent. The continuity of the intraembryonic coelom, as well as the communication of its right and left limbs with the extraembryonic coelom, are indicated by arrows. *B,* Transverse section through the embryo at the level shown in *A.*

forming a partial diaphragm (partition) between them.

After embryonic folding, the caudal part of the foregut, the midgut, and hindgut are suspended in the peritoneal cavity from the posterior abdominal wall by the *dorsal mesentery*[2] (Fig. 10–2F). Transiently, the dorsal and ventral mesenteries divide the peritoneal cavity into right and left halves, but the ventral mesentery soon disappears except where it is attached to the caudal part of the foregut (primordium of the stomach and proximal part of the duodenum). The peritoneal cavity then becomes a continuous space (Fig. 10–3). The arteries supplying the primitive gut (i.e., the celiac [foregut], the superior mesenteric [midgut], and the inferior mesenteric [hindgut]) pass between the layers of the dorsal mesentery (see Figs. 13–1 and 13–2).

Division of the Embryonic Body Cavity

The pericardioperitoneal canals lie lateral to the foregut (future esophagus) and dorsal to the septum transversum (Fig. 10–3B). Partitions form at both ends of these canals and separate the pericardial cavity from the pleural cavities and the pleural cavities from the peritoneal cavity.

---

[2] A mesentery is a double layer of peritoneum.

The *pleuropericardial membranes* (Fig. 10–4) will separate the pericardial cavity from the pleural cavities. Initially, these membranes appear as ridges or bulges of mesenchyme (embryonic connective tissue) that contain the *common cardinal veins* (Fig. 10–4A). These veins drain the primitive venous system into the *sinus venosus* of the primitive heart (see Figs. 15–3 and 15–5). At first the pleuropericardial membranes are free and project into the cranial ends of the *pericardioperitoneal canals* (Fig. 10–4A and B); however, after expansion of the pleural cavities, the pleuropericardial membranes fuse with one another and the mesoderm (primitive mediastinum) ventral to the esophagus (Fig. 10–4C). The right *pleuropericardial opening* closes slightly earlier than the left one, probably because the right common cardinal vein is larger than the left one and produces a larger pleuropericardial membrane.

The *pleuroperitoneal membranes* will separate the pleural cavities from the peritoneal cavity (Fig. 10–5). This pair of membranes is produced as the developing lungs and pleural cavities expand by invading the body wall (see Figs. 10–4 and 12–6). They are attached dorsolaterally to the body wall, and their crescentic free edges initially project into the caudal ends of the pericardioperitoneal canals (Fig. 10–5B). Later, they fuse with other diaphragmatic components to form the diaphragm (Fig. 10–5C to E), thereby separating the pleural cavities from the peritoneal cavity. The *pleuroperitoneal opening* on the right side closes slightly before the left one.

Text continued on page 148

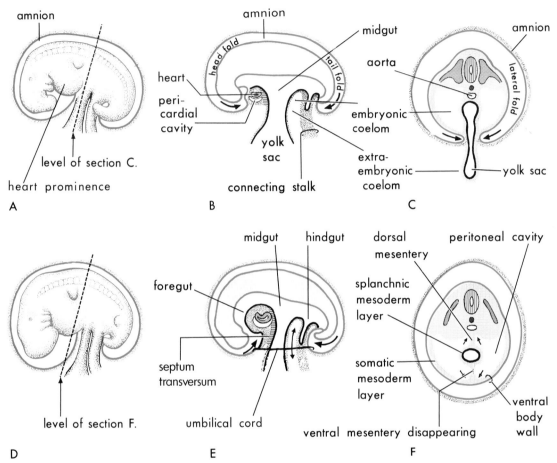

Figure 10–2. Drawings illustrating folding of the embryo and its effects on the intraembryonic coelom and other structures. *A,* Lateral view of an embryo of about 26 days. *B,* Schematic sagittal section of this embryo showing the head and tail folds. *C,* Transverse section at the level shown in *A,* indicating how fusion of the lateral folds gives the embryo a cylindrical form. *D,* Lateral view of a 28-day embryo. *E,* Schematic sagittal section of this embryo showing the reduced communication between the intraembryonic and extraembryonic coeloms (double-headed arrow). *F,* Transverse section as indicated in *D,* illustrating formation of the ventral body wall and disappearance of the ventral mesentery. The arrows indicate the junction of the somatic and splanchnic layers of mesoderm. The somatic mesoderm layer will become the parietal peritoneum, which lines the abdominal wall, and the splanchnic mesoderm layer will become the visceral peritoneum covering the abdominal organs (e.g., the stomach).

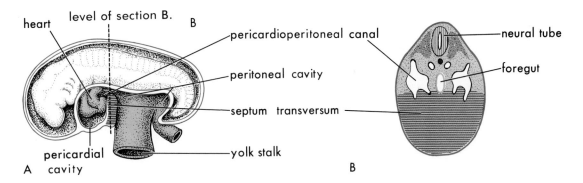

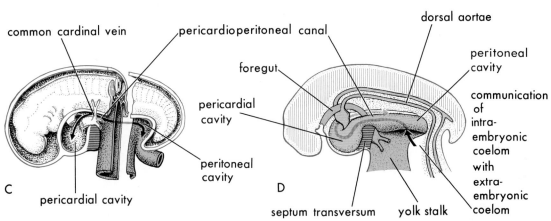

Figure 10–3. Schematic drawings of a four-week embryo (about 24 days). *A,* The lateral wall of the pericardial cavity has been removed to show the heart. *B,* Transverse section of the embryo, illustrating the relationship of the pericardioperitoneal canals to the septum transversum (primordium of the central part of the diaphragm) and the foregut. *C,* Lateral view of the embryo with the heart removed. The embryo has also been sectioned transversely to show the continuity of the intraembryonic and extraembryonic coeloms. *D,* Sketch showing the pericardioperitoneal canals arising from the dorsal wall of the pericardial cavity and passing on each side of the foregut to join the peritoneal cavity. The *arrows* show the communication of the extraembryonic coelom with the intraembryonic coelom and the continuity of the intraembryonic coelom at this stage.

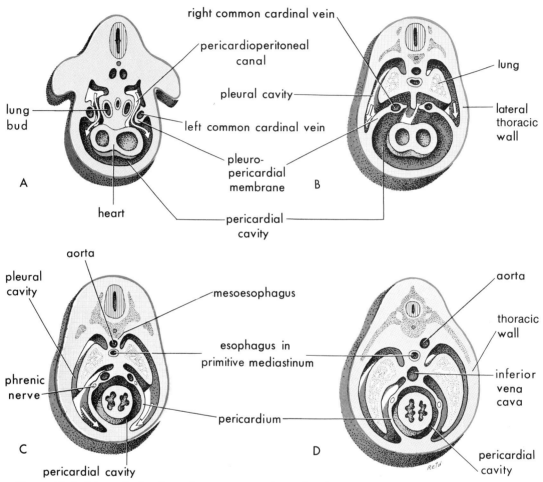

Figure 10–4. Schematic drawings of transverse sections of embryos cranial to the septum transversum, illustrating successive stages in the separation of the pleural cavities from the pericardial cavity. Growth and development of the lungs, expansion of the pleural cavities, and formation of the fibrous pericardium are also shown. *A,* Five weeks. The arrows indicate the communications between the pericardioperitoneal canals and the pericardial cavity. *B,* Six weeks. The arrows indicate development of the pleural cavities as they expand into the body wall. *C,* Seven weeks. Expansion of the pleural cavities ventrally around the heart is shown. The pleuropericardial membranes are now fused in the median plane with each other and with the mesoderm ventral to the esophagus. *D,* Eight weeks. Continued expansion of the lungs and pleural cavities and formation of the fibrous pericardium and chest wall are illustrated.

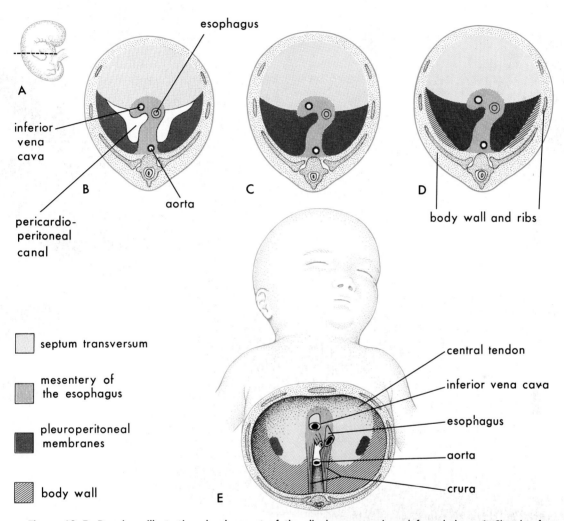

Figure 10–5. Drawings illustrating development of the diaphragm as viewed from below. *A*, Sketch of a lateral view of an embryo during the fifth week (actual size), indicating the level of the sections. *B*, Transverse section showing the unfused pleuroperitoneal membranes. *C*, Similar section at the end of the sixth week after fusion of the pleuroperitoneal membranes with the other two diaphragmatic components. *D*, Transverse section through a 12-week embryo after ingrowth of the fourth diaphragmatic component from the body wall. *E*, View of the diaphragm of a newborn infant, indicating the probable embryological origin of its components.

The reason for this is uncertain, but it may be related to the relatively large right lobe of the liver at this stage of development (see Fig. 13–6).

DEVELOPMENT OF THE DIAPHRAGM[3]

The diaphragm is a dome-shaped, musculotendinous partition that separates the thoracic and abdominal cavities. It has a complex embryonic origin. *The diaphragm develops from four structures* (Fig. 10–5): the septum transversum, the pleuroperitoneal membranes, the dorsal mesentery of the esophagus, and the lateral body walls (Fig. 10–5).

THE SEPTUM TRANSVERSUM (Figs. 10–2*E*, 10–3, and 10–5). This transverse septum, composed of mesoderm, initially forms a thick, incomplete partition or diaphragm between the pericardial and peritoneal cavities. It later fuses dorsally with the mesoderm ventral to the esophagus and the pleuroperitoneal membranes. It is the primordium of the *central tendon of the diaphragm* (Fig. 10–5*E*).

THE PLEUROPERITONEAL MEMBRANES (Fig. 10–5). These membranes fuse with the dorsal mesentery of the esophagus and the septum transversum. This completes the partition between the thoracic and abdominal cavities and forms the *primitive diaphragm.* Although the pleuroperitoneal membranes form large portions of the primitive diaphragm, they represent relatively small portions of the infant's diaphragm (Fig. 10–5*E*).

THE DORSAL MESENTERY OF THE ESOPHAGUS (Figs. 10–4 and 10–5). This mesentery constitutes the median portion of the diaphragm. The *crura of the diaphragm*[4] develop from myoblasts (developing muscle cells) that grow into the dorsal mesentery of the esophagus.

THE LATERAL BODY WALLS (Figs. 10–4 and 10–5). As the lungs grow during the ninth to twelfth weeks, the pleural cavities enlarge and "burrow" into the lateral body walls. During this "excavation" process, the body-wall tissue is split into two layers: (1) an external layer that will form part of the definite body wall, and (2) an internal layer that contributes muscle to peripheral portions of the diaphragm external to the parts derived from the pleuroperitoneal membranes.

Further extension of the pleural cavities into the lateral body walls forms the right and left *costodiaphragmatic recesses* (Fig. 10–6), establishing the characteristic, dome-shaped configuration of the diaphragm. After birth the costodiaphragmatic recesses become alternately smaller and larger as the lungs move in and out of them during inspiration and expiration (Moore, 1992).

Positional Changes and Innervation of the Diaphragm

During the fourth week the septum transversum lies opposite the third, fourth, and fifth *cervical somites* (Fig. 10–7*A*). During the fifth week, myoblasts (primitive muscle cells) from the *myotomes* of these somites migrate into the developing diaphragm and bring their nerves with them. Thus, the nerve supply of the diaphragm is from the third, fourth, and fifth cervical nerve roots, which join to form the **phrenic nerves.** These nerves pass to the septum transversum via the pleuropericardial membranes. This explains why the phrenic nerves subsequently come to lie on the fibrous pericardium, the adult derivative of the pleuropericardial membranes (Fig. 10–4*C* and *D*).

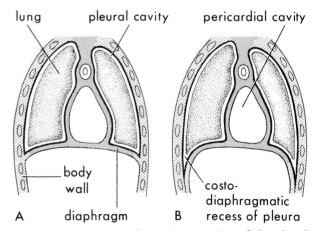

Figure 10–6. Diagrams illustrating extension of the pleural cavities into the body walls to form peripheral portions of the diaphragm, the costodiaphragmatic recesses, and the establishment of the characteristic, dome-shaped configuration of the diaphragm. Note that body wall tissue is added peripherally to the diaphragm as the lungs and pleural cavities enlarge.

---

[3] The diaphragm is a sheet of muscle with a large central tendon. For a description of its clinical anatomy, see Moore (1992).

[4] The crura (a leglike pair of diverging bundles of muscle) cross in the median plane anterior to the aorta (Moore, 1992).

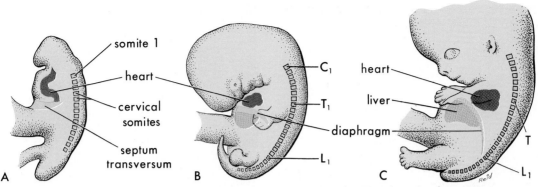

Figure 10-7. Diagrams illustrating positional changes of the developing diaphragm. *A*, About 24 days. The septum transversum is at the level of the third, fourth, and fifth cervical segments. *B*, About 41 days. *C*, About 52 days.

Rapid growth of the dorsal part of the embryo's body results in an apparent migration or *descent of the diaphragm*. By the sixth week the developing diaphragm is at the level of the thoracic somites (Fig. 10–7*B*). The phrenic nerves now take a descending course; and, as the diaphragm "moves" relatively farther caudally in the body, these nerves are correspondingly lengthened[5]. By the beginning of the eighth week, the dorsal part of the diaphragm lies at the level of the first lumbar vertebra (Fig. 10–7*C*).

As the four parts of the diaphragm fuse (Fig. 10–5), mesenchyme in the septum transversum extends into the other three parts and the myoblasts differentiate into the muscle of the diaphragm; hence, the motor nerve supply to the diaphragm is from the phrenic nerves (ventral rami of C3, C4, and C5). The phrenic nerve is also sensory to the central region of the diaphragm, but its costal rim, which develops from the body wall (Fig. 10–5*E*), receives sensory nerves from the lower intercostal nerves.

Congenital Diaphragmatic Defects

Despite the rather complex embryological development of the diaphragm, developmental abnormalities are relatively uncommon.

CONGENITAL DIAPHRAGMATIC HERNIA (CDH). *Posterolateral defect of the diaphragm* is a relatively common developmental abnormality (Figs. 10–8 and 10–9). It occurs about once in 2200 newborn infants (Harrison, 1991) and results from failure of the pleuroperitoneal membrane on the affected side to fuse with the other diaphragmatic components. The defect, usually on the left side, consists of a large opening in the posterolateral region of the diaphragm[6], usually in the region of the kidney. There is free communication between the abdominal and pleural cavities. As a result, the intestines and

---

[6] Sometimes referred to clinically as the foramen of Bochdalek.

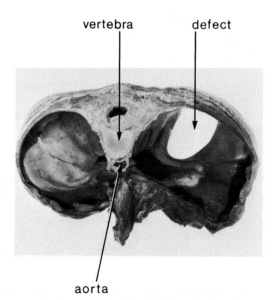

Figure 10-8. Photograph of a transverse section through the thoracic region of a stillborn infant, viewed from the thorax. Note the large, left, posterolateral defect of the diaphragm, which permitted herniation of abdominal contents into the thorax (CDH). Half actual size.

---

[5] The phrenic nerves in the adult are about 30 cm long (Moore, 1992).

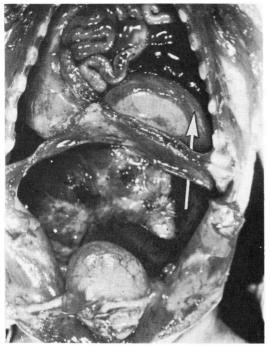

Figure 10–9. Photograph of the thoracic and abdominopelvic cavities of an infant with a large left posterolateral diaphragmatic defect similar to that shown in Figure 10–8. The thoracic and abdominal cavities were opened at autopsy to show the intestines and other viscera in the thoracic cavity (CHD). The liver has been removed to show that only distal parts of the large intestine have remained in the abdominal cavity. The arrow passes through the diaphragmatic defect. (Courtesy of Dr. Jan Hoogstraten, Children's Centre, Winnipeg, Canada.)

other abdominal organs pass into the thorax, producing a CDH (Fig. 10–9). Life-threatening breathing difficulties are usually present because of the presence of the abdominal viscera in the chest. The heart is pushed anteriorly and the lungs are compressed. Ultrasonography of the thorax is used to confirm the diagnosis.

The severity of the pulmonary developmental abnormalities depends on when and to what extent the abdominal viscera herniate into the thorax (i.e., on the timing and degree of compression of the fetal lungs). The effect on the ipsilateral (same side) lung is greater, but the contralateral lung also shows morphological changes (Harrison, 1991). If the abdominal viscera are in the thoracic cavity at birth, the initiation of respiration is likely to be impaired. At birth the intestines dilate with swallowed air and compromise the functioning of the heart and lungs. Because the abdominal organs are most often in the left side of the thorax, the heart and mediastinum are usually displaced to the right.

The lungs in infants with CHD are often hypoplastic and greatly reduced in size. The lungs are often aerated and achieve their normal size after reduction (repositioning) of the herniated viscera and repair of the defect in the diaphragm, but the mortality rate is high, approximately 76 per cent (Harrison, 1991). Most babies with CDH die not because there is a defect in the diaphragm or viscera in the chest, but because the lungs are hypoplastic due to compression during development (Harrison, 1991). For a description of other congenital defects of the diaphragm, see Moore and Persaud (1993).

SUMMARY

The *intraembryonic coelom* (the primordium of the embryonic body cavities) begins to develop near the end of the third week. By the beginning of the fourth week, it appears as a horseshoe-shaped cavity in the cardiogenic and lateral mesoderm. The curve of the "horseshoe" represents the future pericardial cavity; and its limbs represent the future pleural and peritoneal cavities.

During folding of the embryonic disc in the fourth week, lateral parts of the intraembryonic coelom are brought together on the ventral aspect of the embryo. When the caudal part of the ventral mesentery disappears, the right and left parts of the intraembryonic coelom merge to form the *peritoneal cavity.* As the peritoneal portions of the intraembryonic coelom merge, the splanchnic mesoderm encloses the primitive gut and suspends it from the dorsal body wall by a double-layered membrane known as the *dorsal mesentery.*

Until the seventh week, the embryonic pericardial cavity communicates with the peritoneal cavity through paired *pericardioperitoneal canals.* During the fifth and sixth weeks, partitions or membranes form at the cranial and caudal ends of these canals. The cranial *pleuropericardial membranes* separate the pericardial cavity from the pleural cavities, and the caudal *pleuroperitoneal membranes* separate the pleural cavities from the peritoneal cavity.

The diaphragm develops from four structures: (1) the septum transversum, (2) the pleuroperitoneal membranes, (3) the dorsal mesentery of the esophagus, and (4) the lateral body walls.

A posterolateral defect in the diaphragm results in the common type of *congenital dia-phragmatic hernia* (CDH). It is associated with herniation of abdominal viscera into the thoracic cavity and interference with the functioning of the heart and lungs. CDH occurs five times more often on the left side than on the right and results from failure of the pleuroperitoneal membrane on the affected side to fuse with the other diaphragmatic components, thereby separating the pleural and peritoneal cavities.

Commonly Asked Questions

1. I heard about a baby who was born with its liver in its chest. Is this possible?
2. Can a baby with most of its abdominal viscera in its chest survive? I have heard that diaphragmatic defects can be operated on before birth. Is this true?
3. Do the lungs develop normally in babies who are born with CDHs?
4. A friend of mine had a routine chest x-ray about a year ago and was told that a small part of his small intestine was in his chest. He is the type that has never been sick a day in his life. Is it possible for him to have a CDH without being aware of it? Would his lung on the affected side be normal?

The answers to these questions are given on page 331.

REFERENCES

Behrman RE: *Nelson Textbook of Pediatrics,* 14th ed. Philadelphia, WB Saunders, 1992.

Goldstein RB, Callen PW: Ultrasound evaluation of the fetal thorax and abdomen. *In* Callen PW: *Ultrasonography in Obstetrics and Gynecology,* 2nd ed. Philadelphia, WB Saunders, 1988.

Harrison MR: The fetus with a diaphragmatic hernia: pathophysiology, natural history, and surgical management. *In* Harrison MR, Golbus MS, Filly RA (eds): *The Unborn Patient. Prenatal Diagnosis and Treatment,* 2nd ed. Philadelphia, WB Saunders, 1991.

McNamara JJ, Eraklis AJ, Gross RE: Congenital posterolateral diaphragmatic hernia in the newborn. *J Thorac Cardiovasc Surg* 55:55, 1968.

Moore KL: *Clinically Oriented Anatomy,* 3rd ed. Baltimore, Williams & Wilkins, 1992.

Moore KL, Persaud TVN: *The Developing Human. Clinically Oriented Embryology,* 5th ed. Philadelphia, WB Saunders, 1993.

Reynolds M: Diaphragmatic anomalies. *In* Raffensperger JG (ed): *Swenson's Pediatric Surgery,* 5th ed. Norwalk, Appleton & Lange, 1990.

Taeusch HW, Ballard RA, Avery ME (eds): *Schaffer and Avery's Diseases of the Newborn,* 6th ed. Philadelphia, WB Saunders, 1991.

Wells LJ: Development of the human diaphragm and pleural sacs. *Contr Embryol Carneg Instn* 35:107, 1954.

11

THE BRANCHIAL OR PHARYNGEAL APPARATUS[1]

This consists of: (1) branchial (pharyngeal) arches, (2) pharyngeal pouches, (3) branchial (pharyngeal) grooves, and (4) branchial (pharyngeal) membranes (Figs. 11–1 and 11–2). The derivatives of the branchial apparatus contribute greatly to the formation of the head and neck. Most congenital anomalies in these regions originate during transformation of the branchial (pharyngeal) apparatus into its adult derivatives. *Branchial anomalies* (p. 161) result from persistence of parts of the branchial apparatus that normally disappear.

THE BRANCHIAL (PHARYNGEAL) ARCHES

These arches begin to develop early in the fourth week as *neural crest cells* migrate into the future head and neck regions (p. 51). The arches appear as obliquely disposed, rounded ridges on each side of the future head and neck

regions (Figs. 11–1 and 11–2). The arches (numbered in a craniocaudal sequence) are separated from each other by branchial (pharyngeal) grooves (Fig. 11–1D). The primordium of the mouth initially appears as a slight depression of the surface ectoderm called the *stomodeum* (Figs. 11–1D to G and 11–2). At first this cavity is separated from the primordial pharynx by a bilaminar membrane, the *oropharyngeal membrane* (buccopharyngeal membrane). This membrane ruptures at about 24 days, bringing the digestive tract into communication with the amniotic cavity (Fig. 11–1F and 11–1J).

Initially, each branchial or pharyngeal arch is composed of a core of mesenchyme that is covered externally by ectoderm and internally by endoderm (Fig. 11–3). Cells from the *neural crest* (see Fig. 5–6) migrate into the arches and surround the central core of mesenchymal cells derived from the intraembryonic mesoderm. It is the migration of *neural crest cells* into the arches that causes them to enlarge (Figs. 11–1 and 11–2). With the exception of the skeletal musculature and the vascular endothelium, most of the skeletal and connective tissue structures of the head and neck region are derived from neural crest cells.

Contents of a Branchial (Pharyngeal) Arch

A typical arch contains: (1) an *aortic arch* (artery) that runs around the primitive pharynx to

---

[1] The cranial region of an early human embryo somewhat resembles a fish embryo of a comparable stage. This explains why the adjective *branchial* is used to describe this apparatus. The Greek term *branchia* means "gill." By the end of the embryonic period, these primitive branchial structures have either been rearranged and adapted to new functions or they have disappeared. In fish and larval amphibians, the branchial apparatus forms a system of gills for exchanging oxygen and carbon dioxide between the blood and water. The branchial arches support the gills. Although a branchial apparatus develops in human embryos, no gills form.

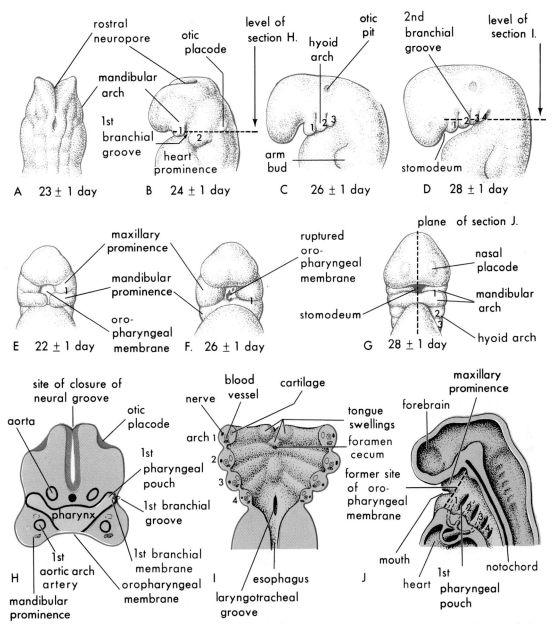

Figure 11-1. Drawings illustrating the human branchial or pharyngeal apparatus. *A,* Dorsal view of the cranial part of an early embryo. *B* to *D,* Lateral views showing later development of the branchial arches. *E* to *G,* Ventral views illustrating the relationship of the first or mandibular arch to the stomodeum or primitive mouth. *H,* Transverse section through the cranial region of an embryo. *I,* Horizontal section through the cranial region of an embryo, illustrating the branchial arch components and the floor of the primitive pharynx. *J,* Sagittal section of the cranial region of an embryo, illustrating the openings of the pharyngeal pouches in the lateral wall of the primitive pharynx.

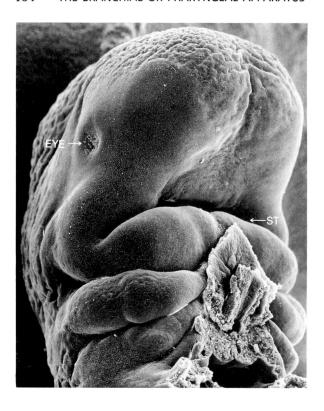

Figure 11–2. Scanning electron micrograph of the head and neck regions of a human embryo (oblique view) of about 32 days (Stage 14, 6.8 mm). If necessary, see Figure 10–1*A* to *F* for identification of the parts of the head and neck. Observe the arches, eye, and large stomodeum (ST) or primitive mouth. (Courtesy of Professor K. Hinrichsen, Ruhr-Universität Bochum, Federal Republic of Germany).

the dorsal aorta (Fig. 11–3*B*), (2) a *cartilaginous rod* that forms the skeleton of the arch, (3) a *muscular component* that forms muscles in the head and neck, and (4) a *nerve* that supplies the mucosa and muscles derived from the arch (Fig. 11–3; Table 11–1). The nerves that grow into the arches are derived from neuroectoderm of the primitive brain.

Fate of the Branchial (Pharyngeal) Arches

The **first branchial arch,** often called the *mandibular arch,* is involved with development of the face (described on p. 168). It develops two elevations called the *mandibular and maxillary prominences.* The mandibular prominence forms the lower jaw or *mandible* (Fig. 11–4*G*), and the maxillary prominence forms the upper jaw or *maxilla,* the zygomatic bone, and the squamous part of the temporal bone (see Fig. 16–8).

During the fifth week, the **second branchial arch,** often called the *hyoid arch,* overgrows the third and fourth arches, forming a deep ectodermal depression known as the *cervical sinus* (Fig. 11–4*A* to *D*). During the sixth and seventh

weeks, the second to fourth branchial (pharyngeal) grooves and the cervical sinus are obliterated, giving the neck a smooth contour (Fig. 11–4*F* and *G*). The branchial arches caudal to the second one make little contribution to the skin of the neck (Fig. 11–4*G*).

Derivatives of the Branchial (Pharyngeal) Arch Arteries

The transformation of the arteries in the arches, called *aortic arches* (Fig. 11–3*B*), into the adult arterial pattern is described with the circulatory system in Chapter 15 (p. 242). In fishes, these arteries supply blood to the capillary network of the gills. In human embryos, the blood supplies the arches and then enters the dorsal aorta.

DERIVATIVES OF THE BRANCHIAL (PHARYNGEAL) ARCH CARTILAGES (Fig. 11–5; Table 11–1). The dorsal end of the *first arch cartilage* (Meckel's cartilage) becomes ossified to form two middle ear bones, the *malleus* and *incus.* The intermediate portion of the cartilage regresses, and its perichondrium forms the *anterior ligament of the malleus* and the *sphenomandibular ligament.* The ventral portion of the first arch cartilage largely

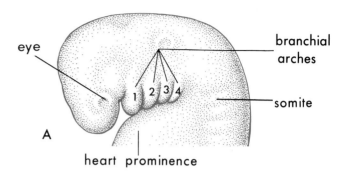

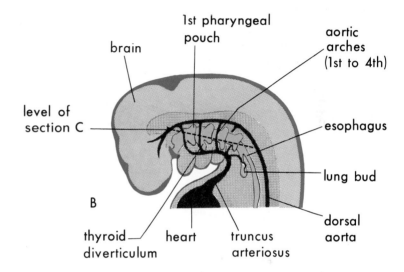

Figure 11–3. *A*, Drawing of the head and neck region of a 28-day embryo, illustrating the human branchial (pharyngeal) apparatus. *B*, Schematic drawing showing the pharyngeal pouches and aortic arches exposed by removal of the ectoderm and mesoderm. *C*, Horizontal section through the embryo, illustrating the germ layer of origin of the branchial arch components.

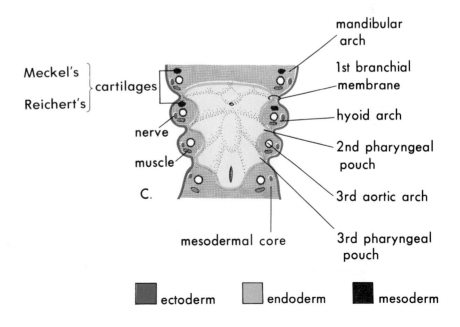

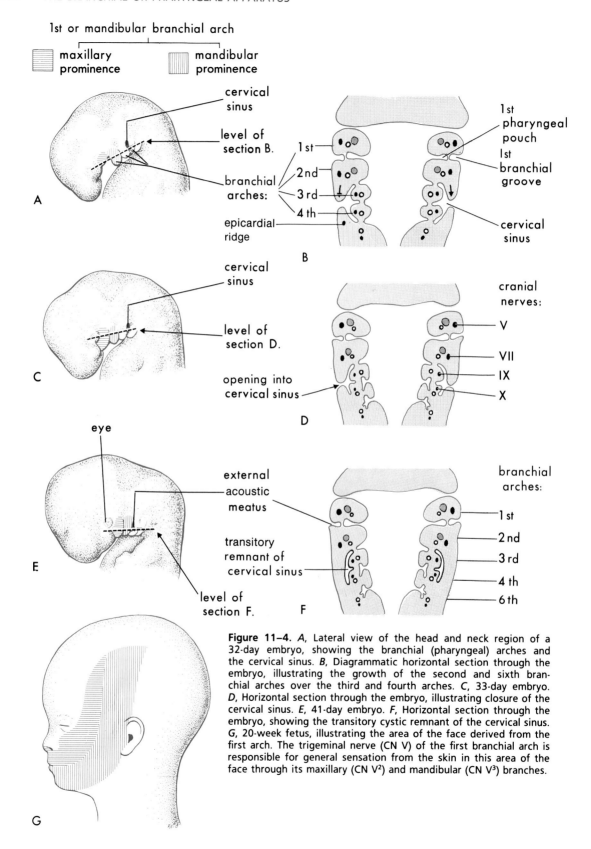

Figure 11–4. *A,* Lateral view of the head and neck region of a 32-day embryo, showing the branchial (pharyngeal) arches and the cervical sinus. *B,* Diagrammatic horizontal section through the embryo, illustrating the growth of the second and sixth branchial arches over the third and fourth arches. *C,* 33-day embryo. *D,* Horizontal section through the embryo, illustrating closure of the cervical sinus. *E,* 41-day embryo. *F,* Horizontal section through the embryo, showing the transitory cystic remnant of the cervical sinus. *G,* 20-week fetus, illustrating the area of the face derived from the first arch. The trigeminal nerve (CN V) of the first branchial arch is responsible for general sensation from the skin in this area of the face through its maxillary (CN V²) and mandibular (CN V³) branches.

Table 11–1. STRUCTURES DERIVED FROM BRANCHIAL (PHARYNGEAL) ARCH COMPONENTS*

Arch	Nerve	Muscles	Skeletal Structures	Ligaments
First (mandibular)	Trigeminal† (V)	Muscles of mastication‡ Mylohyoid and anterior belly of digastric Tensor tympani Tensor veli palatini	Malleus Incus	Anterior ligament of malleus Sphenomandibular ligament
Second (hyoid)	Facial (VII)	Muscles of facial expression§ Stapedius Stylohyoid Posterior belly of digastric	Stapes Styloid process Lesser cornu of hyoid Upper part of body of the hyoid bone	Stylohyoid ligament
Third	Glossopharyngeal (IX)	Stylopharyngeus	Greater cornu of hyoid Lower part of body of the hyoid bone	
Fourth and Sixth‖	Superior laryngeal branch of vagus (X) Recurrent laryngeal branch of vagus (X)	Cricothyroid Levator veli palatini Constrictors of pharynx Intrinsic muscles of larynx Striated muscles of the esophagus	Thyroid cartilage Cricoid cartilage Arytenoid cartilage Corniculate cartilage Cuneiform cartilage	

* The derivatives of the aortic arch arteries are described in Chapter 15 (see Fig. 15–17).
† The ophthalmic division does not supply any branchial components.
‡ Temporalis, masseter, medial and lateral pterygoids.
§ Buccinator, auricularis, frontalis, platysma, orbicularis oris and oculi.
‖ The fifth branchial arch is often absent. When present, it is rudimentary and usually has no recognizable cartilage bar. The cartilaginous components of the fourth and sixth arches fuse to form the cartilages of the larynx.

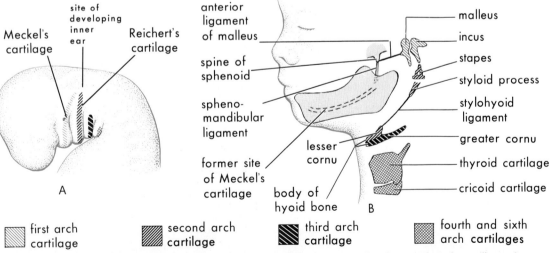

Figure 11–5. *A,* Schematic lateral view of the head and neck region of a four-week embryo, illustrating the location of the branchial (pharyngeal) arch cartilages. *B,* Similar view of a 24-week fetus, illustrating the adult derivatives of the arch cartilages. Note that the mandible is formed by intramembranous ossification of the mesenchymal tissue surrounding Meckel's cartilage. This cartilage acts as a template or guide but does not contribute much to the formation of the mandible.

disappears as the mandible develops around it by intramembranous ossification. For details on the development of the mandible, see Sperber (1989).

The dorsal end of the *second arch cartilage* (Reichert's cartilage) also ossifies and forms the *stapes* of the middle ear and the *styloid process* of the temporal bone. The portion of cartilage between the styloid process and the hyoid bone regresses, and its perichondrium forms the *stylohyoid ligament*. The ventral end of the second arch cartilage ossifies to form the *lesser cornu* (L., horn) of the *hyoid bone* and the superior part of the body of the hyoid bone (Fig. 11–5).

The *third arch cartilage* also contributes to the formation of the *hyoid bone*. It is located in the ventral portion of the arch where it ossifies to form the *greater cornu* and inferior part of the body of the hyoid bone. The *fourth and sixth arch cartilages* also persist in the ventral regions of the arches. They fuse to form the *laryngeal cartilages*. The rudimentary fifth arch has no recognizable adult derivative.

DERIVATIVES OF THE BRANCHIAL (PHARYNGEAL) ARCH MUSCLES (Fig. 11–6; Table 11–1). The muscular components of the arches form various striated muscles in the head and neck (e.g., the muscles of facial expression).

DERIVATIVES OF THE BRANCHIAL (PHARYNGEAL) ARCH NERVES (Table 11–1). Each arch is supplied by its own cranial nerve. The cranial nerves supplying the branchial muscles are classified as *branchial motor or efferent nerves*. Because mesenchyme from the branchial arches contributes to the dermis and mucous membranes of the head and neck, these areas are supplied with branchial sensory or *afferent nerves*.

The facial skin is supplied by the fifth cranial nerve *(trigeminal nerve)*; however, only its caudal two branches *(maxillary and mandibular)* supply derivatives of the first arch (Fig. 11–4). CN V is the principal sensory nerve of the head and neck and is the motor nerve for the muscles of mastication. Its sensory branches innervate the face, teeth, and mucous membranes of the nasal cavities, palate, mouth, and tongue.

The seventh cranial nerve *(facial nerve)*, the ninth cranial nerve *(glossopharyngeal nerve)*, and the tenth cranial nerve *(vagus nerve)* supply the second, third, and caudal (fourth to sixth) arches, respectively. The fourth arch is supplied by the superior laryngeal branch of the vagus

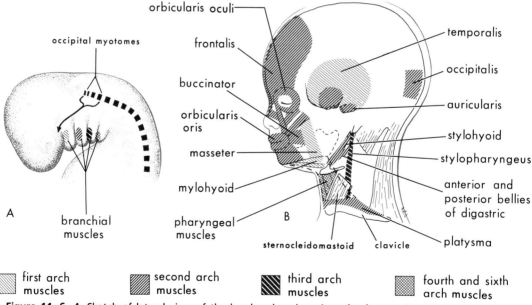

Figure 11–6. *A*, Sketch of lateral view of the head and neck region of a four-week embryo, showing the branchial muscles. The arrow shows the pathway taken by myoblasts from the occipital myotomes to form the tongue musculature. *B*, Sketch of the head and neck of a 20-week fetus, dissected to show the muscles derived from the branchial arches. Parts of the platysma and sternocleidomastoid muscles have been removed to show the deeper muscles. Note that myoblasts from the second branchial arch migrate from the neck region to the head and give rise to the muscles of facial expression. Thus, these muscles are supplied by the facial nerve, the nerve of the second branchial arch.

(CN X) and the sixth arch by its recurrent laryngeal branch. The nerves of the second to sixth arches have little cutaneous distribution, but they innervate the mucous membranes of the tongue, pharynx, and larynx.

THE PHARYNGEAL POUCHES

The *primitive pharynx*, derived from the foregut, is wide cranially and narrow caudally. The endoderm of the pharynx lines the internal surfaces of the branchial or pharyngeal arches and passes into balloonlike outgrowths called *pharyngeal pouches* (Figs. 11–1H to J and 11–3B and C). The pouches develop in a craniocaudal sequence between the arches, e.g., the first pharyngeal pouch lies between the first and second arches. There are four, well-defined pairs of pharyngeal pouches. The fifth pharyngeal pouches are absent or rudimentary.

Derivatives of the Pharyngeal Pouches

Because these pouches give rise to several important organs, the fate of each pouch is discussed separately.

THE FIRST PHARYNGEAL POUCH (Fig. 11–7). This pouch expands into an elongated *tubotympanic recess*, which forms the *tympanic cavity* and *mastoid antrum*. Its connection with the pharynx gradually elongates to form the *auditory tube* (eustachian tube). More details about the developing ear are given in Chapter 18.

THE SECOND PHARYNGEAL POUCH (Fig. 11–7). The endoderm of this pouch proliferates and forms buds that grow into the underlying mesenchyme. The central parts of these buds break down, forming the *tonsillar crypts* (pitlike depressions). The pouch endoderm forms the surface epithelium and the lining of the crypts of the **palatine tonsil**. The mesenchyme surrounding the crypts differentiates into lymphoid tissue which soon becomes organized into *lymphatic nodules*. Although it is largely obliterated as the palatine tonsil develops, part of the cavity of the second pouch remains as the *intratonsillar cleft* (tonsillar fossa).

THE THIRD PHARYNGEAL POUCH (Fig. 11–7). This pouch expands into a solid, dorsal bulbar portion and a hollow, ventral elongated portion. Each dorsal bulbar portion differentiates into an *inferior parathyroid gland*. The elongated ventral portions form two masses that eventually meet and fuse to form the bilobed *thymus*.[2] The thymus and parathyroid glands migrate caudally. Later, the parathyroid glands separate from the thymus and come to lie on the dorsal surface of the thyroid gland, which has descended from the foramen cecum of the tongue into the neck (see Fig. 11–11).

THE FOURTH PHARYNGEAL POUCH (Fig. 11–7). This pouch also expands into a dorsal bulbar portion and an elongated ventral portion. Each dorsal portion develops into a *superior parathyroid gland*. The elongated ventral portion of each fourth pouch develops into an *ultimobranchial body*, which becomes incorporated into the thyroid gland and gives rise to its *parafollicular* or *C cells*. These cells produce *calcitonin*, a hormone involved in the regulation of the normal calcium level in body fluids. The C cells differentiate from *neural crest cells* that migrate into the branchial (pharyngeal) arches.

THE FIFTH PHARYNGEAL POUCH. This rudimentary structure, if present, is partially incorporated into the fourth pouch.

THE BRANCHIAL (PHARYNGEAL) GROOVES

The neck region of human embryos exhibits four branchial grooves on each side from the fourth to sixth weeks (Figs. 11–1, 11–2, and 11–4). These grooves separate the branchial (pharyngeal) arches externally. Only one pair of grooves contributes to adult structures. The ectoderm of the first groove persists as the epithelium of the *external acoustic meatus* (Fig. 11–7C). The other branchial grooves come to lie in a slitlike depression called the *cervical sinus*. These are normally obliterated with this sinus as the neck develops (Figs. 11–4 and 11–7).

THE BRANCHIAL (PHARYNGEAL) MEMBRANES

Four of these membranes appear in the bottoms of the branchial (pharyngeal) grooves on each side of the future neck region of the human embryo during the fourth week (Figs. 11–1H and 11–3C). These membranes form where the epithelia of a branchial groove and a

---

[2] For details on the histogenesis of the thymus and parathyroid glands, see Moore and Persaud (1993).

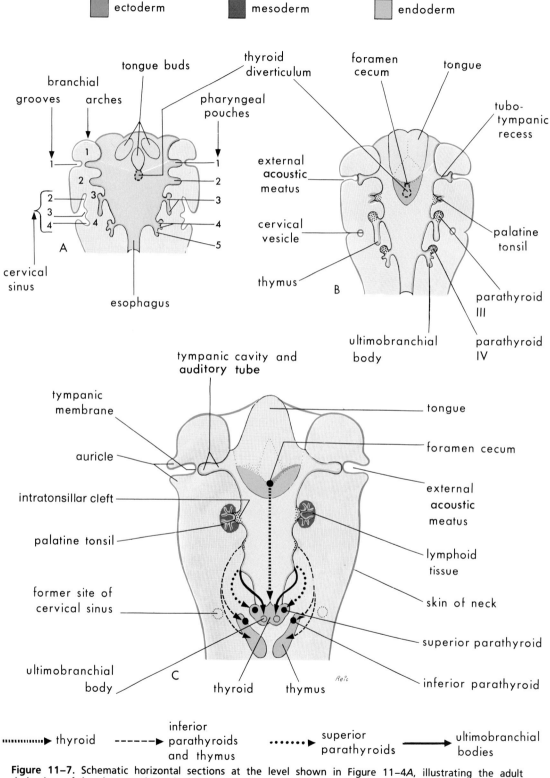

Figure 11–7. Schematic horizontal sections at the level shown in Figure 11–4A, illustrating the adult derivatives of the pharyngeal pouches. A, Five weeks. B, Six weeks. C, Seven weeks.

pharyngeal pouch approach each other. They are temporary structures in the human embryo. The endoderm of the pouches and the ectoderm of the grooves are soon separated by mesenchyme. Only one pair of membranes contributes to the formation of adult structures. The first branchial (pharyngeal) membrane, along with the intervening layer of mesoderm, gives rise to the *tympanic membrane* or eardrum (Fig. 11–7C); see also Chapter 18.

BRANCHIAL (PHARYNGEAL) ANOMALIES

Congenital anomalies of the head and neck mainly originate during transformation of the branchial or pharyngeal apparatus into adult structures (Fig. 11–7). Most of these abnormalities represent *remnants of the branchial apparatus* that normally disappear as these structures develop. Most branchial anomalies are uncommon (Stricker et al., 1990).

CONGENITAL AURICULAR SINUSES AND CYSTS (Fig. 11–8F). Small blind sinuses (pits) and cysts in the skin are commonly found in a triangular area anterior to the ear, but they may occur in other sites around the auricle or in its lobule. Most auricular sinuses and cysts are remnants of the first branchial (pharyngeal) groove.

BRANCHIAL SINUSES (Figs. 11–7D and 11–9). These *lateral cervical sinuses* are uncommon, and almost all that open externally on the side of the neck result from failure of the second branchial or pharyngeal groove and the cervical sinus to obliterate. The blind sinus that remains typically opens along the anterior border of the sternocleidomastoid muscle in the inferior third of the neck.

External branchial sinuses are commonly detected during infancy due to the discharge of mucus from their orifices on the neck (Fig. 11–9). Branchial sinuses are bilateral in about ten per cent of cases and are commonly associated with auricular sinuses (described previously).

Internal branchial sinuses opening into the pharynx are uncommon (Fig. 11–8D). Because they usually open into the intratonsillar cleft or near the palatopharyngeal arch, almost all these sinuses result from persistence of part of the second pharyngeal pouch.

BRANCHIAL FISTULA (Fig. 11–8E). An abnormal canal that opens on the side of the neck and in the pharynx is called a branchial fistula. It results from persistence of parts of the second branchial groove and second pharyngeal pouch. The fistula ascends from its opening on the neck through the subcutaneous tissue, platysma muscle, and deep fascia to reach the carotid sheath (Moore, 1992). It then passes between the internal and external carotid arteries and opens in the intratonsillar cleft (tonsillar fossa).

Recent studies suggest that *piriform sinus fistulas* are the result of persistence of remnants of the ultimobranchial body (Miyauchi et al., 1992) and that the fistulas trace the migration route of this embryonic body to the thyroid gland (Fig. 11–7C).

BRANCHIAL CYSTS (Figs. 11–4B and 11–8F). The third and fourth branchial (pharyngeal) arches are normally buried in the *cervical sinus*. Remnants of the cervical sinus and/or the second branchial (pharyngeal) groove may persist and form spherical or elongated cysts. Although they may be associated with branchial sinuses and drain through them, these cysts often lie free in the neck just inferior to the angle of the mandible. They may, however, develop anywhere along the anterior border of the sternocleidomastoid muscle. Branchial cysts often do not become apparent until late childhood or early adulthood when they produce a slowly enlarging, painless swelling in the neck. The cysts enlarge due to the accumulation of fluid and cellular debris derived from desquamation of their epithelial linings.

Branchial cysts have also been observed in the parathyroid glands and may arise from cystic degeneration and accumulation of secretions in embryological remnants that normally disappear (Chetty and Forder, 1991).

BRANCHIAL VESTIGES (Fig. 11–8F). Normally, the branchial (pharyngeal) arch cartilages disappear except for parts that form ligaments or bones (Fig. 11–5B). In unusual cases, cartilaginous or bony remnants of branchial arch cartilages appear under the skin on the side of the neck. These are usually found anterior to the inferior third of the sternocleidomastoid muscle.

THE FIRST ARCH SYNDROME (Fig. 11–10). Maldevelopment of components of the first branchial (pharyngeal) arch results in various congenital defects of the eyes, ears, mandible, and palate that together constitute the first arch syndrome. These symptoms result from insufficient migration of cranial neural crest cells into the first arch during the fourth week. There are two main manifestations of the first arch syndrome: the *Treacher Collins syndrome* and the *Pierre Robin syndrome* (Behrman, 1992).

DEVELOPMENT OF THE THYROID GLAND

The thyroid gland appears during the fourth week (about 24 days) as a median endodermal

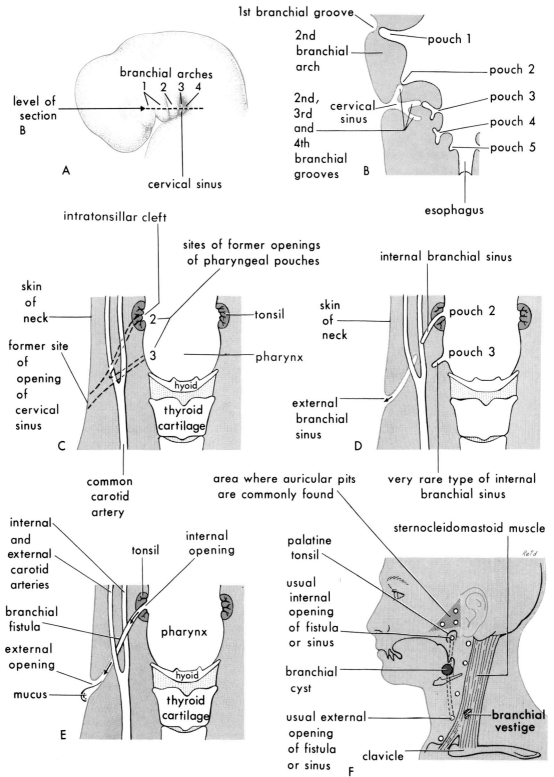

Figure 11-8. *A,* Drawing of the head and neck region of a five-week embryo. *B,* Horizontal section through the embryo, illustrating the relationship of the cervical sinus to the branchial (pharyngeal) arches and pharyngeal pouches. *C,* Diagrammatic sketch of the adult neck region, indicating the former sites of openings of the cervical sinus and the pharyngeal pouches. The broken lines indicate possible courses of branchial fistulas. *D,* Similar sketch, showing the embryological basis of various types of branchial sinus. *E,* Drawing of a branchial fistula resulting from persistence of parts of the second branchial groove and the second pharyngeal pouch. *F,* Sketch showing possible sites of branchial cysts and openings of branchial sinuses and fistulas. A branchial vestige is also illustrated.

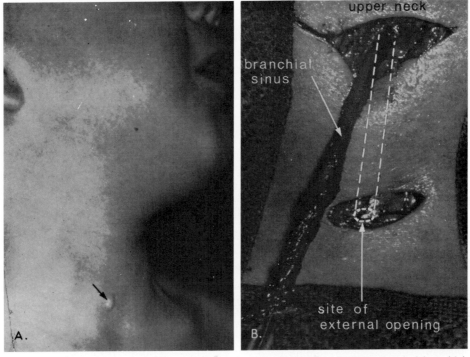

Figure 11–9. *A,* Photograph of a child's neck showing mucus dripping from an external branchial sinus *(arrow). B,* Photograph of a branchial sinus taken during excision. The external opening in the skin of the neck and the original course of the sinus in the subcutaneous tissue are indicated by broken lines. (From Swenson O: *Pediatric Surgery,* 1958. Courtesy of Appleton-Century-Crofts.)

Figure 11–10. Photograph of an infant with the first arch syndrome, a pattern of abnormalities resulting from insufficient migration of neural crest cells into the first branchial (pharyngeal) arch. Note the following: deformed auricle of the external ear, preauricular appendage, defect in cheek between the ear and the mouth, hypoplasia of the mandible, and large mouth.

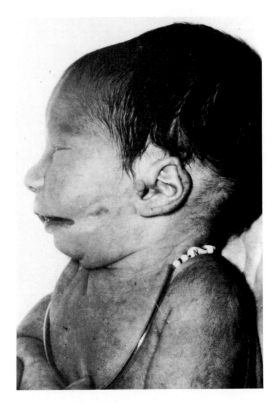

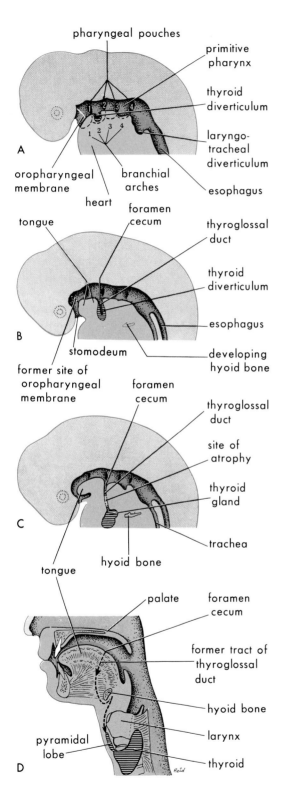

Figure 11–11. *A*, *B*, and *C*, Schematic sagittal sections of the head and neck region of embryos at four, five, and six weeks, respectively, illustrating successive stages of development of the thyroid gland. *D*, Similar section of an adult head, showing the path taken by the thyroid gland during its descent and the former tract of the thyroglossal duct.

thickening in the floor of the primitive pharynx (Figs. 11–7 and 11–11). It is *the first endocrine gland to form* in the embryo. The thickening indicating the thyroid gland soon forms a downgrowth known as the *thyroid diverticulum.* As the developing thyroid descends in the neck, it retains its connection to the tongue by a narrow *thyroglossal duct.* By seven weeks the thyroid gland has usually reached its final site in the neck, and the thyroglossal duct has disappeared. The original opening of the thyroglossal duct persists as a vestigial pit, the *foramen cecum of the tongue* (see Figs. 11–11D and 11–13C).[3]

Congenital Anomalies of the Thyroid Gland

THYROGLOSSAL DUCT CYSTS AND SINUSES (Fig. 11–12). Cysts may form anywhere along the course followed by the thyroglossal duct during descent of the primordium of the thyroid gland from the tongue. Normally, the thyroglossal duct atrophies and disappears, but a remnant of it may persist and give rise to a cyst in the tongue or in the midline of the neck, usually just inferior to the hyoid bone. The swelling produced by a cyst usually develops as a painless, progressively enlarging, and movable mass. In some cases following infection of a cyst, an

---

[3] For a description of the histogenesis of the thyroid gland, see Moore and Persaud (1993).

opening through the skin exists due to perforation following infection of the cyst. This forms a *thyroglossal duct sinus* that usually opens in the median plane of the neck anterior to the laryngeal cartilages (Fig. 11–12A).

ECTOPIC THYROID GLAND AND ACCESSORY THYROID TISSUE. Uncommonly, the thyroid fails to descend, resulting in a *lingual thyroid.* Incomplete descent may result in the thyroid gland appearing high in the neck, at or just inferior to the hyoid bone. *Accessory thyroid tissue* results from remnants of the thyroglossal duct. This glandular tissue may be functional, but it is often of insufficient size to maintain normal function if the thyroid gland is removed. Accessory thyroid tissue may be found anywhere from the tongue to the usual site of the thyroid gland in the neck.

DEVELOPMENT OF THE TONGUE

The first indication of tongue development appears around the end of the fourth week as a median elevation, the *median tongue bud* (tuberculum impar), in the floor of the primitive pharynx just rostral to the foramen cecum (Fig. 11–13A). Soon, two oval *distal tongue buds* (lateral lingual swellings) develop on each side of the median tongue bud. The distal tongue buds rapidly increase in size, merge with each other, and overgrow the median tongue bud. The fused distal tongue buds form the anterior two thirds

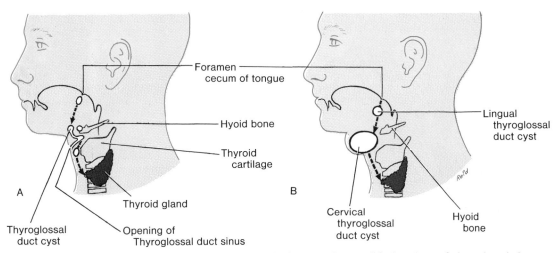

Figure 11–12. *A,* Diagrammatic sketch of the head, showing the possible locations of thyroglossal duct cysts. A thyroglossal duct sinus is also illustrated. The broken line indicates the course taken by the thyroglossal duct during descent of the thyroid gland from the foramen cecum in the tongue to its final position in the anterior part of the neck. *B,* A similar sketch illustrating lingual and cervical thyroglossal duct cysts. Most cysts are located close to or in the median plane near the hyoid bone.

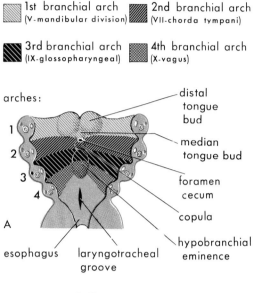

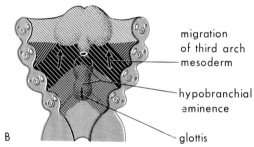

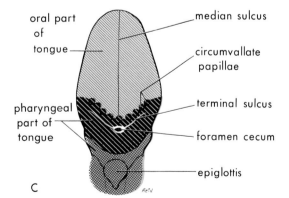

Figure 11–13. *A* and *B*, Schematic horizontal sections of the pharynx at the level shown in Figure 11–4*A*, showing successive stages in the development of the tongue during the fourth and fifth weeks. *C*, Adult tongue showing the branchial arch derivation of the nerve supply of the mucosa.

or *oral part of the tongue* (Fig. 11–13C). The plane of fusion of the distal tongue buds is indicated by the *median sulcus (groove) of the tongue.* The median tongue bud forms no identifiable adult derivative.

The posterior third or pharyngeal part of the tongue is initially indicated by two elevations that develop caudal to the foramen cecum (Fig. 11–13A). One elevation, called the *copula* (L., bond), forms by fusion of the ventromedial parts of the second branchial (pharyngeal) arches. The other elevation, called the *hypobranchial eminence,* develops caudal to the copula from mesoderm in the ventromedial parts of the third and fourth arches.

As the tongue develops, the copula is gradually overgrown by the hypobranchial eminence and disappears (Fig. 11–13B and C). As a result, *the posterior third of the tongue develops from the rostral part of the hypobranchial eminence.* The line of fusion of the anterior and posterior parts of the tongue is roughly indicated by the V-shaped groove called the *terminal sulcus* (Fig. 11–13C).

Branchial arch mesenchyme forms the connective tissue and the lymphatic and blood vessels of the tongue. Most of the tongue musculature is derived from myoblasts that migrate from the *myotomes of the occipital somites* (Fig. 11–6A). These myoblasts (primitive muscle cells) migrate into the tongue where they differentiate into muscle fibers. The hypoglossal nerve (CN XII) accompanies the myoblasts during their migration and innervates the tongue muscles as they develop. The entire tongue is in the mouth at birth; its posterior third descends into the pharynx by 4 years of age (Sperber, 1989).

Taste buds develop during weeks 11 to 13 by inductive interaction between the epithelial cells of the tongue and invading gustatory nerve cells from the chorda tympani, glossopharyngeal, and vagus nerves (Sperber, 1989). Most taste buds form on the dorsal surface of the tongue, and some develop on the palatoglossal arches, palate, posterior surface of the epiglottis, and the posterior wall of the oropharynx.

Congenital Anomalies of the Tongue

Abnormalities of the tongue are uncommon except for the fissures and hypertrophy of the lingual papillae, which are features of infants with *Down syndrome* (see Chapter 9).

CONGENITAL LINGUAL CYSTS AND FISTULAS (Fig. 11–12). Cysts in the tongue, often just superior to the hyoid bone, are usually derived from *remnants of the thyroglossal duct.* They may enlarge and produce symptoms of pharyngeal discomfort and/or *dysphagia* (difficulty in swallowing). Fistulas in the tongue are derived from persistence of the thyroglossal duct, and they open through the *foramen cecum* into the oral cavity.

ANKYLOGLOSSIA (TONGUE-TIE). The lingual frenulum normally connects the inferior surface of the anterior part of the tongue to the floor of the mouth (Moore, 1992). In tongue-tie, the frenulum extends to the tip of the tongue and interferes with its free protrusion. Usually the frenulum stretches with time so that surgical correction of the anomaly is not necessary.

MACROGLOSSIA. An excessively large tongue is not common. It results from generalized hypertrophy of the tongue. These cases usually result from lymphangioma or muscular hypertrophy.

MICROGLOSSIA. An abnormally small tongue is extremely rare and is usually associated with *micrognathia* (underdeveloped mandible with recession of the chin) and limb defects.

BIFID OR CLEFT TONGUE. Incomplete fusion of the distal tongue buds posteriorly results in a deep median groove or *cleft of the tongue;* usually, the cleft does not extend to the tip of the tongue. Complete failure of fusion of the distal tongue buds results in a cleft in the oral part of the tongue. This uncommon anomaly is referred to as *bifid tongue.*

DEVELOPMENT OF SALIVARY GLANDS

During the sixth and seventh weeks, these glands begin as solid epithelial proliferations or buds from the primitive oral cavity (Fig. 11–7C). The club-shaped ends of these epithelial buds grow into the underlying mesenchyme. The connective tissue in the glands is derived from *neural crest cells.* All parenchymal (secretory) tissue arises by proliferation of the oral epithelium.

The *parotid glands* are the first to appear (early in the sixth week). They develop from buds that arise from the oral ectodermal lining near the angles of the stomodeum (primitive mouth). These buds grow toward the ears and branch to form solid cords with rounded ends. Later these cords are canalized (i.e., develop lumina) and become ducts by about ten weeks. The rounded ends of the cords differentiate into acini. Secretions commence at 18 weeks (Sperber, 1989). The capsule and connective tissue develop from the surrounding mesenchyme.

The *submandibular glands* appear late in the sixth week. They develop from endodermal buds from the oral epithelium in the floor of the stomodeum. Solid cellular processes grow posteriorly, lateral to the developing tongue. Later they branch and differentiate. Acini begin to form at 12 weeks and secretory activity begins at 16 weeks (Sperber, 1989). Growth of the submandibular glands continues after birth with the formation of mucous acini. Lateral to the tongue, a linear groove forms that closes over to form the *submandibular duct.*

The *sublingual glands* appear in the eighth week, two weeks later than the other salivary glands. They develop from multiple endodermal epithelial buds in the paralingual sulcus or groove. These buds branch and canalize to form 10 to 12 ducts that open independently into the floor of the mouth.

DEVELOPMENT OF THE FACE

The five facial primordia appear around the rather large *stomodeum*, the primordium of the mouth early in the fourth week (Figs. 11–1E, 11–2, 11–14, and 11–15A). The large *frontonasal prominence* (FNP) constitutes the cranial boundary of the stomodeum. The paired *maxillary prominences* of the first branchial arch form the lateral boundaries of the stomodeum, and the paired *mandibular prominences* of this same arch constitute the caudal boundary of the stomodeum.

Bilateral oval-shaped thickenings of the surface ectoderm called *nasal placodes* develop on each side of the caudal part of frontonasal elevation (Fig. 11–15B). Horseshoe-shaped *medial and lateral nasal prominences* develop at the margins of the nasal placodes (Fig. 11–15C and D). As a result, the nasal placodes lie in depressions called *nasal pits* (Fig. 11–15C). The maxillary prominences grow rapidly and soon approach each other and the medial nasal prominences (Fig. 11–15D and E).

The face mainly develops between the fourth and eighth weeks. By the end of this period, the face has an unquestionably human appearance. Facial proportions develop during the fetal period (Fig. 11–15H and I). During the sixth and seventh weeks, the medial nasal prominences merge with each other and the maxillary prominences (Fig. 11–15F and G). As the medial nasal prominences merge with each other, they form the *intermaxillary segment* of the maxilla (Fig.

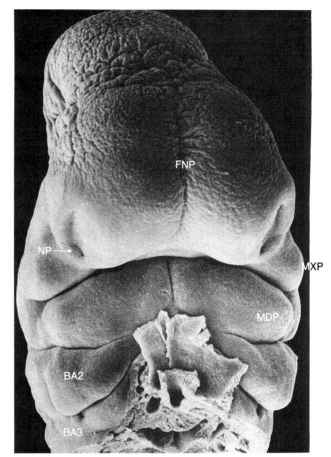

Figure 11–14. Scanning electron micrograph of a ventral view of a human embryo of about 33 days. Observe the prominent frontonasal process (FNP) surrounding the telencephalon (forebrain). Also observe the nasal pits (NP) located in the ventrolateral regions of the frontonasal prominence. Medial and lateral nasal prominences surround these pits. The cuneiform, wedge-shaped, maxillary prominences (MXP) form the lateral boundaries of the primitive oral cavity or stomodeum. The fusing mandibular prominences (MDP) are located just caudal to the stomodeum. The second branchial or pharyngeal arch (BA2) is clearly visible and shows overhanging margins (opercula). The third branchial or pharyngeal arch (BA3) is also clearly visible. (From Hinrichsen K: The early development of morphology and patterns of the face in the human embryo. *In: Advances in Anatomy, Embryology and Cell Biology,* vol. 98. New York, Springer-Verlag, 1985.)

11–15H). This segment gives rise to: (1) the ventral groove of the upper lip called the *philtrum*, (2) the premaxillary part of the maxilla and its associated gingiva (gum), and (3) the *primary palate*. The lateral parts of the upper lip, most of the maxilla, and the *secondary palate* form from the maxillary prominences (Figs. 11–15H and I and 11–16). These prominences merge laterally with the mandibular prominences.

The *frontonasal prominence* (Fig. 11–15) forms the forehead and the dorsum and apex of the nose. The sides of the nose are derived from the lateral nasal prominences (Fig. 11–15H and I). The *mandibular prominences* merge with each other in the fourth week, and the groove between them disappears before the end of the fifth week (Fig. 11–15D). The *mandibular prominences* give rise to the mandible (lower jaw), lower lip, and the inferior part of the face. Final development of the face occurs slowly and results mainly from changes in the proportion and relative position of the facial components.

> The smallness of the face at birth results from: (1) the rudimentary upper and lower jaws, (2) the unerupted teeth, and (3) the small size of the nasal cavities and maxillary sinuses.

DEVELOPMENT OF NASAL CAVITIES

As the face develops, the *nasal placodes* are gradually surrounded by the *nasal prominences;* they then form the floors of depressions called *nasal pits* (Fig. 11–15C). Growth of the surrounding mesenchyme results in deepening of the nasal pits and formation of *nasal sacs.* These sacs are the primordia of the nasal cavities (Fig. 11–16). At first the nasal sacs are separated from the oral cavity by the *oronasal membrane* (Fig. 11–11A and B). This membrane soon ruptures, bringing the nasal and oral cavities into communication. The regions of continuity are the *primitive choanae* (openings between the nasal cavity and nasopharynx), which lie posterior to the primary palate. After the *secondary palate* develops, the choanae are located at the junction of the nasal cavity and nasopharynx. This occurs when the lateral palatine processes fuse with each other and the nasal septum (Fig. 11–16E and G).

While these changes are occurring, the *superior, middle, and inferior conchae* develop as elevations on the lateral walls of the nasal cavities (Fig. 11–16E). Concurrently, the ectodermal epithelium in the roof of each nasal cavity becomes specialized to form the olfactory epithelium. Some epithelial cells differentiate into *olfactory receptor cells* (neurons). The axons of these cells constitute the *olfactory nerves,* which grow into the *olfactory bulbs* of the brain (Fig. 11–16E).

THE PARANASAL SINUSES. Some paranasal (air) sinuses develop during late fetal life; the remainder develop after birth. They form as outgrowths or diverticula of the walls of the nasal cavities and become air-filled extensions of the nasal cavities in the adjacent bones (e.g., the maxillae). Growth of the *paranasal sinuses* is important in altering the size and shape of the face during infancy and childhood and in adding resonance to the voice during adolescence. Most of these sinuses develop after birth.

DEVELOPMENT OF THE PALATE

The palate develops from two primordia: the *primary palate* and the *secondary palate.* Although palatogenesis begins toward the end of the fifth week, fusion of its parts is not complete until the twelfth week.

THE PRIMARY PALATE (Fig. 11–16). The primary palate or *median palatine process* begins to develop early in the sixth week from the innermost part of the *intermaxillary segment* of the maxilla. It forms a wedge-shaped mass of mesoderm between the maxillary prominences of the developing maxilla.

THE SECONDARY PALATE (Fig. 11–16). The secondary palate develops from two internal projections from the maxillary prominences called the *lateral palatine processes* (palatal shelves). These shelflike structures initially project inferomedially on each side of the tongue (Fig. 11–16C). As the jaws develop, the tongue moves inferiorly, and the lateral palatine processes gradually grow toward each other and fuse (Fig. 11–16E and G). They also fuse with the primary palate and the *nasal septum* (Fig. 11–16D to H).

Fusion of the palatal processes begins anteriorly during the ninth week and ends posteriorly in the region of the *uvula* by the twelfth week. The uvula (L., little grape) is the last part of the palate to form. The *palatine raphe* indicates the line of fusion of the lateral palatine processes (Fig. 11–16H).

Bone gradually develops in the primary palate (Fig. 11–16E and G), forming the *premaxillary part of the maxilla,* which lodges the incisor teeth. Concurrently, bone extends from the maxillae and palatine bones into the lateral palatine processes (shelves) to form the *hard palate* (Fig. 11–16). The posterior portions of the lateral palatine processes do not become ossified. They extend beyond the nasal septum and fuse

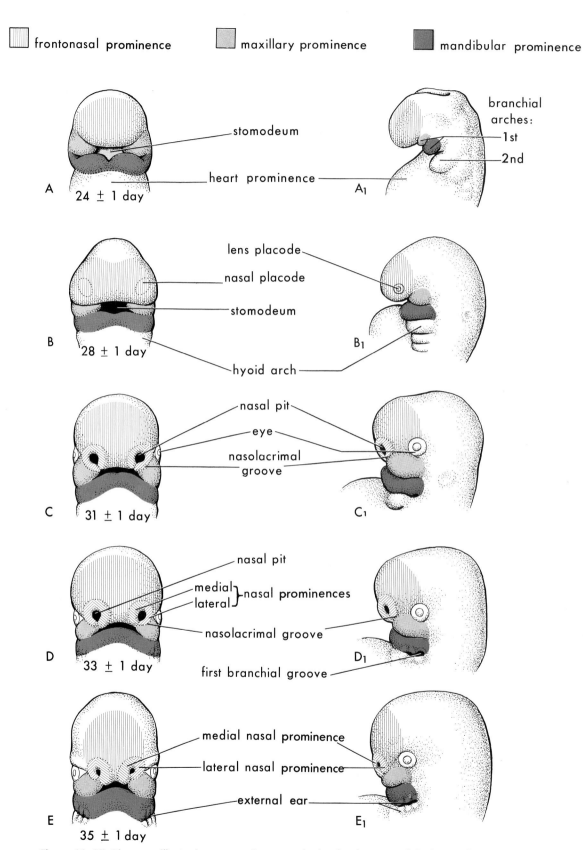

Figure 11–15. Diagrams, illustrating progressive stages in the development of the human face.

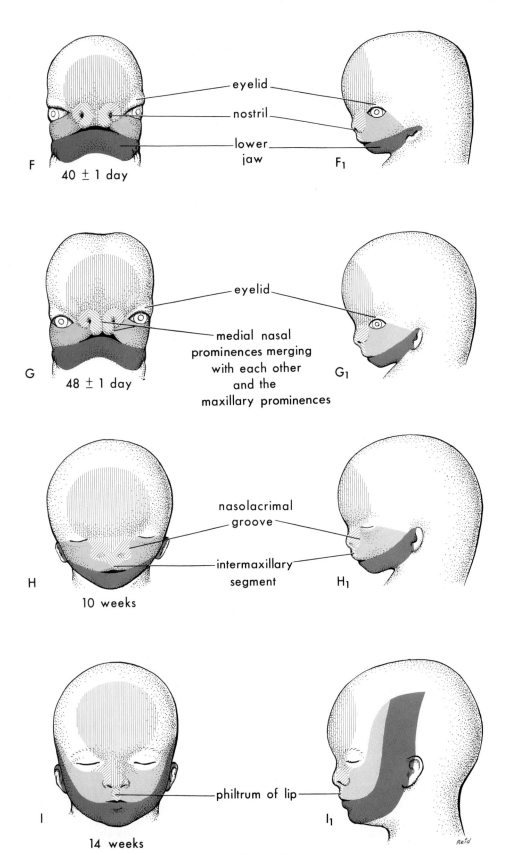

F   40 ± 1 day   F₁

eyelid

nostril

lower jaw

G   48 ± 1 day   G₁

eyelid

medial nasal prominences merging with each other and the maxillary prominences

H   10 weeks   H₁

nasolacrimal groove

intermaxillary segment

I   14 weeks   I₁

philtrum of lip

Figure 11–15. *Continued*

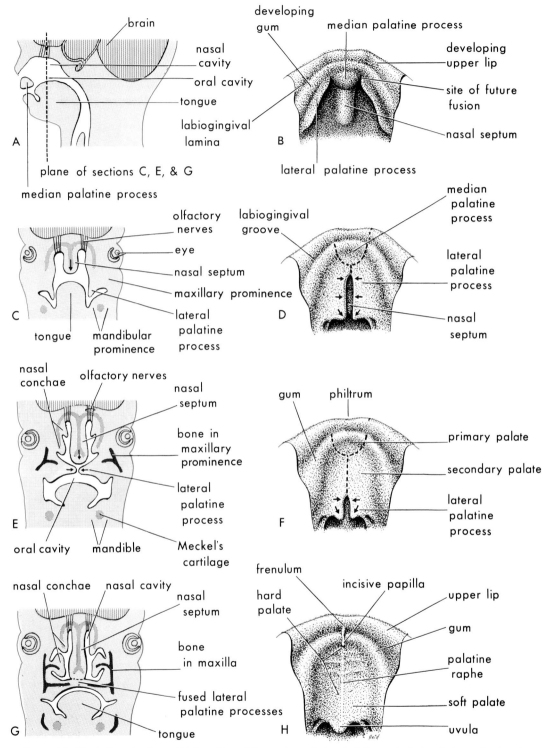

Figure 11–16. *A,* Sketch of a sagittal section of the embryonic head at the end of the sixth week, showing the primary palate. *B, D, F,* and *H,* Drawings of the roof of the mouth from the sixth to twelfth weeks, illustrating development of the palate. The broken lines in *D* and *F* indicate sites of fusion of the palatine processes; the arrows indicate medial and posterior growth of the lateral palatine processes (palatal shelves). *C, E,* and *G,* Drawings of frontal sections of the head, illustrating fusion of the lateral palatine processes with each other and the nasal septum and separation of the nasal and oral cavities.

to form the *soft palate* and its conical projection called the *uvula* (Fig. 11–16*D, F,* and *H*).

A small *nasopalatine canal* persists in the median plane of the palate between the premaxillary part of the maxilla and the palatine processes of the maxillae. This canal is represented in the adult hard palate by the *incisive fossa*, which is the common opening for the right and left incisive canals (Moore, 1992). An irregular suture runs from the incisive fossa to the alveolar process of the maxilla, between the lateral incisor and canine teeth on each side. It is visible in the anterior region of the palates of young persons. This suture indicates where the embryonic primary and secondary palates fused and where clefts of the anterior palate occur (see Fig. 11–19).

Cleft Lip and Palate

Cleft lip and cleft palate are common anomalies of the face and palate. Although often associated, cleft lip and palate are embryologically and etiologically distinct anomalies. They originate at different times during development and involve different developmental processes.

CLEFT LIP (Figs. 11–17 to 11–21). This defect of the upper lip, with or without cleft palate, occurs about once in 1000 births. The defect may be unilateral or bilateral and is *more common in males.* The clefts vary from a small notch in the lip (Fig. 11–17*B*) to complete division of the lip and alveolar part of the maxilla. This defect is also inappropriately called a "harelip."

Unilateral cleft lip results from failure of the maxillary prominence on the affected side to unite with the merged medial nasal prominences (Fig. 11–18).

Bilateral cleft lip results from failure of the maxillary prominences to meet and merge with the medial nasal prominences. In complete bilateral cleft of the upper lip and alveolar part of the maxilla, the intermaxillary segment hangs free (Fig. 11–17*C* and *D*). The defects may be

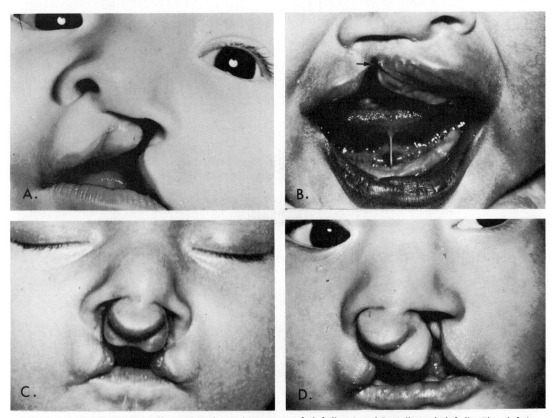

Figure 11–17. Photographs illustrating the various types of cleft lip. *A* and *B*, Unilateral cleft lip. The cleft in *B* is incomplete; the arrow indicates a band of tissue (Simonart's band) connecting the parts of the lip. *C* and *D*, Bilateral cleft lip. Note that the intermaxillary segment of the maxilla protrudes between the clefts in the lip. Deformed, supernumerary, or absent teeth are often associated abnormalities. (Courtesy of Dr. D. A. Kernahan, The Children's Memorial Hospital, Chicago.)

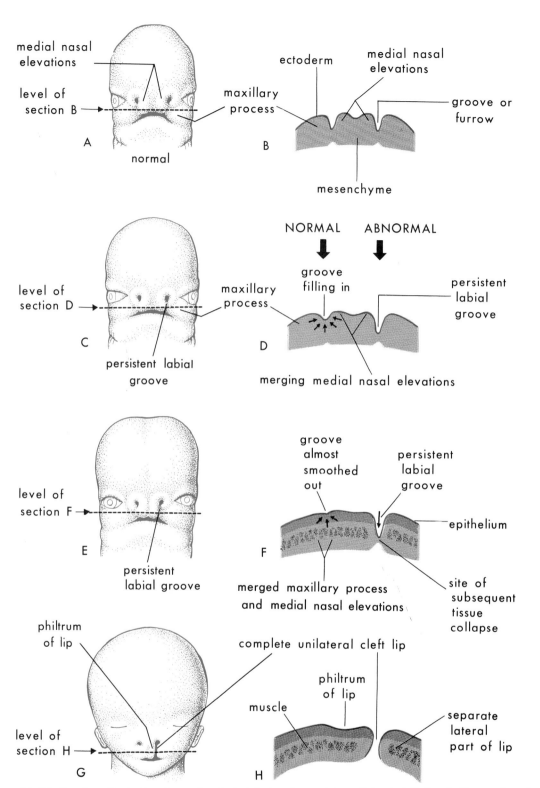

Figure 11–18. Drawings illustrating the embryological basis of complete unilateral cleft lip. *A*, Five-week embryo. *B*, Horizontal section through the head, illustrating the grooves between the maxillary prominences and the merging medial nasal prominences. *C*, Six-week embryo, showing a persistent labial groove on the left side. *D*, Horizontal section through the head, showing the groove gradually filling in on the right side because of proliferation of mesenchyme *(arrows)*. *E*, Seven-week embryo. *F*, Horizontal section through the head, showing that the epithelium on the right has almost been pushed out of the groove between the maxillary prominence and medial nasal prominence. *G*, Ten-week fetus with a complete unilateral cleft lip. *H*, Horizontal section through the head after stretching of the epithelium and breakdown of the tissues in the floor of the persistent labial groove on the left side, forming a complete unilateral cleft lip.

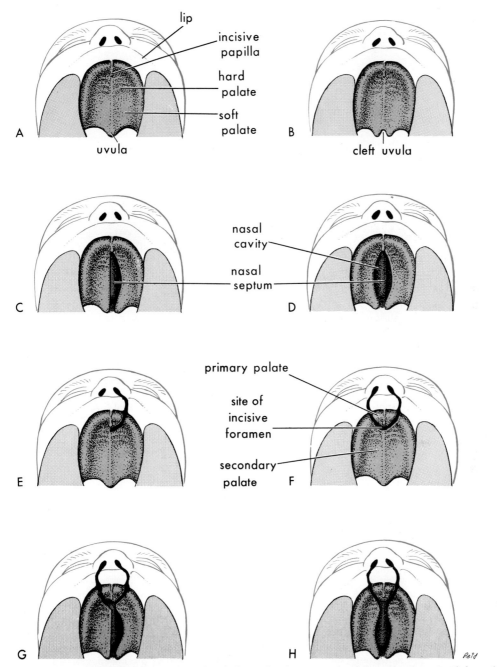

Figure 11–19. Drawings of various types of cleft lip and palate. *A,* Normal lip and palate. *B,* Cleft uvula. *C,* Unilateral cleft of the posterior or secondary palate. *D,* Bilateral cleft of the posterior palate. *E,* Complete unilateral cleft of the lip and alveolar process of the maxilla with a unilateral cleft of the anterior or primary palate. *F,* Complete bilateral cleft of the lip and alveolar process with bilateral cleft of the anterior palate. *G,* Complete bilateral cleft of the lip and alveolar process with bilateral cleft of the anterior palate and unilateral cleft of the posterior palate. *H,* Complete bilateral cleft of the lip and alveolar process with complete bilateral cleft of the anterior and posterior parts of the palate.

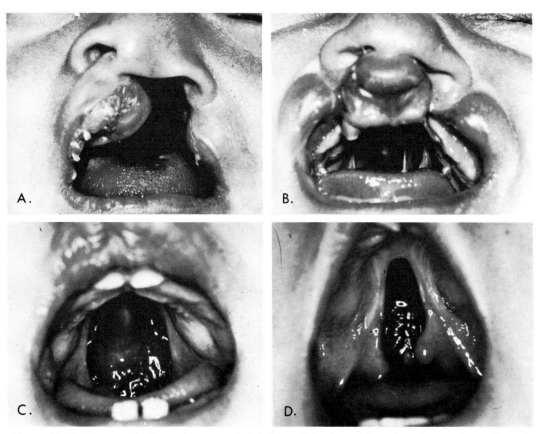

Figure 11–20. Photographs illustrating congenital defects of the lip and/or palate. *A*, Complete unilateral cleft of the lip and alveolar process of the maxilla. *B*, Complete bilateral cleft of the lip and alveolar processes of the maxillae with bilateral cleft of the anterior palate. Note the protruding intermaxillary segment between the clefts in the lip. *C* and *D*, Bilateral cleft of the posterior or secondary palate.

similar or dissimilar, with varying degrees of defect on each side.

Median cleft lip, resulting from incomplete merger of the medial nasal prominences, is very uncommon (Fig. 11–21).

CLEFT PALATE (Figs. 11–19 and 11–20). Cleft palate, with or without cleft lip, occurs about once in 2500 births. The clefts may be unilateral or bilateral and are *more common in females*. A cleft may involve only the uvula or it may extend through the soft and hard regions of the palate. In severe cases associated with cleft lip, the cleft in the anterior and posterior regions of the palate extends through the alveolar part of the maxilla and the lip on both sides.

The embryological basis of cleft palate is failure of the mesenchymal masses of the lateral palatine processes (palatal shelves) to meet and fuse with each other, the nasal septum, and/or with the median palatine process (primary palate).

Most cases of cleft lip and palate are determined by multiple factors, genetic and nongenetic, each causing only a minor developmental disturbance. This is called *multifactorial inheritance* (p. 139). These factors seem to operate by influencing the number of neural crest cells that migrate into the embryonic facial primordia. If the number is insufficient, clefting of the lip and/or palate occurs. Studies of twins indicate that genetic factors are of more importance in cleft lip, with or without cleft palate, than in cleft palate alone. A sibling of a child with a cleft palate has an elevated risk of having a cleft palate but no increased risk of having a cleft lip.

Facial Clefts

Various types of facial cleft occur, but they are all uncommon. Severe facial clefts are usually associated with gross anomalies of the head. In *median cleft of the lower lip and mandible*

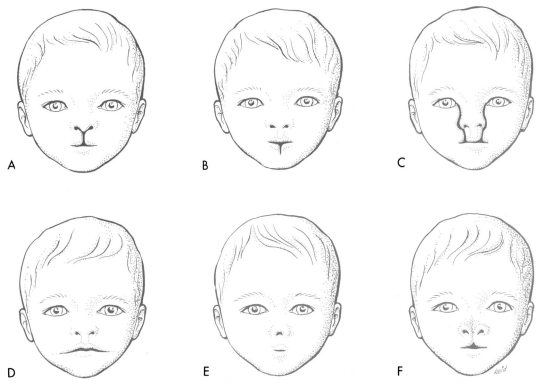

Figure 11–21. Drawings of uncommon anomalies of the face. *A,* Median cleft of the upper lip. *B,* Median cleft of the lower lip and jaw. *C,* Bilateral oblique facial clefts with complete bilateral cleft lip. *D,* Macrostomia or lateral facial cleft. *E,* Single nostril and microstomia; these anomalies are not usually associated. *F,* Bifid nose and incomplete median cleft of the upper lip.

(Fig. 11–21*B*), there is a deep cleft resulting from failure of the mandibular prominences of the first branchial or pharyngeal arch to merge completely with each other.

Oblique facial clefts are often bilateral and extend from the upper lip to the medial margin of the eye (Fig. 11–21*C*). They result from failure of the maxillary prominences to merge with the lateral and medial nasal prominences. Lateral or *transverse facial clefts* run from the mouth toward the external ear. Bilateral clefts result in a very large mouth, a condition called *macrostomia* (Fig. 11–21*D*).

Congenital microstomia (small mouth) results from excessive merging of the maxillary and mandibular prominences of the first arch (Fig. 11–21*E*). A *single nostril* results when only one nasal placode forms (Fig. 11–21*E*). *Bifid nose* results from failure of the medial nasal prominences to merge completely (Fig. 11–21*F*). In mild forms of bifid nose, a small groove is present in the tip of the nose.

SUMMARY

During the fourth and fifth weeks the primitive pharynx is bounded laterally by barlike branchial (pharyngeal) arches. Each arch consists of a core of mesenchymal tissue, which is covered externally by surface ectoderm and internally by endoderm. Each arch also contains an artery called an aortic arch, a cartilage bar, a nerve, and a muscle component. Externally between the arches, are branchial (pharyngeal) grooves. Internally between the arches, are extensions of the pharynx called pharyngeal pouches. Branchial membranes are formed where the ectoderm of each branchial groove contacts the endoderm of each pharyngeal pouch. The pharyngeal pouches and the branchial (pharyngeal) arches, grooves, and membranes make up the branchial (pharyngeal) apparatus.

Development of the tongue, face, lips, jaws, palate, pharynx, and neck largely involves transformation of the branchial apparatus into adult structures. The branchial grooves disappear except for the first pair, which persists as the external acoustic meatus. The branchial membranes also disappear, except for the first pair, which becomes the tympanic membranes.

The first pharyngeal pouch gives rise to the tympanic cavity, mastoid antrum, and auditory tube. The second pharyngeal pouch is associated with development of the palatine tonsil. The *thymus* is derived from the third pair of pharyngeal pouches, and the parathyroid glands are formed from the third and fourth pairs of pharyngeal pouches. The *thyroid gland* develops from a downgrowth from the floor of the pharynx in the region where the tongue develops.

Most congenital anomalies of the head and neck originate during transformation of the branchial apparatus into adult structures. Branchial cysts, sinuses, and fistulas may develop from parts of the second branchial groove, the cervical sinus, or the second pharyngeal pouch, which fail to obliterate. An ectopic thyroid gland results when the thyroid gland fails to descend or only partially descends from its site of origin in the tongue.

The thyroglossal duct may persist, or remnants of it may give rise to thyroglossal duct cysts; these cysts, if infected, may perforate and form thyroglossal duct sinuses, which open anteriorly in the median plane of the neck.

Cleft lip is the most common congenital birth defect of the face. Although frequently associated with cleft palate, cleft lip and cleft palate are etiologically distinct anomalies, which involve different developmental processes that occur at different times. *Cleft lip* results from failure of mesenchymal masses of the medial nasal prominences and maxillary prominences to merge; whereas, *cleft palate* results from failure of the mesenchymal masses of the palatine processes to fuse.

Most cases of cleft lip, with or without cleft palate, are caused by a combination of genetic and environmental factors *(multifactorial inheritance)*. These factors appear to act by interfering with the migration of *neural crest cells* into the maxillary prominences of the first branchial arch. If the number of cells is insufficient, clefting of the lip and/or palate may occur.

Commonly Asked Questions

1. My mother said that my uncle had a "harelip." What kind of lip defect is this?
2. I was told that embryos have cleft lips and that this common facial anomaly represents a persistence of this embryonic condition. Are these statements accurate?
3. Neither my husband nor I have a cleft lip or palate, and no one in our families is known to have or to have had these anomalies. What are our chances of having a child with a cleft lip with or without cleft palate?
4. I have a son with cleft lip and cleft palate. My brother has a similar defect of his lip and palate. Although I do not plan to have any more children, my husband says that I am entirely to blame for our son's birth defects. Was the defect likely inherited only from my side of the family?
5. My sister's son has minor anomalies of his external ears, but he does not have hearing abnormalities or facial malformations. Would the ear abnormalities be considered *branchial defects?*

The answers to these questions are given on page 331.

REFERENCES

Behrman RE (ed): *Nelson Textbook of Pediatrics*, 14th ed. Philadelphia, WB Saunders, 1992.

Chetty R, Forder MD: Parathyroiditis associated with hyperthyroidism and branchial cysts. *Am J Clin Path* 96:348, 1991.

Ferguson MWJ: Palate development. *Development* 103 (Suppl):41, 1988.

Fraser FC: The genetics of cleft lip and palate: yet another look. *In* Pratt RM, Christiansen RL (eds): *Current Research Trends in Prenatal Craniofacial Development.* New York, Elsevier North-Holland, 1980.

Gorlin RJ, Cohen Jr, MM, Levin LS: *Syndromes of the Head and Neck*, 3rd ed. New York, Oxford Univ Press, 1990.

Greene RM: Signal transduction during craniofacial development. *Critical Rev in Toxicol* 20:153, 1989.

Hall BK: Mechanisms of craniofacial development. *In* Vig KWL, Burdi AR (eds): *Craniofacial Morphogenesis and Dysmorphogenesis.* Ann Arbor, The University of Michigan, 1988.

Hinrichsen K: The Early Development of Morphology and Patterns of the Face in the Human Embryo. *Advances in Anatomy, Embryology and Cell Biology* 98:1, New York, Springer-Verlag, 1985.

Jones KL: *Smith's Recognizable Patterns of Human Malformation*, 4th ed. Philadelphia, WB Saunders, 1988.

Kendall MD: Functional anatomy of the thymic microenvironment. *J Anat* 177:1, 1991.

Kirby MF, Bockman DE: Neural crest and normal development: a new perspective. *Anat Rec* 209:1, 1984.

Miyauchi A, Matsuzuka F, Kuma K, Katayama S: Piriform sinus fistula and the ultimobranchial body. *Histopath* 20:221, 1992.

Moore KL: *Clinically Oriented Anatomy*, 3rd ed. Baltimore, Williams & Wilkins, 1992.

Moore KL, Persaud TVN: *The Developing Human. Clinically Oriented Embryology*, 5th ed. Philadelphia, WB Saunders, 1993.

Morris HL, Bardach J: Cleft lip and palate and related disorders: issues for future research of high priority. *Cleft Palate J* 26:141, 1989.

Niermeyer MF, Van der Meulen J: Genetics of craniofacial malformations. *In* Stricker M, Van der Meulen JC, Raphael B, Mazzola R (eds): *Craniofacial Malformations.* Edinburgh, Churchill Livingstone, 1990.

Noden DM: New views on old problems. *Anat Rec* 208:1, 1984.

Pfeifer G (ed): *Craniofacial Abnormalities and Clefts of the Lip, Alveolus and Palate.* New York, Georg Thieme Verlag, 1991.

Poswillo D: The aetiology and pathogenesis of craniofacial deformity. *Development* 103(Suppl):213, 1988.

Raffensperger JG (ed): *Swenson's Pediatric Surgery*, 5th ed. Philadelphia, WB Saunders, 1990.

Ross RB, Johnston MC: *Cleft Lip and Palate.* Baltimore, Williams & Wilkins, 1972.

Schubert J, Schmidt R, Raupach H-W: New findings explaining the mode of action in prevention of facial clefting and first clinical experience. *J Cranio-Max Fac Surg* 18:343, 1990.

Shepard TH: Development of the thyroid gland. *In* Gardner LI (ed): *Endocrine and Genetic Diseases of Childhood and Adolescence*, 2nd ed. Philadelphia, WB Saunders, 1975.

Slavkin HC: Cellular and molecular determinants during craniofacial development. *In* Stricker M, Van der Meulen JC, Raphael B, Mazzola R (eds): *Craniofacial Malformations.* Edinburgh, Churchill Livingstone, 1990.

Sperber GH: *Craniofacial Embryology*, 4th ed. London, Butterworth, 1989.

Steinmann GG: Changes of the human thymus during ageing. *In* Müller-Hermelink HK (ed): *The Human Thymus. Histophysiology and Pathology. Current Topics in Pathology*, 75. Berlin, Springer-Verlag, 1986.

Stricker M, Raphael B, Van der Meulen J, Mazzola R: Craniofacial growth and development. *In* Stricker M, Van der Meulen JC, Raphael B, Mazzola R (eds): *Craniofacial Malformations.* Edinburgh, Churchill Livingstone, 1990.

Sulik KK, Cook CS, Webster WS: Teratogens and craniofacial malformations: relationships to cell death. *Development* 103(Suppl):213, 1988.

Taeusch HW, Ballard RA, Avery ME (eds): *Schaffer and Avery's Diseases of the Newborn*, 6th ed. Philadelphia. WB Saunders, 1991.

Thompson MW, McInnes RR, Willard HF: *Thompson & Thompson Genetics in Medicine*, 5th ed. Philadelphia, WB Saunders Co, 1991.

van der Meulen J, Mozzola B, Stricker M, Raphael B: Classification of craniofacial malformations. *In* Stricker M, Van der Meulen JC, Raphael B, Mazzola R (eds): *Craniofacial Malformations.* Edinburgh, Churchill Livingstone, 1990.

Vanderas AP: Incidence of cleft lip, cleft palate, and cleft lip and palate among races: a review. *Cleft Palate J* 24:216, 1987.

Vermeij-Keers C: Craniofacial embryology and morphogenesis: normal and abnormal. *In* Stricker M, Van der Meulen JC, Raphael B, Mazzola R (eds): *Craniofacial Malformations.* Edinburgh, Churchill Livingstone, 1990.

Wedden SE, Ralphs JR, Tickle C: Pattern formation in the facial primordia. *Development* 103(Suppl):31, 1988.

12

THE RESPIRATORY SYSTEM

The development of the *upper respiratory system* (nose, nasal cavities, paranasal sinuses, nasopharynx, and oropharynx) is described in Chapter 11. The *lower respiratory system* (larynx, trachea, bronchi, and lungs) begins to form during the fourth week (26 to 27 days). The respiratory primordium is first indicated by a median **laryngotracheal groove** that develops in the caudal end of the ventral wall of the primitive pharynx (Fig. 12–1). This groove soon deepens to form *laryngotracheal diverticulum*, an outpouching ventral to the primitive pharynx (Fig.

12–2*A*). As this diverticulum grows ventrocaudally, it is invested with splanchnic mesenchyme, and its distal end enlarges to form a globular *lung bud*.

The laryngotracheal diverticulum gradually separates from the pharynx; however, it maintains open communication with the pharynx through the *primordial or primitive laryngeal aditus* (Fig. 12–2*C*), the future inlet of the larynx. *Tracheoesophageal folds* develop within the laryngotracheal diverticulum and soon grow toward each other and fuse to form a partition

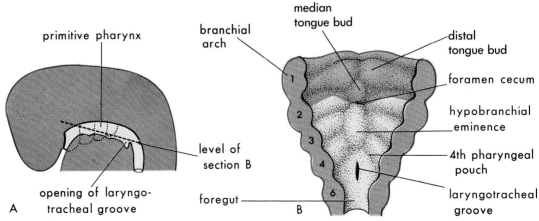

Figure 12–1. *A,* Diagrammatic sagittal section of the cranial half of a human embryo (about 26 days), showing the laryngotracheal groove in the caudal end of the floor of the primitive pharynx. *B,* Horizontal section at the level shown in *A,* illustrating the floor of the primitive pharynx and the location of the laryngotracheal groove.

180

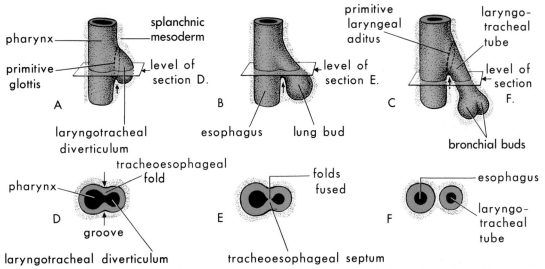

Figure 12–2. Drawings illustrating successive stages in the development of the tracheoesophageal septum during the fourth week. *A*, *B*, and *C*, Lateral views of the caudal part of the primitive pharynx, illustrating partitioning of the foregut into the esophagus and laryngotracheal tube. *D*, *E*, and *F*, Transverse sections illustrating development of the tracheoesophageal septum and division of the cranial part of the foregut into the laryngotracheal tube and esophagus.

known as the *tracheoesophageal septum* (Fig. 12–2*E*). This septum divides the cranial part of the foregut into two parts, the *laryngotracheal tube* and the primordium of the oropharynx and *esophagus* (Fig. 12–2*F*). The laryngotracheal tube is the primordium of the larynx, trachea, bronchi, and lungs.

DEVELOPMENT OF THE LARYNX

The endodermal lining of the cranial end of the laryngotracheal tube and the surrounding mesenchyme from the fourth and sixth pairs of branchial (pharyngeal) arches develop into the larynx. The *laryngeal cartilages* are derived from the fourth and sixth pairs of branchial (pharyngeal) arch cartilages (see Fig. 11–5). These cartilages are derived from *neural crest cells* surrounding the original mesoderm in these arches. The epiglottis develops from the caudal half of the *hypobranchial eminence* (see Fig. 11–13). Folds of mucous membrane of the larynx become the *vocal folds* (cords). The *laryngeal muscles* develop from myoblasts in the fourth and sixth pairs of branchial (pharyngeal) arches.

DEVELOPMENT OF THE TRACHEA

The endodermal lining of the laryngotracheal tube distal to the larynx differentiates into the epithelium and glands of the trachea, and the pulmonary epithelium (Fig. 12–3). The cartilage, connective tissue, and muscle of the trachea are derived from the surrounding splanchnic mesenchyme.

TRACHEOESOPHAGEAL FISTULA (Fig. 12–4). An abnormal communication or fistula connecting the trachea and esophagus occurs about once in every 2500 births; most affected infants are males. Tracheoesophageal fistula is usually associated with *esophageal atresia;* in all cases, there is an abnormal communication between the trachea and the esophagus (Fig. 12–4). Tracheoesophageal fistula, the most common anomaly of the lower respiratory tract, results from incomplete division of the cranial part of the foregut into respiratory and digestive portions during the fourth week. Incomplete fusion of the tracheoesophageal folds produces a *defective tracheoesophageal septum* and an abnormal communication between the trachea and esophagus.

Four types of tracheoesophageal fistula may develop. The most common abnormality is for the cranial portion of the esophagus to end blindly *(esophageal atresia)* and for the caudal portion to join the trachea near its bifurcation (Fig. 12–4*A*). Other varieties of this anomaly are illustrated in Figure 12–4*B* to *D*.

Infants with esophageal atresia and tracheoesophageal fistula cough and choke on swallowing due to accumulation of excessive amounts of saliva in the mouth and upper respiratory tract.

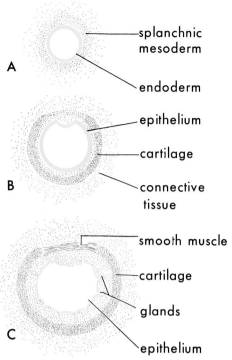

splanchnic
mesoderm

endoderm

epithelium

cartilage

connective
tissue

smooth muscle

cartilage

glands

epithelium

Figure 12–3. Drawings of transverse sections through the laryngotracheal tube, illustrating progressive stages of development of the trachea. *A,* Four weeks. *B,* Ten weeks. *C,* Eleven weeks.

When the infant swallows milk, it rapidly fills the esophageal pouch and is regurgitated. Some of this milk passes into the trachea, resulting in gagging, coughing, and *respiratory distress.* Gastric contents may also reflux through the fistula into the trachea and lungs from the stomach. This causes choking and may result in pneumonia or *pneumonitis* (inflammation of the lungs).

Normal fetuses swallow amniotic fluid, which is absorbed through their intestines into their blood. It then passes via the placenta into the maternal blood via the placenta (see Chapter 8) and is excreted by the maternal kidneys. An excess of amniotic fluid *(polyhydramnios)* may be associated with esophageal atresia and tracheoesophageal fistula. This condition occurs because amniotic fluid cannot pass to the stomach and intestines for absorption and subsequent placental transfer to the mother's blood for disposal.

DEVELOPMENT OF BRONCHI AND LUNGS

The bulb-shaped *lung bud* that develops at the caudal end of the laryngotracheal tube during the fourth week (Fig. 12–5A) soon divides into two knoblike *bronchial buds* (Fig. 12–5B). These endodermal buds grow laterally into the *pericardioperitoneal canals,* the primordia of the pleural cavities (Fig. 12–6A). Together with the surrounding splanchnic mesenchyme, the bronchial

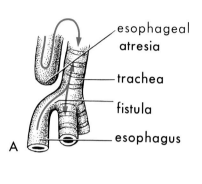

esophageal
atresia

trachea

fistula

esophagus

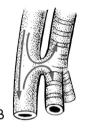

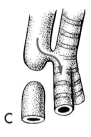

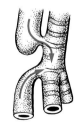

Figure 12–4. Sketches illustrating the four main types of tracheoesophageal fistula. Possible direction of flow of contents is indicated by arrows. Esophageal atresia, as illustrated in *A,* occurs in more than 85 per cent of cases. The abdomen rapidly becomes distended as the intestines fill with air. In *C,* air cannot enter the lower esophagus and stomach.

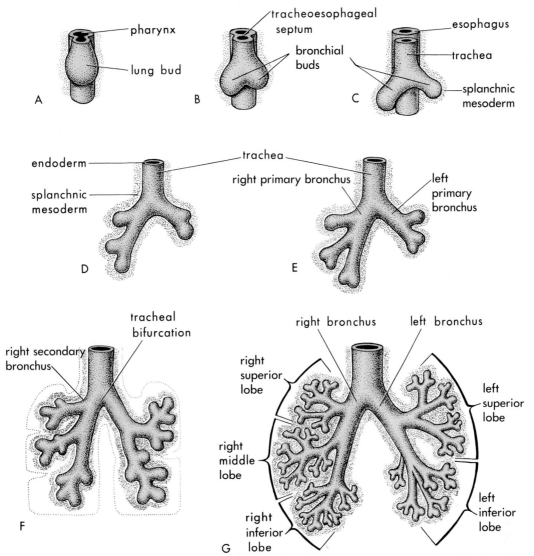

Figure 12–5. Drawings of ventral views, illustrating successive stages in the development of the bronchi and lungs. *A* to *C*, Four weeks. *D* and *E*, Five weeks. *F*, Six weeks. *G*, Eight weeks.

Figure 12–6. Diagrams illustrating growth of the developing lungs into the splanchnic mesoderm of the medial walls of the pericardioperitoneal canals (primitive pleural cavities). The development of the layers of the pleura is also shown. *A*, Five weeks. *B*, Six weeks.

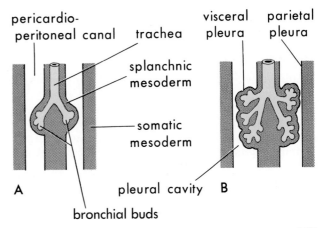

buds differentiate into the bronchi and their ramifications in the lungs.

The bronchial buds enlarge during the fifth week to form the primordia of the *primary bronchi.* Soon, the primary bronchi subdivide into *secondary bronchi* (Fig. 12–5C to F). On the right, the superior secondary bronchus will supply the superior lobe of the lung; whereas, the inferior secondary bronchus soon subdivides into two bronchi, one to the middle lobe of the right lung and the other to the inferior lobe. On the left, the two secondary bronchi supply the superior and inferior lobes of the lung (Fig. 12–5G).

Each secondary bronchus subsequently undergoes progressive branching; each branch bifurcates repeatedly into branches. Tertiary or *segmental bronchi,* ten in the right lung and eight or nine in the left, begin to form by the seventh week. As this occurs, the surrounding mesenchymal tissue also divides. Each tertiary or segmental bronchus with its surrounding mass of mesenchyme will form a *bronchopulmonary segment*[1].

About 17 orders of branches have formed by 24 weeks, and the respiratory bronchioles are present (Fig. 12–7A). Additional orders of airways develop after birth. As the bronchi develop, cartilaginous plates develop from the surrounding mesenchyme. This splanchnic mesenchyme also gives rise to the bronchial smooth musculature and connective tissue and to the pulmonary connective tissue and capillaries. As the lungs develop, they acquire a layer of *visceral pleura* from the splanchnic mesenchyme (Fig. 12–6B). With expansion, the lungs and pleural cavities grow caudally into the mesenchyme of the body wall and soon come to lie close to the heart (see Fig. 10–4). The thoracic body wall becomes lined by a layer of *parietal pleura* derived from the somatic mesoderm (Fig. 12–6B).

Maturation of the Lungs

Lung development can be divided into four stages.

THE PSEUDOGLANDULAR PERIOD (5 to 17 Weeks). Microscopically, the developing lung somewhat resembles an exocrine gland. The air-conducting system develops during this period, but respira-

---

[1] For a description of the adult anatomy of these clinically important segments, see Moore (1992).

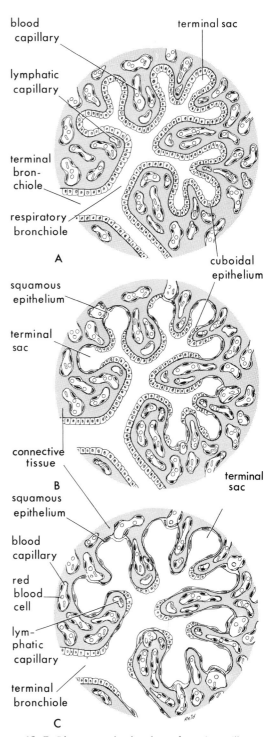

Figure 12–7. Diagrammatic sketches of sections, illustrating progressive stages of lung development. *A*, 24 weeks (late canalicular period). *B*, 26 weeks (early terminal sac period). *C*, Newborn infant (early alveolar period).

tion is not possible; hence, embryos or fetuses born during this period cannot survive.

THE CANALICULAR PERIOD (16 to 25 Weeks). This period overlaps the pseudoglandular period because cranial segments of the lung develop faster than caudal ones. During the canalicular period, the lumina of the bronchi and terminal bronchioles enlarge, and the lung tissue becomes highly vascular. Each terminal bronchiole gives rise to two or more *respiratory bronchioles* (Fig. 12–7A). Each of these then divides into three to six tubular passages called *alveolar ducts*. Toward the end of this period, the lining cells of these ducts become attenuated, permitting the blood capillaries to project as capillary loops into the future air spaces.

Respiration is possible toward the end of the canalicular period because some thin-walled *terminal sacs* (primitive alveoli) have developed at the ends of the respiratory bronchioles, and these regions are *well vascularized* (Fig. 12–7A). Although a fetus born toward the end of this period may survive if given intensive care (see Fig. 7–8), death often occurs because the respiratory and other systems are still immature.

THE TERMINAL SAC PERIOD (24 Weeks to birth). The alveolar ducts give rise to clusters of thin-walled terminal air sacs or primitive *pulmonary alveoli* (Fig. 12–7B and C). The capillary network proliferates rapidly in the mesenchyme around the developing alveoli, and some capillaries bulge into these thin-walled air sacs. There is concurrent active development of lymphatic capillaries. By 28 weeks, sufficient terminal air sacs are usually present to permit survival of a prematurely born infant. The development

of an adequate pulmonary vasculature is critical to the survival of premature infants.

During the terminal sac period, the type **II** alveolar epithelial cells or pneumocytes produce **pulmonary surfactant,** a complex mixture of phospholipids that covers the internal walls of the alveoli before birth (Whitsett, 1991). It is capable of lowering the surface tension at the air-alveolar interface, thereby maintaining patency of the alveoli and facilitating expansion of the lungs at birth.

THE ALVEOLAR PERIOD (late fetal period to childhood). The lining of the terminal air sacs becomes extremely thin, thus forming *characteristic pulmonary alveoli* (Fig. 12–7C). About one sixth of the adult number of alveoli are present at birth; their number increases until about the eighth year. The lungs at birth are about half inflated with liquid derived from the lungs, amniotic cavity, and tracheal glands; consequently, aeration of the lungs at birth involves rapid replacement of intra-alveolar fluid by air.

RESPIRATORY DISTRESS SYNDROME (RDS). Infants born prematurely are most susceptible to RDS. Shortly after birth these infants develop rapid and labored breathing. A deficiency of pulmonary surfactant is a major cause of *hyaline membrane disease* (HMD), a common cause of death in the perinatal period. The lungs are underinflated, and the alveoli contain a fluid of high protein content that resembles a hyaline (glassy) membrane.

Congenital anomalies of the lungs are uncommon. For a description of them, see Moore and Persaud (1993). Abnormal fissures or lobes are occasionally observed, but they are usually clinically unimportant.

SUMMARY

The lower respiratory system begins to develop around the middle of the fourth week from a median *laryngotracheal groove* in the floor of the primitive pharynx. This groove deepens to produce a *laryngotracheal diverticulum,* which soon becomes separated from the foregut by a *tracheoesophageal septum.* This results in the formation of the esophagus and the *laryngotracheal tube.* The endodermal lining of the laryngotracheal tube gives rise to the epithelium of the lower respiratory organs and the tracheobronchial glands. The splanch-

nic mesenchyme surrounding this tube forms the connective tissue, cartilage, muscle, and blood and lymphatic vessels of these organs.

Branchial (pharyngeal) arch mesenchyme contributes to the formation of the epiglottis and the connective tissue of the larynx. The laryngeal muscles and the cartilage skeleton of the larynx are derived from mesenchyme in the caudal branchial arches.

During the fourth week the laryngotracheal tube develops a lung bud which divides at its termination into two *bronchial buds* (lung buds). Each bud soon enlarges to form a *primary bronchus,* and then each of these gives rise to two new bronchial buds, which develop into *secondary bronchi.* The right inferior secondary bronchus soon divides into two bronchi. The secondary bronchi supply the lobes of the developing lungs. Each secondary bronchus undergoes progressive branching, forming tertiary or *segmental bronchi.* Branching continues until about 17 orders of branches have formed. Additional airways are formed after birth until about 24 orders of branches are formed.

Lung development is divided into four stages: (1) the *pseudoglandular period,* 5 to 17 weeks, when the bronchi and terminal bronchioles form, (2) the *canalicular period,* 16 to 25 weeks, when the lumina of the bronchi and terminal bronchioles enlarge, the respiratory bronchioles and alveolar ducts develop, and the lung tissue becomes highly vascular, (3) the *terminal sac period,* 24 weeks to birth, when the alveolar ducts give rise to terminal air sacs (primitive alveoli), and (4) the final stage of lung development, the *alveolar period,* from the late fetal period to about eight years of age when the characteristic pulmonary alveoli develop.

The respiratory system develops so that it is capable of immediate function at birth. To be capable of respiration, the lungs must acquire an *alveolocapillary membrane* that is sufficiently thin, and an adequate amount of *pulmonary surfactant* must be present. Surfactant is formed by secretory epithelial cells or type II pneumocytes.

Major congenital anomalies of the lower respiratory system are uncommon except for *tracheoesophageal fistula,* which is usually associated with esophageal atresia. These anomalies result from faulty partitioning of the foregut into the esophagus and trachea during the fourth and fifth weeks.

Commonly Asked Questions

1. I recently read in the newspaper about *fetal breathing.* Does the fetus breathe before birth?
2. What stimulates the baby to start breathing when it is born? Is "slapping the buttocks" necessary?
3. My sister's baby died about 72 hours after birth from *hyaline membrane disease* (HMD). What is this condition? Is its cause genetic or environmental?
4. Can an infant born 22 weeks after fertilization survive?

The answers to these questions are given on page 332.

REFERENCES

Ballard PL: Hormonal control of lung maturation. *Bailliere's Clin Endocrin Metabol* 3:723, 1989.

Behrman RE (ed): *Nelson Textbook of Pediatrics,* 14th ed. Philadelphia, WB Saunders, 1992.

Boyden EA: Development and growth of the airways. *In* Hodson WA (ed): *Development of the Lung.* New York, Marcel Dekker, 1977.

Chernick V, Kryger MH: Pediatric lung disease. *In* Kryger MH (ed): *Introduction to Respiratory Medicine,* 2nd ed. New York, Churchill Livingstone, 1990.

Cormack DH: *Essential Histology.* Philadelphia, JB Lippincott, 1993.

Crelin ES: Development of the lower respiratory system. *Clin Symp* 27(4), 1975.

Crelin ES: Development of the upper respiratory system. *Clin Symp* 28(3), 1976.

De Vries PA, De Vries CR: Embryology and development. *In* Othersen Jr, HB (ed): *The Pediatric Airway.* Philadelphia, WB Saunders, 1991.

Fowler CL, Pokorny WJ, Wagner ML, Kessler MS: Review of bronchopulmonary foregut malformations. *J Pediatr Surg* 23:793, 1988.

Harrison MR: The fetus with a diaphragmatic hernia: Pathology, natural history, and surgical management. *In* Harrison MR, Golbus MS, Filly RA: *The Unborn Patient. Prenatal Diagnosis and Treatment,* 2nd ed. Philadelphia, WB Saunders, 1991.

Hast HM: Developmental anatomy of the larynx. *In* Hinchcliffe R, Harrison D (eds): *Scientific Foundations of Otolaryngology.* London, W Heinemann, 1976.

Herbst JL: Esophagus. *In* Behrman RE (ed): *Nelson Textbook of Pediatrics,* 14th ed. Philadelphia, WB Saunders, 1992.

Hodson WA (ed): *Development of the Lung.* New York, Marcel Dekker, 1977.

Kozuma S, Nemoto A, Okai T, Mizuno M: Maturational sequence of fetal breathing movements. *Biol Neonate* 60 (suppl 1):36, 1991.

Landing BH: Pathogenetic considerations of respiratory tract malformations in humans. *In* Persaud TVN (ed): *Advances in the Study of Birth Defects. Cardiovascular, Respiratory, Gastrointestinal and Genitourinary Malformations,* Vol 6. New York, Alan R. Liss, 1982.

Moore KL: *Clinically Oriented Anatomy,* 3rd ed. Baltimore, Williams & Wilkins, 1992.

Moore KL, Persaud TVN: *The Developing Human: Clinically Oriented Embryology,* 5th ed. Philadelphia, WB Saunders, 1993.

O'Rahilly R, Boyden E: The timing and sequence of events in the development of the human respiratory system during the embryonic period proper. *Z Anat Entwicklungsgesch 141*:237, 1973.

O'Rahilly R, Müller F: *Developmental Stages in Human Embryos.* Carnegie Instn Wash Publ 637, Washington, DC, 1987.

O'Rahilly R, Tucker JA: The early development of the larynx in staged human embryos. Part 1. Embryos of the first five weeks (to stage 15). *Ann Otol Rhinol Laryngol 82 (suppl 7)*:1, 1973.

Patrick J, Gagnon R: Fetal breathing and body movement. *In* Creasy RK, Resnik R (eds): *Maternal-Fetal Medicine. Principles and Practice,* 2nd ed. Philadelphia, WB Saunders, 1989.

Salzberg AM: Congenital malformations of the lower respiratory tract. *In* Kendig EL, Jr, Chernick V (eds): *Disorders of the Respiratory Tract in Children,* 4th ed. Philadelphia, WB Saunders 1983.

Scarpelli EM (ed): *Pulmonary Physiology: Fetus, Newborn, Child and Adolescent,* 2nd ed. Philadelphia, Lea and Febiger, 1990.

Wells LJ, Boyden EA: The development of the bronchopulmonary segments in human embryos of horizons XVII and XIX. *Am J Anat 95*:163, 1954.

Whitsett JA: Molecular aspects of the pulmonary surfactant system in the newborn. *In* Chernick V, Mellins RB (eds): *Basic Mechanisms of Pediatric Respiratory Disease: Cellular and Integrative.* Philadelphia, BC Decker, 1991.

13

THE DIGESTIVE SYSTEM

The **primordium of the gut** (primitive gut) forms during the fourth week as the head, tail, and lateral folds incorporate the dorsal part of the yolk sac into the embryo (see Fig. 6–1). The endoderm of the primordial gut gives rise to most of the epithelium and glands of the digestive tract. The epithelium at the cranial and caudal extremities of the tract is derived from ectoderm of the *stomodeum* (primordium of the mouth) and *proctodeum* (anal pit), respectively (Fig. 13–1). The muscular, connective tissue, and other layers of the digestive tract are derived from the splanchnic mesenchyme surrounding the endoderm of the primitive gut. For descriptive purposes, the primordial gut is divided into three parts: foregut, midgut, and hindgut (Fig. 13–1).

THE FOREGUT

The adult derivatives of the foregut are: the pharynx and its derivatives (oral cavity, pharynx, tongue, tonsils, salivary glands, and upper respiratory system [discussed in Chapter 11]), lower respiratory system (described in Chapter 12), the esophagus, and stomach, the proximal part of the duodenum, the liver, biliary apparatus (gallbladder and bile duct system), and pancreas.

Development of the Esophagus

The partitioning of the trachea from the esophagus by the *tracheoesophageal septum* is described in Chapter 12 and is illustrated in Figure 12–2. Initially, the esophagus is short (Fig. 13–1), but it elongates rapidly, mainly due to the growth and descent of the lungs. The esophagus reaches its final relative length by the seventh week. The smooth muscle of the esophagus develops from the surrounding splanchnic mesenchyme. The epithelium of the esophagus and the esophageal glands are derived from endoderm. The epithelium of the esophagus proliferates and partly or completely obliterates the lumen, but recanalization of the esophagus normally occurs by the end of the embryonic period.

ESOPHAGEAL ATRESIA (see Fig. 12–4A). Esophageal atresia occurs in about one of 3000 to 4500 live births (Herbst, 1992) and is usually associated with *tracheoesophageal fistula*. About one third of affected infants are born prematurely. It may occur as a separate anomaly, but this is uncommon. Esophageal atresia is the result of deviation of the *tracheoesophageal septum* in a posterior direction (see Fig. 12–2); as a result, there is incomplete separation of the esophagus from the laryngotracheal tube.

When there is esophageal atresia, amniotic fluid cannot pass to the intestines for absorption and transfer via the placenta to the maternal blood for disposal; consequently, there is *polyhydramnios*, the accumulation of an excessive amount of amniotic fluid (p. 109). Newborn infants with esophageal atresia usually appear healthy, and their first swallows are normal. Suddenly, fluid returns through the nose and

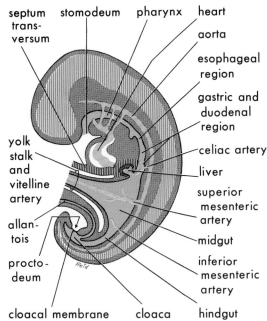

Figure 13–1. Drawing of a median section of a four-week embryo, showing the primitive gut and its blood supply. The blood vessels of the gut are derived from those that originally supplied the yolk sac.

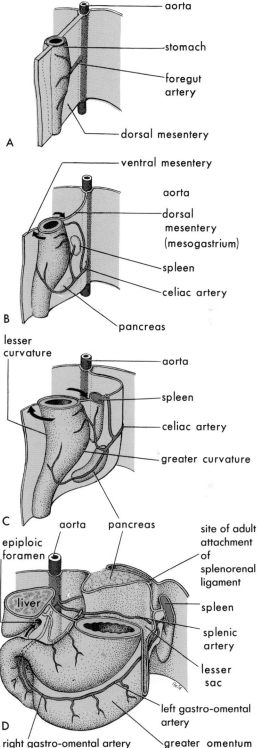

Figure 13–2. Drawings illustrating development and rotation of the stomach and formation of the greater omentum. *A*, About 30 days. *B*, About 35 days. *C*, About 40 days. *D*, About 48 days.

mouth, and *respiratory distress* occurs. Confirmation of the presence of esophageal atresia can be made by demonstrating that a radiopaque catheter cannot pass into the stomach. Surgical repair of esophageal atresia results in survival rates of more than 85 per cent.

ESOPHAGEAL STENOSIS. Narrowing of the esophagus is usually present in the distal third of the esophagus, either as a web or a long segment of esophagus with only a threadlike lumen. Esophageal stenosis is the result of incomplete recanalization of the esophagus during the eighth week of development.

Development of the Stomach

The stomach first appears as a fusiform dilatation of the caudal part of the foregut (Figs. 13–1 and 13–2A). This primordium soon enlarges and broadens ventrodorsally (Fig. 13–2B). During the next two weeks the dorsal border grows faster than the ventral border; this demarcates the *greater curvature of the stomach* (Fig. 13–2C). As it acquires its adult shape, the stomach rotates 90 degrees in a clockwise direction around its longitudinal axis.

The stomach is suspended from the dorsal wall of the abdominal cavity by a dorsal mesentery called the *dorsal mesogastrium* (Fig. 13–2A).

This mesentery is carried to the left during rotation of the stomach and formation of a cavity known as the *omental bursa* or lesser sac of peritoneum (Fig. 13–2A to C). The omental bursa communicates with the main peritoneal cavity or *greater peritoneal sac* through a small opening called the *omental (epiploic) foramen* (Fig. 13–2D).

A ventral mesentery or *ventral mesogastrium* (Fig. 13–2B) persists only in the region of the inferior end of the esophagus, stomach, and superior part of the duodenum. It attaches the stomach and duodenum to the developing liver and the ventral abdominal wall (Fig. 13–2D).

CONGENITAL HYPERTROPHIC PYLORIC STENOSIS. Anomalies of the stomach are uncommon except for hypertrophic pyloric stenosis. It affects one in every 150 male infants and one in every 750 females. Infants with this abnormality have a *marked thickening of the pylorus,* the distal sphincteric region of the stomach. The circular and, to a lesser degree, the longitudinal muscle in the pyloric region are hypertrophied. This results in severe narrowing *(stenosis)* of the pyloric canal and obstruction to the passage of food. As a result, the stomach becomes greatly distended, and the infant expels the stomach's contents with considerable force. This is referred to as *projectile vomiting.* Surgical relief of the pyloric obstruction is the usual treatment. Although the cause of congenital pyloric stenosis is unknown, the high incidence of the condition in both infants of monozygotic twins suggests the involvement of genetic factors. Multifactorial inheritance is likely (Shandling, 1992).

Development of the Duodenum

The duodenum begins to develop during the early part of the fourth week from the caudal part of the foregut, the cranial part of the midgut, and the splanchnic mesenchyme associated with these endodermal parts of the primitive gut. These parts grow rapidly and form a C-shaped loop that projects ventrally (Fig. 13–3B to D). The junction of the two embryonic parts of the duodenum is just distal to the entrance of the developing *bile duct* (common bile duct). During the fifth and sixth weeks, the lumen of the duodenum becomes reduced and is temporarily obliterated by epithelial cells, but it normally recanalizes by the end of the embryonic period.

DUODENAL STENOSIS. Narrowing of the duodenal lumen usually results from incomplete recanalization of the embryonic duodenum (Fig. 13–4A and B_3). Most stenoses involve the horizontal (third) and/or ascending (fourth) parts of the duodenum. The vomitus usually contains bile.

DUODENAL ATRESIA. Blockage of the lumen of the duodenum is not common (Fig. 13–4B) except in premature infants and in those with Down syndrome (see Fig. 9–4). During the solid stage of duodenal development, the lumen is completely filled with epithelial cells. If reformation of the lumen fails to occur by a process of vacuolization (Fig. 13–4D), a short segment of the duodenum is occluded. In infants with duodenal atresia, vomiting begins within a few hours of birth and *the vomitus almost always contains bile.* Most atresias involve the descending (second) and horizontal (third) parts of the duodenum and are located distal to the opening of the bile duct. Investigation of families with duodenal atresia suggests an autosomal recessive inheritance (Best et al., 1989).

Development of the Liver and Biliary Apparatus

The liver, gallbladder, and biliary duct system arise as a ventral outgrowth from the most caudal part of the foregut early in the fourth week (Fig. 13–3A). The *hepatic diverticulum* grows into the septum transversum[1] and later between the layers of the ventral mesentery where it rapidly enlarges and divides into two parts (Fig. 13–3B). The larger cranial part of the hepatic primordium becomes the liver. The endodermal cells form interlacing cords of *hepatic cells,* which soon become arranged in a series of branching and anastomosing plates. The fibrous and *hemopoietic (hematopoietic) tissue* and the *Kupffer cells* of the liver are derived from the splanchnic mesenchyme of the septum transversum (Fig. 13–1).

The liver grows rapidly and, from the fifth to tenth weeks, fills most of the abdominal cavity (see Fig. 6–10B). *Hemopoiesis* (formation and development of blood cells) begins during the sixth week. This activity is mainly responsible for the relatively large size of the liver (Fig. 13–3D). By nine weeks the liver represents

---

[1] A mass of splanchnic mesoderm between the developing heart and midgut (Fig. 13–1).

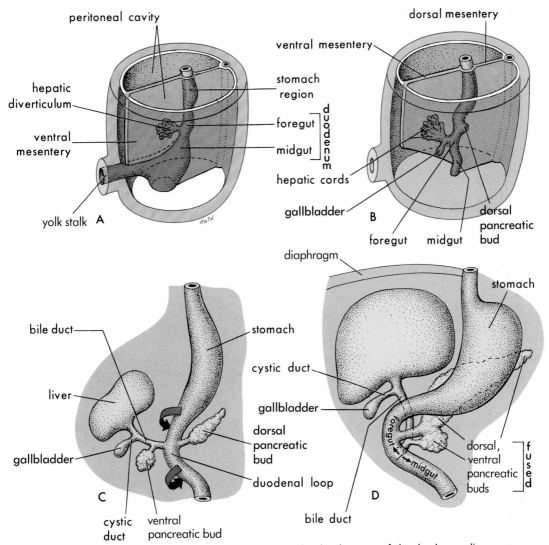

Figure 13–3. Drawings illustrating progressive stages in the development of the duodenum, liver, pancreas and extrahepatic biliary apparatus. *A,* Four weeks. *B* and *C,* Five weeks. *D,* Six weeks. The pancreas develops from dorsal and ventral buds that fuse to form the pancreas. Note that, as the result of the positional changes of the duodenum, the entrance of the bile duct into the duodenum gradually shifts from its initial position to a posterior one. This explains why the bile duct in the adult passes posterior to the duodenum and the head of the pancreas.

about ten per cent of the total weight of the fetus. *Bile formation* by the hepatic cells begins during the twelfth week.

The smaller caudal portion of the hepatic diverticulum expands to form the *gallbladder,* and its stalk becomes the *cystic duct* (Fig. 13–3C). The stalk connecting the hepatic and cystic ducts to the duodenum becomes the *bile duct.* Initially, the extrahepatic biliary apparatus is occluded with epithelial cells, but it is later recan-

alized due to vacuolization resulting from degeneration of the epithelial cells.

ANOMALIES OF THE LIVER. Minor variations of liver lobulation are common, but congenital anomalies of the liver are rare. Variations of the hepatic ducts, bile duct, and cystic duct are common and clinically significant (Moore, 1992). *Accessory hepatic ducts* may be present, and awareness of their possible presence is of

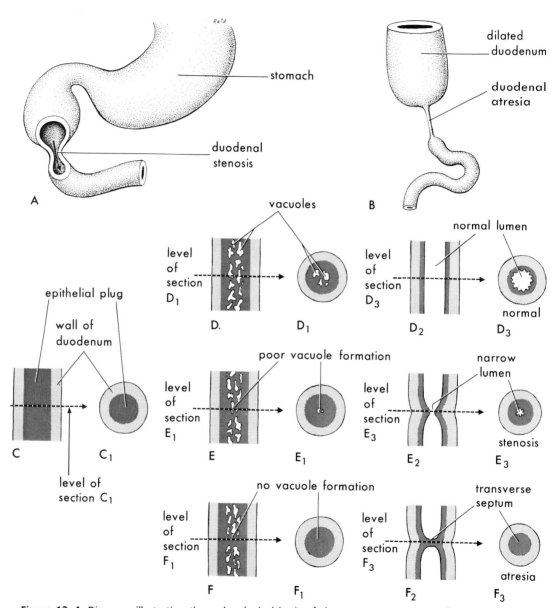

Figure 13–4. Diagrams illustrating the embryological basis of the two common types of congenital intestinal obstruction. *A,* Duodenal stenosis. *B,* Duodenal atresia. *C* to *F,* Diagrammatic longitudinal and transverse sections of the duodenum showing: (1) normal recanalization (*D* to D_3), (2) stenosis (*E* to E_3), and (3) atresia (*F* to F_3).

surgical importance. These accessory ducts are narrow channels running from the right lobe of the liver into the anterior surface of the body of the gallbladder. In some cases, the cystic duct opens into an accessory hepatic duct rather than into the common hepatic duct.

EXTRAHEPATIC BILIARY ATRESIA. This is the most serious anomaly of the extrahepatic biliary system and occurs in 1:10,000 to 1:15,000 live births. The most common form of extrahepatic biliary atresia is obstruction of the ducts at or superior to the *porta hepatis*.[2] Failure of the bile ducts to canalize often results from persistence of the solid stage of duct development. It also could result from liver infection during late fetal development. *Jaundice*[3] occurs soon after birth. When biliary atresia cannot be corrected surgically, the child may die if a liver transplant is not performed.

Development of the Pancreas

The pancreas develops from dorsal and ventral *pancreatic buds* of endodermal cells that arise from the caudal part of the foregut (Fig. 13–5A). As the duodenum grows and rotates to the right (clockwise), the ventral bud is carried dorsally and fuses with the dorsal bud (Fig. 13–5D and G). As the pancreatic buds fuse, their ducts anastomose. The fetal pancreas begins to secrete *insulin* at ten weeks (Moore and Persaud, 1993).

Development of the Spleen

Development of the spleen is mentioned here because this organ is derived from a mass of mesenchymal cells located between the layers of the dorsal mesentery of the stomach (Fig. 13–2). The spleen, a large vascular, lymphatic organ, acquires its characteristic shape early in the fetal period.

THE MIDGUT

The derivatives of the midgut are the small intestines, including most of the duodenum, the cecum, vermiform appendix, ascending colon, and the right half to two thirds of the transverse colon.

---

[2] The porta hepatis is a deep transverse fissure on the visceral surface of the liver, about 5 cm long in adults (Moore, 1992).

[3] Yellowish staining of the skin, sclerae, and deeper tissues with bile pigments.

Rotation and Fixation of the Midgut

At first the midgut communicates widely with the yolk sac (Fig. 13–1), but this connection soon becomes reduced to the narrow *yolk stalk* (Fig. 13–6A). As the midgut elongates it forms a ventral, U-shaped *midgut loop,* which projects into the proximal part of the umbilical cord (Fig. 13–6A). This "herniation" is a normal migration of the midgut into the extraembryonic coelom in the cord, which occurs because there is not enough room in the abdomen. The space shortage is caused mainly by the relatively massive liver and kidneys.

Within the umbilical cord, the midgut loop rotates counterclockwise, as viewed from the ventral aspect of the embryo (Fig. 13–6B), around the axis of the *superior mesenteric artery.* This brings the cranial limb of the midgut loop to the right and the caudal limb to the left (Fig. 13–6B and B_1). During the tenth week, the intestines return to the abdomen, the so-called *"reduction of the midgut hernia."* As the intestines return, they undergo further rotation (Fig. 13–6C_1 and D_1).

The decrease in the relative size of the liver and kidneys and enlargement of the abdominal cavity are likely important factors related to the return of the intestines to the abdomen. When the colon returns to the abdominal cavity, its cecal end rotates to the right side and enters the lower right quadrant of the abdomen (Fig. 13–6D and E).

Fixation of the Intestines

Lengthening of the proximal part of the colon gives rise to the *hepatic flexure* and the ascending colon (Fig. 13–6D and E). As the ascending colon assumes its final position, its mesentery is pressed against the posterior abdominal wall and gradually disappears. The other derivatives of the midgut loop retain their mesenteries.

The Cecum and Vermiform Appendix

The primordium of the cecum and appendix is the *cecal diverticulum.* This conical pouch appears during the sixth week on the caudal limb of the midgut loop (Fig. 13–6B). The distal end or apex of this blind sac does not grow as rapidly as the rest of it; thus, the appendix is initially a small diverticulum of the cecum (Fig. 13–6D). By birth, it is a long blind tube that is longer than in the adult.

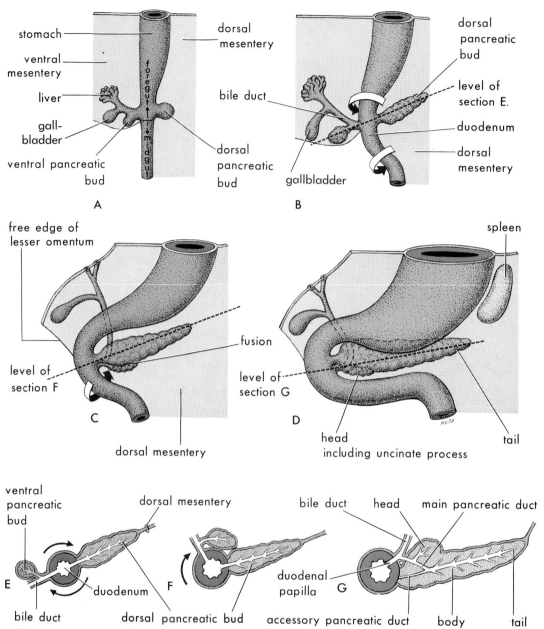

Figure 13–5. *A* to *D*, Schematic drawings showing successive stages in the development of the pancreas from the fifth to the seventh weeks. *E* to *G*, Diagrammatic transverse sections through the duodenum and developing pancreas. Growth and rotation *(arrows)* of the duodenum bring the ventral pancreatic bud toward the dorsal bud where they subsequently fuse. Note that the bile duct initially attaches to the ventral aspect of the duodenum and that it is carried around to the dorsal aspect as the duodenum rotates.

Figure 13–6. Drawings showing rotation of the midgut as seen from the left. *A*, Beginning of the sixth week, showing the midgut loop partially within the umbilical cord. Note the elongated, double-layered dorsal mesentery containing the superior mesenteric artery. *A₁*, Transverse section through the midgut loop, illustrating the initial relationship of the limbs of the midgut to the artery. *B*, Later stage, showing the beginning of midgut rotation. *B₁*, Illustrates the 90-degree counterclockwise rotation, which carries the cranial limb to the right. *C*, About ten weeks, showing the intestines returning to the abdomen. *C₁*, Illustrates a further rotation of 90 degrees. *D*, Slightly later, following return of intestines to the abdomen. *D₁*, Shows there has been a further 90-degree rotation of the gut, making a total of 270 degrees. *E*, Late fetal period, after rotation of the cecum to its normal position in the lower right quadrant of the abdomen and fixation of the gut.

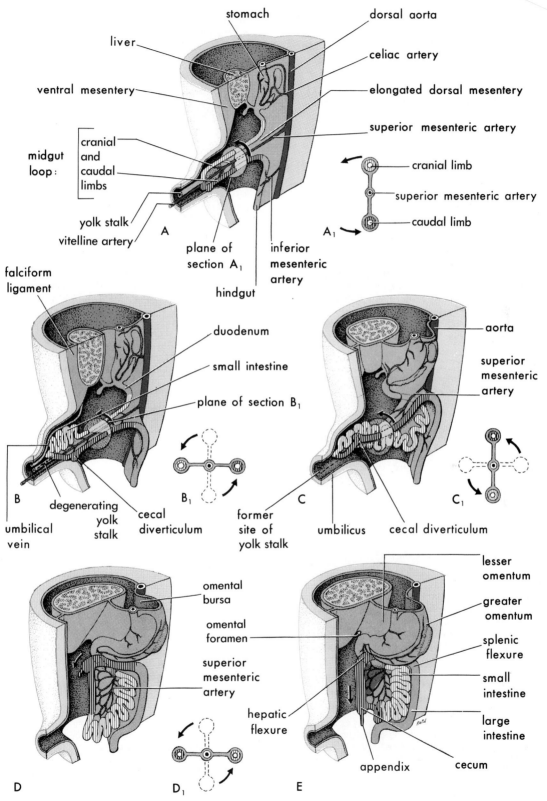

Figure 13-6. *See legend on opposite page.*

Anomalies of the Midgut

Congenital abnormalities of the intestine are common; most of them are anomalies of rotation and fixation of the gut.

CONGENITAL OMPHALOCELE (Fig. 13–7). This condition occurs once in about 5000 births and results from failure of the intestines to return to the abdomen during the tenth week. The hernia may consist of a single loop of bowel or it may contain most of the intestines. The covering of the hernial sac is the epithelium of the umbilical cord, which is formed by the amnion (see Figs. 8–12 and 8–15).

UMBILICAL HERNIA. When the intestines return normally to the abdominal cavity and then herniate either prenatally or postnatally through an *inadequately closed umbilicus,* an umbilical hernia forms. An umbilical hernia differs from an omphalocele in that the protruding mass (e.g., loop of bowel) is covered by subcutaneous tissue and skin. The hernia usually does not reach its maximum size until the end of the first month after birth. It ranges in size from that of a marble to a grapefruit.

NONROTATION OF THE MIDGUT (Fig. 13–8A). This relatively common condition, sometimes called "left-sided colon," is generally asymptomatic, but twisting of the intestine *(volvulus)* may occur. Nonrotation occurs when the midgut loop does not rotate as it enters the abdomen; as a result, the caudal limb of the loop returns to the abdomen first, and the small intestine lies on the right side of the abdomen and the entire large intestine on the left. When volvulus occurs, the superior mesenteric artery may be obstructed by the twisting. This results in infarction and gangrene of the bowel supplied by it.

MIXED ROTATION AND VOLVULUS (Fig. 13–8B). In this condition, the cecum lies just inferior to the pylorus of the stomach and is fixed to the posterior abdominal wall by peritoneal bands that pass over the duodenum. These bands and the frequent presence of volvulus of the intestines usually cause *duodenal obstruction.* This

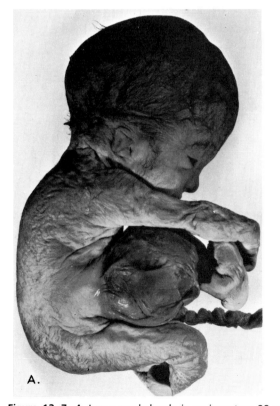

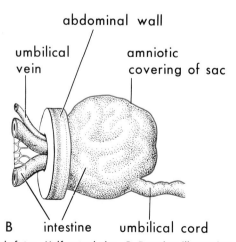

Figure 13–7. *A,* Large omphalocele in an immature 28-week fetus. Half actual size. *B,* Drawing illustrating the structure and contents of the hernial sac. This condition results when the intestines do not return to the abdominal cavity from the umbilical cord during the tenth week.

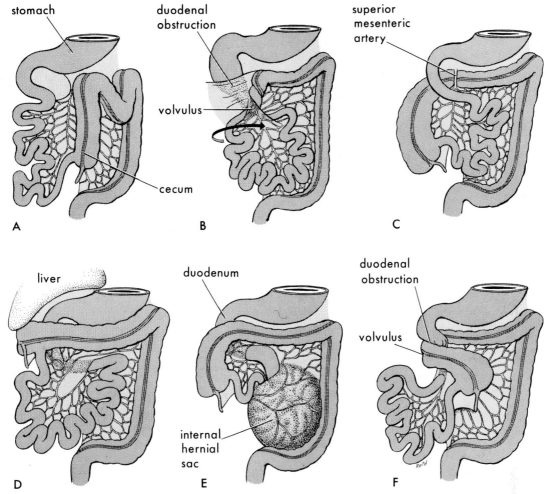

Figure 13–8. Drawings illustrating various abnormalities of midgut rotation. *A,* Nonrotation. *B,* Mixed rotation and volvulus (twisting) of the intestines. *C,* Reversed rotation. *D,* Subhepatic cecum. *E,* Paraduodenal hernia. *F,* Midgut volvulus.

type of malrotation results from failure of the midgut loop to complete the final 90 degrees of rotation (Fig. 13–6*D*); consequently, the terminal part of the ileum returns to the abdomen first.

SUBHEPATIC CECUM AND APPENDIX (Fig. 13–8*D*). Failure of the proximal part of the ascending colon to elongate during the third stage of rotation results in the cecum remaining near the liver as the abdomen enlarges. More common in males, this condition occurs in about six per cent of fetuses and results in the cecum and appendix being located in the subcostal region near the inferior surface of the liver. Some elongation of the colon occurs during childhood; hence, a subhepatic cecum is not common in adults.

MOBILE CECUM. In about ten per cent of people the cecum has an unusual amount of freedom. It may even herniate through the right inguinal canal. This condition results from incomplete fixation of the ascending colon.

MIDGUT VOLVULUS (Fig. 13–8*F*). In this condition the small bowel fails to enter the abdominal cavity normally; as a result, the mesentery fails to undergo normal fixation. Twisting of the intestine commonly occurs with incomplete rotation of the midgut loop. Because of the twisting of the intestines, *intestinal obstruction* and occlusion of the superior mesenteric artery frequently occur.

INTESTINAL STENOSIS AND ATRESIA (Fig. 13–4). Narrowing (stenosis) and complete obstruction (atresia) of the intestinal lumen occur most often in the duodenum and the ileum. The length of the area affected varies. Failure of an adequate number of vacuoles to form during recanalization leaves a transverse membrane or diaphragm, producing a so-called *diaphragmatic atresia*. Most jejunoileal atresias are probably caused by infarction of the fetal bowel due to impairment of its blood supply. This probably occurs during the tenth week when the intestines are returning to the abdomen. Malfixation of the gut predisposes it to strangulation and impairment of its blood supply due to *volvulus*.

ILEAL DIVERTICULUM (Fig. 13–9). This diverticulum of the ileum is one of the most common anomalies of the digestive tract. It occurs in two to four per cent of people and is three to five times more prevalent in males than in females. *An ileal (Meckel) diverticulum is of clinical significance* because it sometimes becomes inflamed and causes symptoms mimicking appendicitis. The wall of the diverticulum contains all layers of the ileum and may contain gastric and pancreatic tissues. The gastric mucosa often secretes acid, producing ulceration.

This type of ileal diverticulum represents the remnant of the proximal portion of the yolk stalk. It appears typically as a fingerlike pouch, 3 to 6 cm long, that arises from the antimesenteric border of the ileum 40 to 50 cm from the ileocecal junction. The diverticulum may be connected to the umbilicus by a fibrous cord or a fistula (Fig. 13–9C to F). For a discussion of other anomalies of the midgut, see Moore and Persaud (1993).

THE HINDGUT

The derivatives of the hindgut are: (1) The left one third to one half or distal part of the transverse colon, the descending colon and sigmoid colon, the rectum and superior portion of

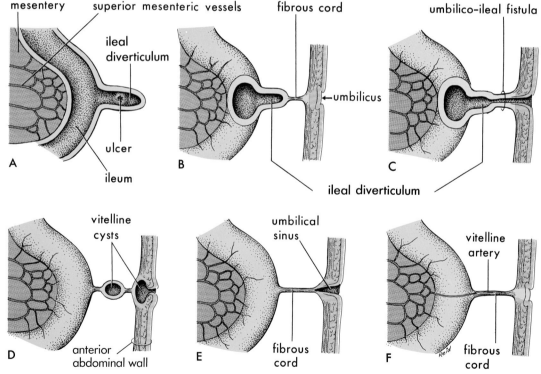

Figure 13–9. Drawings illustrating ileal (Meckel) diverticula and other remnants of the yolk stalk. *A*, Section of the ileum and a diverticulum with an ulcer. *B*, An ileal diverticulum connected to the umbilicus by a fibrous cord. *C*, Umbilico-ileal fistula resulting from persistence of the entire intra-abdominal portion of the yolk stalk. *D*, Vitelline cysts at the umbilicus and in a fibrous remnant of the yolk stalk. *E*, Umbilical sinus resulting from the persistence of the yolk stalk near the umbilicus. The sinus is not always connected to the ileum by a fibrous cord as illustrated. *F*, The yolk stalk has persisted as a fibrous cord connecting the ileum with the umbilicus. A persistent vitelline artery extends along the fibrous cord to the umbilicus.

the anal canal, (2) The epithelium of the urinary bladder and most of the urethra (see Chapter 14).

The hindgut extends from the midgut to the *cloacal membrane* (Fig. 13–10A and B). This membrane is composed of endoderm of the cloaca and ectoderm of the *proctodeum* or anal pit (Fig. 13–10D). The expanded terminal part of the hindgut called the *cloaca* receives the allantois ventrally (Figs. 13–1 and 13–10A).

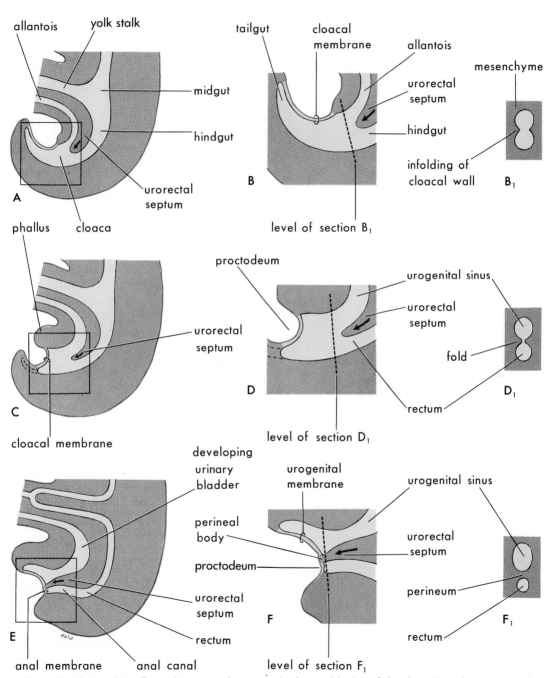

Figure 13–10. Drawings illustrating successive stages in the partitioning of the cloaca into the rectum and urogenital sinus by the urorectal septum. *A, C,* and *E,* Views from the left side at four, six, and seven weeks, respectively. *B, D,* and *F* are enlargements of the cloacal region. *B₁, D₁,* and *F₁* are transverse sections through the cloaca at the levels shown in *B, D,* and *F.*

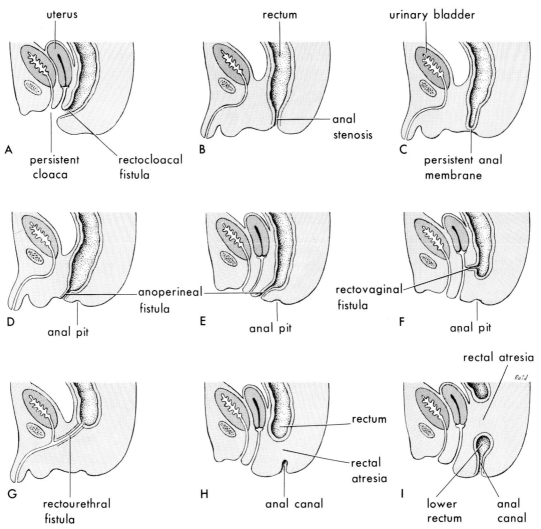

Figure 13–11. Drawings illustrating various anorectal anomalies. *A*, Persistent cloaca. Note the common outlet for the intestinal, urinary, and reproductive tracts. *B*, Anal stenosis. *C*, Membranous atresia (covered anus). *D* and *E*, Anal agenesis with fistula. *F*, Anorectal agenesis with rectovaginal fistula. *G*, Anorectal agenesis with rectourethral fistula. *H* and *I*, Rectal atresia. Sometimes the two segments of bowel are connected by a fibrous cord.

Partitioning of the Cloaca

The cloaca is divided by a coronal wedge of mesenchyme called the *urorectal septum*, which develops in the angle between the allantois and the hindgut (Fig. 13–10*B*). As this septum grows toward the cloacal membrane, infoldings of the lateral walls of the cloaca form (Fig. 13–10*B₁*). These folds grow toward each other and fuse, dividing the cloaca into two parts: (1) the *rectum* and cranial part of the *anal canal* dorsally, and (2) the *urogenital sinus* ventrally (Fig. 13–10*D* and *F*). By the seventh week, the urorectal sep-

tum has fused with the cloacal membrane, dividing it into a dorsal *anal membrane* and a larger ventral *urogenital membrane* (Fig. 13–10*E* and *F*). The anal membrane ruptures at the end of the eighth week, thus establishing the *anal canal*.

The area of fusion of the urorectal septum with the cloacal membrane is represented in the adult by the *perineal body*, the tendinous center of the perineum (Moore, 1992). This fibromuscular node is the *landmark of the perineum* where several muscles converge and insert. The urorectal septum also divides the *cloacal sphincter* into anterior and posterior parts. The posterior part becomes the external anal sphincter, and the anterior part develops into the superficial transverse perineal, bulbospongiosus, and ischiocavernosus muscles, and the urogenital diaphragm (Moore, 1992). This developmental fact explains why one nerve, the pudendal nerve, supplies all these muscles.

Imperforate Anus and Related Anomalies

Imperforate anus occurs once in about 5000 births; it is more common in males. *Most anorectal anomalies are the result of abnormal development of the urorectal septum,* resulting in incomplete separation of the cloaca into urogenital and anorectal portions (Fig. 13–10). If the urorectal septum fails to develop, a *persistent cloaca* remains (Fig. 13–11A). This is an uncommon anomaly.

ANAL AGENESIS WITH OR WITHOUT FISTULA (Fig. 13–11D and E). The anal canal may end blindly, but more often it has an abnormal opening *(ectopic anus)* or a fistula that opens into the perineum. The fistula may, however, open into the vulva in females or the urethra in males. Anal agenesis with fistula is the result of incomplete separation of the cloaca by the urorectal septum.

ANAL STENOSIS (Fig. 13–11B). The anus is in the normal position, but the anal canal is narrow. This anomaly probably results from a slight dorsal deviation of the urorectal septum as it grows caudally to fuse with the cloacal membrane. Sometimes only a small probe can be inserted into the anal canal.

MEMBRANOUS ATRESIA OF THE ANUS (Fig. 13–11C). The anus is in the normal position, but a thin layer of tissue separates the anal canal from the exterior. This condition results from failure of the anal membrane to perforate at the end of the eighth week.

ANORECTAL AGENESIS WITH OR WITHOUT FISTULA (Fig. 13–11F and G). The rectum ends blindly, superior to the puborectalis muscle (Moore, 1992). This is the most common type of anorectal anomaly, which accounts for about two thirds of anorectal defects. Although the rectum may end blindly, there is usually a fistula (communication) to the urethra in males or the vagina in females. Anorectal agenesis has an embryological basis similar to that of anal agenesis (i.e., incomplete separation of the cloaca by the urorectal septum).

RECTAL ATRESIA (Fig. 13–11H and I). The anal canal and rectum are present but they are separated. Sometimes the atretic (blocked) segment of rectum is represented by a fibrous cord. The cause of rectal atresia is abnormal recanalization or defective blood supply, as discussed with atresia of the small intestines (p. 197).

SUMMARY

The **primordium of the gut** forms during the fourth week by incorporation of the dorsal part of the yolk sac into the embryo. The primordial gut consists of three parts: foregut, midgut, and hindgut.

The **foregut** gives rise to the pharynx and lower respiratory system, the esophagus, stomach, duodenum (as far distally as the bile duct), pancreas, liver, and biliary apparatus. The *hepatic diverticulum* is an outgrowth of the endodermal epithelial lining of the foregut. The epithelial liver cords and primordia of the biliary system, which develop from the hepatic diverticulum, grow into the septum transversum. Between the layers of the ventral mesentery derived from the septum transversum, these primordial cells differentiate into the parenchyma of the liver and the lining of the ducts of the biliary system.

The *pancreas* is formed by dorsal and ventral pancreatic buds that originate from the endodermal lining of the foregut. When the duodenum rotates to the right, the ventral pancreatic bud moves dorsally and fuses with the dorsal pancreatic bud. The *ventral pancreatic bud* forms most of the head of the pancreas including the uncinate process. The *dorsal pancreatic bud* forms the remainder of the pancreas.

The **midgut** gives rise to the duodenum (distal to the bile duct), jejunum, ileum, cecum, appendix, ascending colon, and right or proximal half to two thirds of the transverse colon. The midgut herniates into the umbilical cord during the fifth week because of inadequate room in the abdomen. During the tenth week, the intestines return to the abdomen.

Omphaloceles, malrotations, and abnormalities of fixation result from failure of or abnormal return of the intestines to the abdomen. Because the gut is normally occluded at one stage, *stenosis* (narrowing), *atresia* (obstruction), and duplications may result if recanalization fails to occur or occurs abnormally. Various remnants of the yolk stalk may persist; an *ileal (Meckel) diverticulum* is common and is clinically significant.

The **hindgut** gives rise to the left or distal one third to half of the transverse colon, the descending and sigmoid colon, the rectum, and the superior part of the anal canal. The remainder of the anal canal develops from the proctodeum (anal pit). The expanded caudal part of the hindgut forms the **cloaca,** which is divided by the *urorectal septum* into the urogenital sinus and rectum. At first, the rectum is separated from the exterior by the *anal membrane*, but this normally breaks down at the end of the eighth week. Most anorectal anomalies arise from abnormal partitioning of the cloaca by the urorectal septum into anorectal and urogenital parts.

Commonly Asked Questions

1. About two weeks after birth my sister's baby began to vomit shortly after feeding. The unusual thing was that the vomitus was propelled about two feet. The physician told her that the baby had a stomach tumor that resulted in a narrow outlet from its stomach. Is there an embryological basis for this anomaly? Is the tumor malignant?
2. I have heard that infants with *Down syndrome* have an increased incidence of *duodenal atresia*. Is this true? Can the condition be corrected?
3. My friend said that his appendix is on his left side. Is this possible and if so, how could this happen?
4. A nurse told me about a friend of his who supposedly had two appendices and had had separate operations to remove them. Do people ever have two appendices?
5. What is *Hirschsprung's disease?* I have heard that it is a congenital condition resulting from a large bowel obstruction. Is this correct? If so, what is its embryological basis?
6. A nurse friend of mine told me that feces can sometimes be expelled from a baby's umbilicus. She said she has even seen urine dripping from the umbilicus. Was she "pulling my leg?"

The answers to these questions are given on page 332.

REFERENCES

Bear JC: Infantile hypertrophic pyloric stenosis: approaches to liability. *In* Persaud, TVN (ed): Advances in the Study of Birth Defects. vol. 6. *Cardiovascular, Respiratory, Gastrointestinal and Genitourinary Malformations*. New York, Alan R. Liss, 1982.

Beasley SW, Myers NA, Auldist AW (eds): *Oesophageal Atresia*. London, Chapman and Hall, 1991.

Best LG, Wiseman NE, Chudley AE: Familial duodenal atresia: A report of two families and review. *Am J Med Genet* 34:442, 1989.

Brassett C, Ellis H: Transposition of the viscera. *Clin Anat* 4:139, 1991.

Cobb RA, Williamson RCN: Embryology and developmental abnormalities of the large intestine. *In* Phillips SF, Pemberton JH, Shorter RG (eds): *The Large Intestine: Physiology, Pathophysiology, and Disease*. New York, Raven Press, 1991.

Filly RA: Sonographic anatomy of the normal fetus. *In* Harrison MR, Golbus MS, Filly RA (eds): *The Unborn Patient: Prenatal Diagnosis and Treatment*, 2nd ed. Philadelphia, WB Saunders, 1991.

Grand RJ, Watkins JB, Torti FM: Progress in gastroenterology: Development of the human gastrointestinal tract. A review. *Gastroenterology* 70:790, 1976.

Hamilton JR: Stomach and intestines. *In* Behrman RE (ed): *Nelson Textbook of Pediatrics*, 14th ed. Philadelphia, WB Saunders, 1992.

Herbst JJ: Disorders of the esophagus. *In* Behrman RE (ed): *Nelson Textbook of Pediatrics*, 14th ed. Philadelphia, WB Saunders, 1992.

Kleigman RM, Behrman RE: The umbilicus. *In* Behrman RE (ed): *Nelson Textbook of Pediatrics*, 14th ed. Philadelphia, WB Saunders, 1992.

McLean JM: Embryology of the pancreas. *In* Howat HT, Sarles H (eds): *The Exocrine Pancreas*. Philadelphia, WB Saunders, 1979.

Moore KL: *Clinically Oriented Anatomy*, 3rd ed. Baltimore, Williams & Wilkins, 1992.

Moore KL, Persaud TVN: *The Developing Human: Clinically Oriented Embryology,* 5th ed. WB Saunders, 1993.

Noordijk JA: Omphalocele and gastroschisis. *In* Persaud, TVN (ed): Advances in the Study of Birth Defects. vol. 6. *Cardiovascular, Respiratory, Gastrointestinal and Genitourinary Malformations.* New York, Alan R. Liss, 1982.

Raffensperger JF (ed): *Swenson's Pediatric Surgery.* Norwalk, Connecticut, Appleton & Lange, 1990.

Severn CB: A morphological study of the development of the human liver. I. Development of the hepatic diverticulum. *Am J Anat 131:*133, 1971.

Severn CB: A morphological study of the development of the human liver. II. Establishment of liver parenchyma, extrahepatic ducts, and associated venous channels. *Am J Anat 133:*85, 1972.

Shandling B: Congenital and perinatal anomalies of the gastrointestinal tract and intestinal rotation. *In* Behrman RE (ed): *Nelson Textbook of Pediatrics,* 14th ed. Philadelphia, WB Saunders, 1992.

Taeusch HW, Ballard RA, Avery ME (eds): *Schaffer and Avery's Diseases of the Newborn,* 6th ed. Philadelphia, WB Saunders, 1991.

Thompson JC: *Atlas of Surgery of the Stomach, Duodenum, and Small Bowel.* St. Louis, Mosby-Year Book, 1992.

von Dorsche HH: Inselorgan. *In* Hinrichsen KV (ed): *Humanembryologie.* Berlin Springer-Verlag, 1990.

14

THE UROGENITAL SYSTEM

Development of the urinary (excretory) and genital (reproductive) systems is closely associated, and parts of one system are used by the other and vice versa. Both the urinary and genital systems develop from the intermediate mesoderm (Fig. 14–1*B*), which extends along the dorsal body wall of the embryo.

During folding of the embryo in the horizontal plane, the intermediate mesoderm is carried ventrally and loses its connection with the somites. This longitudinal ridge of mesoderm on each side of the primitive aorta is called the *urogenital ridge* (Fig. 14–1*D*). It gives rise to parts of both the urinary and genital systems. The part of the urogenital ridge giving rise to the urinary system is known as the *nephrogenic cord or ridge* (Fig. 14–1*D*), and the part that gives rise to the genital system is known as the *gonadal or genital ridge* (see Fig. 14–10).

Development of the urogenital system is easier to understand when the urinary and genital systems are described separately. Development of the urinary system begins first.

THE URINARY SYSTEM

The urinary system consists of the following structures: (1) the *kidneys*, which excrete urine, (2) the *ureters*, which convey urine to (3) the *urinary bladder* where it is stored temporarily, and (4) the *urethra*, through which the urine is discharged to the exterior.

Development of the Kidneys and Ureters

Three sets of excretory organs develop in human embryos: the pronephros, mesonephros, and metanephros. The third set remains as the permanent kidneys.

The *pronephroi* (plural of pronephros) are transitory, nonfunctional structures that appear early in the fourth week (Figs. 14–2 and 14–3). The pronephroi soon degenerate, but most of their pronephric ducts are utilized by the next pair of kidneys.

Later in the fourth week, the *mesonephroi* (plural of mesonephros) appear caudal to the rudimentary pronephroi (Figs. 14–2 and 14–3). They function as interim kidneys until the permanent kidneys (metanephroi) develop and are able to function. By the end of the embryonic period, the mesonephroi have begun to degenerate and disappear, except for their ducts and a few tubules, which persist as genital ducts in males or vestigial remnants (Moore and Persaud, 1993).

The *metanephroi* (plural of metanephros) become the permanent kidneys. They appear early in the fifth week and begin to function about four weeks later. *Urine formation* continues actively throughout fetal life. The urine is excreted into the amniotic cavity and mixes with the amniotic fluid, which the fetus drinks. This fluid is absorbed by the intestine, and the waste products pass to the placenta for transfer to the

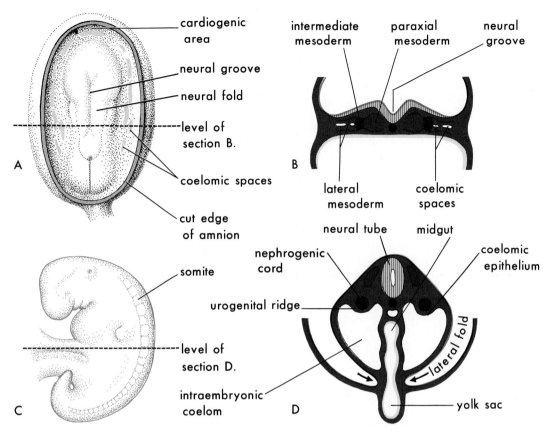

Figure 14–1. *A*, Dorsal view of an embryo during the third week (about 18 days). *B*, Transverse section of the embryo, showing the position of the intermediate mesoderm before folding of the embryo. *C*, Lateral view of an embryo during the fourth week (about 26 days). *D*, Transverse section of the embryo after lateral folding, showing the urogenital ridges produced by the nephrogenic cords of mesoderm.

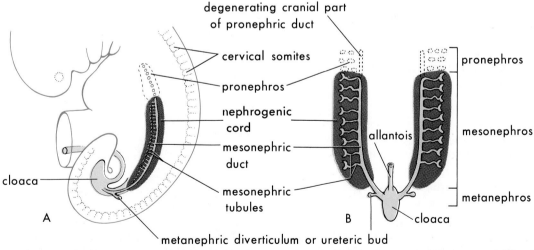

Figure 14–2. Diagrammatic sketches illustrating the three sets of excretory structures present in an embryo during the fifth week. *A*, Lateral view. *B*, Ventral view. The metanephros becomes the permanent kidney. For simplicity, the mesonephric tubules have been pulled to the sides of the mesonephric ducts. The tubules actually lie medial to ducts.

mother's blood and elimination by her kidneys (see Chapter 8, p. 109).

DEVELOPMENT OF THE PERMANENT KIDNEYS (Figs. 14–3 and 14–4). The metanephroi or permanent kidneys develop from two sources: the metanephric diverticulum (ureteric bud) and the metanephric mesoderm. Both primordia of the kidneys are of mesodermal origin. The *metanephric diverticulum* (ureteric bud) is a dorsal outgrowth from the mesonephric duct that grows into a mass of *metanephric mesoderm* (Fig. 14–3*B*). The stalk of the metanephric diverticulum becomes the ureter, and its expanded cranial end forms the *renal pelvis.* The pelvis divides into *major* and *minor calices,* from which collecting tubules soon grow (Fig. 14–3*C* to *E*).

Each collecting tubule undergoes repeated branching, forming successive generations of collecting tubules. Near the blind end of each arched collecting tubule (Fig. 14–4*A*), clusters of mesenchymal cells develop into *metanephric tubules* (Fig. 14–4*C*). The ends of these tubules are invaginated by an ingrowth of fine blood vessels called the *glomerulus,* to form a double-layered cup, the *glomerular capsule* (Bowman capsule). The renal corpuscle (glomerulus and capsule) and its associated tubules form a **nephron.** The distal convoluted tubule of the nephron contacts an arched collecting tubule, and the two tubules become confluent (Fig. 14–4*D*). Cell surface molecules probably play a role in the inductive interaction between the metanephric diverticulum and the metanephric mesoderm (Moore and Persaud, 1993).

The *fetal kidneys* are subdivided into lobes that are visible externally. This lobation diminishes toward the end of the fetal period, but the lobes are still indicated in the kidneys of a newborn infant. The lobation usually disappears during infancy as the nephrons grow. The increase in kidney size after birth mainly results from elongation of the proximal convoluted tubules and loops of Henle as well as an increase in interstitial tissue. Each kidney contains about one million nephrons. It is now believed that nephron formation is complete at birth except in premature infants. Functional maturation of the kidneys occurs after birth.

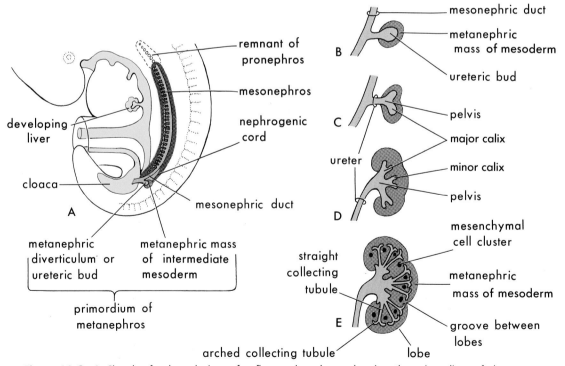

Figure 14–3. *A,* Sketch of a lateral view of a five-week embryo, showing the primordium of the metanephros or permanent kidney. *B* to *E,* Sketches showing successive stages in the development of the metanephric diverticulum (fifth to eighth weeks) into the ureter, renal pelvis, calices (calyces), and collecting tubules. The renal lobes illustrated in *E* are visible in the kidneys of newborn infants. The external evidence of the lobes normally disappears by the end of the first year.

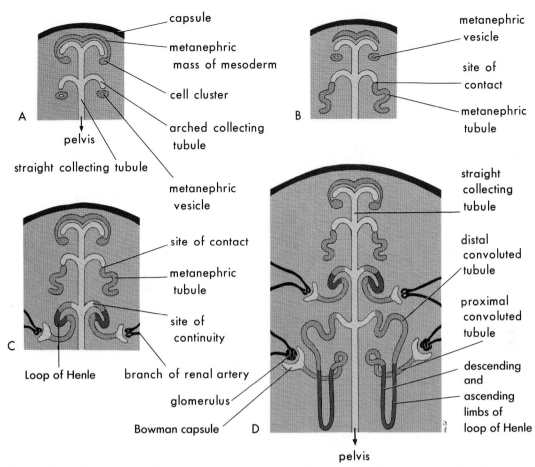

Figure 14–4. Diagrammatic sketches illustrating stages in the development of nephrons. Note that the metanephric tubules, the primordia of the nephrons, become continuous with the collecting tubules to form uriniferous tubules.

POSITIONAL CHANGES OF THE PERMANENT KIDNEYS (Fig. 14–5). Initially the kidneys are in the pelvis but they gradually come to lie in the abdomen. This "migration" is mainly the result of growth of the embryo's body caudal to the kidneys. In effect, the caudal part of the embryo grows away from the kidneys so that they progressively occupy more cranial levels. Eventually, they come to lie retroperitoneal or exterior to the peritoneum on the posterior abdominal wall. As the kidneys move out of the pelvis, they are supplied by arteries at successively higher levels. The caudal arteries normally degenerate as the kidneys ascend and new vessels form.

Congenital Anomalies of the Kidneys and Ureters

Some abnormality of the kidneys and ureters occurs in three to four per cent of newborn infants and includes variations in blood supply, abnormal positions, and urinary tract duplications. Variations in shape and position are most common.

RENAL AGENESIS (Fig. 14–6A). Unilateral absence of a kidney (agenesis) is relatively common, occurring about once in every 1000 newborn infants. *Unilateral renal agenesis* causes no symptoms and is usually not discovered during infancy. The other kidney undergoes compensatory hypertrophy and is able to perform the function of the missing kidney. *Bilateral renal agenesis* occurs about once in 3000 newborn infants and is incompatible with postnatal life. Most infants afflicted with this anomaly die at birth or a few hours later. Because no urine is excreted into the amniotic fluid, *bilateral renal agenesis is associated with oligohydramnios* (a deficiency in the amount of amniotic fluid).

Renal agenesis occurs when the metanephric diverticulum fails to develop or with early de-

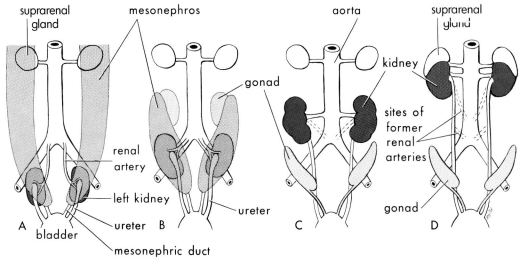

Figure 14–5. Diagrams of ventral views of the abdominopelvic region of embryos and fetuses (sixth to ninth weeks), showing the medial rotation and "ascent" of the kidneys from the pelvis to the abdomen. Note that, as the kidneys ascend, they are supplied by arteries at successively higher levels.

generation of this ureteric bud. Failure of the metanephric diverticulum to penetrate the metanephric mesoderm results in absence of kidney development because no nephrons are induced by the collecting tubules to develop from the metanephric mesoderm.

ECTOPIC KIDNEYS (Fig. 14–6*B* and *E*). One or both kidneys may be in an abnormal position. Usually they are more inferior than usual and have not rotated. Most ectopic kidneys are located in the pelvis, but some are in the inferior part of the abdomen. *Pelvic kidneys* and other forms of ectopic kidney result from failure of the kidneys to "ascend." Pelvic kidneys are close to each other and may fuse to form a round mass known as a discoid or *"pancake kidney"* (Fig. 14–6*E*).

Ectopic kidneys receive their blood supply from blood vessels near them; they are often supplied by multiple vessels. An unusual type of ectopic kidney is a *unilateral fused kidney* (Fig. 14–6*D*). The developing kidneys fuse while in the pelvis, and one kidney "ascends" to its normal position, carrying the other one across the median plane with it.

HORSESHOE KIDNEY (Fig. 14–7). In one in about 500 infants, the kidneys are fused, usually at their inferior poles. About seven per cent of persons with Turner syndrome (p. 122) have horseshoe kidneys (Behrman, 1992). The large, U-shaped kidney is usually located in the hypogastrium (i.e., inferior to the stomach) anterior to the inferior lumbar vertebrae. Normal ascent was prevented because it was caught by the root of the inferior mesenteric artery (Moore, 1992). A *horseshoe kidney usually produces no*

symptoms because the collecting system commonly develops normally, and the ureters enter the bladder. If urinary outflow is impeded, signs and symptoms of obstruction and/or infection may appear.

MULTIPLE RENAL VESSELS. Vascular variations result from persistence of embryonic vessels that normally disappear when the definitive renal arteries form. Variations in the number of renal arteries and in their position with respect to the renal veins are common. About 25 per cent of kidneys have two or more renal arteries. *Supernumerary arteries*, usually two or three, are about twice as common as supernumerary veins, and they usually arise at the level of the kidney. Variations in blood supply are most common in ectopic kidneys. Accessory vessels may arise from the suprarenal artery and pass to the superior pole of the kidney. Polar vessels may also arise from the aorta and pass to the inferior pole of the kidney. Sometimes an accessory renal artery supplying the inferior pole of the kidney compresses and obstructs the ureter at the ureteropelvic junction.

DUPLICATIONS OF THE URINARY TRACT (Fig. 14–6). Duplications of the abdominal part of the ureter and renal pelvis are common, but a *supernumerary kidney* is uncommon. These abnormalities result from division of the metanephric diverticulum (ureteric bud). The extent of ureteral duplication depends on completeness of the division of the diverticulum. Incomplete division results in a divided kidney with a bifid ureter (Fig. 14–6*B*). Complete division of the diverticulum results in a supernumerary (extra) or a *double kidney* with a bifid ureter (Fig.

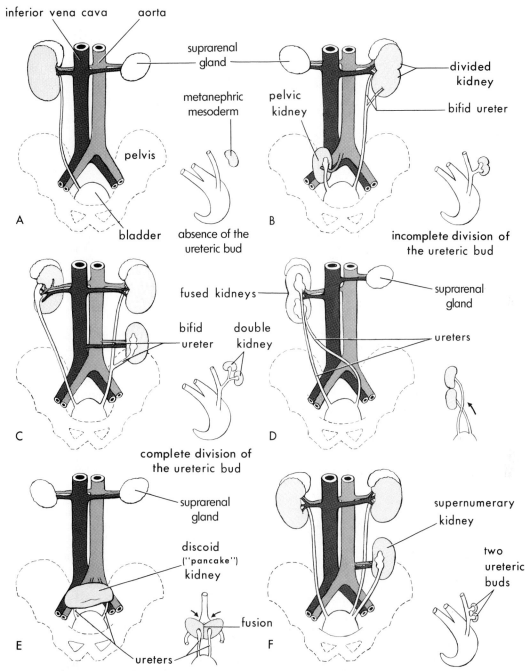

Figure 14–6. Drawings illustrating various congenital anomalies of the urinary system. The small sketch at the lower right of each drawing illustrates the probable embryological basis of the anomaly. *A*, Unilateral renal agenesis. *B*, Right side, pelvic kidney; left side, bifid ureter. *C*, Right side, malrotation of the kidney; left side, bifid ureter and two kidneys. *D*, Crossed renal ectopia. The left kidney crossed to the right side and fused with the right kidney. *E*, "Pancake" or discoid kidney resulting from fusion of the unascended kidneys. *F*, Supernumerary left kidney resulting from the development of two ureteric buds.

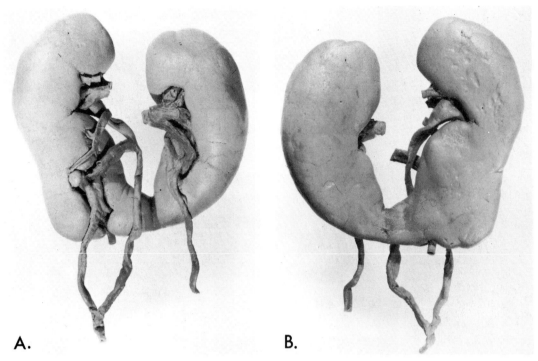

A.   **B.**

Figure 14–7. Photographs of a typical horseshoe kidney resulting from fusion of the inferior poles of the embryonic kidneys early in development. *A,* Anterior view. *B,* Posterior view. Half actual size. The larger right kidney has a bifid ureter.

14–6) or with separate ureters. A supernumerary kidney with its own ureter probably results from the formation of an extra ureteric bud (Fig. 14–6F).

ECTOPIC URETERIC ORIFICES. A ureter that opens anywhere except into the urinary bladder has an ectopic orifice. *Ureteric ectopia* occurs when the ureter is not incorporated into the posterior part of the urinary bladder (Fig. 14–8). In males, an ectopic ureter usually opens into the neck of the bladder or into the prostatic portion of the urethra (Moore, 1992), but it may enter the ductus deferens, prostatic utricle, or a seminal vesicle. In females, ectopic ureteric orifices may be in the bladder neck, urethra, vagina, or vestibule of the vagina (Behrman, 1992). *Incontinence* is the common complaint resulting from an ectopic ureteric orifice because the urine flowing from the ectopic orifice does not enter the bladder; instead, it continually dribbles from the urethra in males and the urethra and/or vagina in females.

Development of the Urinary Bladder

Division of the cloaca by the *urorectal septum* into a dorsal rectum and a ventral urogenital sinus is described in Chapter 13 and illustrated in Figure 14–8. The urinary bladder is derived from the *urogenital sinus* and adjacent splanchnic mesenchyme. As the bladder enlarges, caudal portions of the mesonephric ducts are incorporated into its dorsal wall (Fig. 14–8D). As the mesonephric ducts are absorbed, the ureters come to open separately into the urinary bladder (Fig. 14–8F). In infants and children the urinary bladder, even when empty, is in the abdomen. It begins to enter the pelvis major at about six years of age but does not enter the pelvis minor and become a pelvic organ until after puberty (Moore, 1992).

EXSTROPHY OF THE BLADDER (Fig. 14–9). This severe anomaly occurs only about once in every 10,000 to 40,000 births. It chiefly occurs in males. Exposure and protrusion of the posterior wall of the urinary bladder characterize this congenital anomaly. The trigone of the bladder and the ureteric orifices are exposed, and urine dribbles intermittently from the everted bladder. *Epispadias* (see Fig. 14–17D) and wide separation of the pubic bones are associated with complete exstrophy of the bladder. In some cases the penis or clitoris is divided, and the halves of the scrotum or labia majora are widely separated.

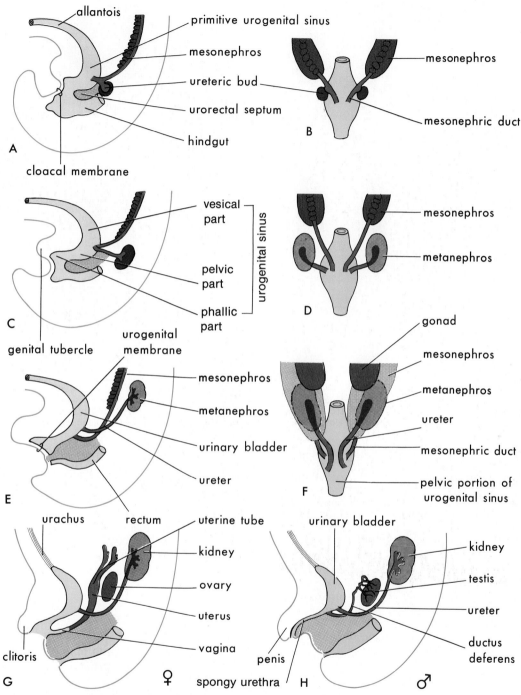

Figure 14–8. Diagrams showing: (1) division of the cloaca into the urogenital sinus and rectum, (2) absorption of the mesonephric ducts, (3) development of the urinary bladder, urethra, and urachus, and (4) changes in the location of the ureters. *A*, Lateral view of the caudal half of a five-week embryo. *B*, *D*, and *F*, Dorsal views. *C*, *E*, *G*, and *H*, Lateral views. The stages shown in *G* and *H* are reached by 12 weeks.

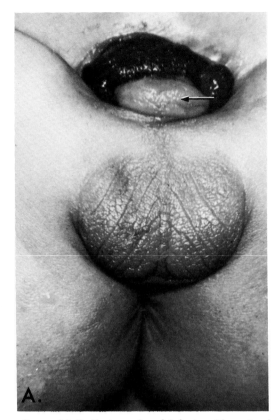 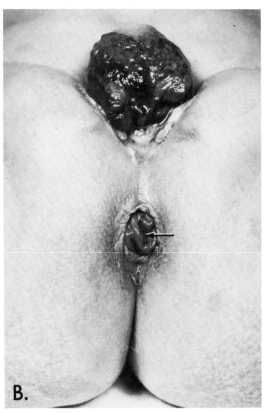

Figure 14–9. Photographs of infants with exstrophy of the urinary bladder. *A,* Male. Epispadias is also present and the penis *(arrow)* is small and flattened. (Courtesy of Dr. Colin C. Ferguson, Children's Centre, Winnipeg, Canada.) *B,* Female. The arrow indicates a slight prolapse of the rectum. (Courtesy of Mr. Innes Williams, Genitourinary Surgeon, The Hospital for Sick Children, Great Ormond Street, London, England.)

Exstrophy of the bladder is caused by incomplete median closure of the inferior part of the anterior abdominal wall. The fissure involves not only the anterior abdominal wall but also the anterior wall of the urinary bladder. The defective closure is due to failure of mesenchymal cells to migrate between the surface ectoderm and the urogenital sinus during the fourth week; as a result, no muscle and connective tissue form in the anterior abdominal wall over the urinary bladder. Later, the thin epidermis and the anterior wall of the bladder rupture, causing a wide communication between the exterior and the mucous membrane of the bladder, as shown in Figure 14–9.

Development of the Urethra

The epithelium of most of the male urethra and the entire female urethra is derived from endoderm of the urogenital sinus (see Figs. 14–8 and 14–14). The distal part of the urethra in the male is derived from the *glandular plate.* This ectodermal plate grows from the tip of the glans penis to meet the part of the spongy urethra derived from the phallic part of the urogenital sinus. The glandular plate becomes canalized and joins the rest of the urethra; consequently, the epithelium of the terminal part of the urethra is derived from surface ectoderm (see Fig. 14–14). The connective tissue and smooth muscle of the urethra in both sexes are derived from the adjacent splanchnic mesenchyme.

THE SUPRARENAL GLANDS[1]

The cortex and medulla of the suprarenal (adrenal) glands have different origins. The *cortex*

---

[1] The *suprarenal (adrenal)* glands are described in this chapter for two reasons: (1) they are closely related to the superior poles of the kidneys, and (2) congenital *adrenal hyperplasia* (CAH) causes virilization (masculinization) of female external genitalia (e.g., enlargement of the clitoris); this *accounts for most cases of female pseudohermaphroditism* (p. 221).

develops from mesoderm and the *medulla* from neural crest cells. The cells that form the medulla are derived from the neural crest, which appears as the neural tube forms (see Chapter 5). The cells that form the *suprarenal cortex* are derived from the coelomic epithelium lining the posterior abdominal wall. During the fifth week, cells migrate from adjacent sympathetic ganglia and form a mass on the medial side of the fetal cortex (Fig. 14–10C). These cells are gradually encapsulated by the fetal cortex as they differentiate into the secretory cells of the suprarenal medulla (Fig. 14–10D). Differentiation of the characteristic suprarenal cortical zones begins during the late fetal period but is not complete until the end of the third year.

> **CONGENITAL ADRENAL HYPERPLASIA (CAH).** Hyperplasia of the fetal suprarenal cortex during the fetal period usually results in *female pseudohermaphroditism* (see Fig. 14–16). The adrenogenital syndrome associated with CAH manifests itself in various clinical forms. *Congenital hyperplasia of the suprarenal glands* is caused by a genetically determined deficiency of suprarenal cortical enzymes that are necessary for the synthesis of various steroid hormones (Thompson et al., 1991). The reduced hormone output results in an increased release of adrenocorticotropic hormone (ACTH), which causes suprarenal hyperplasia and overproduction of androgens by the hyperplastic suprarenal glands. In females, this causes masculinization; in males, the excess androgens may cause precocious sexual development.

THE GENITAL SYSTEM

Although the chromosomal and genetic sex of an embryo is determined at fertilization by the kind of sperm that fertilizes the ovum (p. 29), there is no morphological indication of a sex difference until the seventh week when the *gonads* (future ovaries or testes) begin to acquire sexual characteristics. The early genital system is similar in both sexes; therefore, the period of early genital development is referred to as the *indifferent or undifferentiated stage* of sexual development.

Development of Testes and Ovaries

The gonads (testes and ovaries) are derived from three sources: (1) the *mesothelium* (derived from mesoderm) lining the posterior abdominal wall, (2) underlying *mesenchyme*, and (3) the *primordial germ cells.*

THE INDIFFERENT OR UNDIFFERENTIATED GONADS (Figs. 14–10 and 14–11A). The gonads are first indicated during the fifth week when a thickened area of coelomic epithelium develops on the medial aspect of the mesonephros. Proliferation of these epithelial cells produces a bulge on the medial side of each mesonephros known as the *gonadal ridge*. Fingerlike epithelial cords called *primary sex cords* soon grow from the gonadal ridges into the underlying mesenchyme (Fig. 14–10D). The indifferent gonad now consists of an external *cortex* and an internal *medulla*.

In embryos with an XX sex chromosome complex, the cortex normally differentiates into an ovary and the medulla regresses. In embryos with an XY sex chromosome complex, the medulla normally differentiates into a testis and the cortex regresses. Large spherical primitive sex cells called **primordial germ cells** are visible early in the fourth week on the wall of the yolk sac. These cells later migrate along the dorsal mesentery of the hindgut to the gonadal ridges (Fig. 14–10) and become incorporated in the primary sex cords.

SEX DETERMINATION. Chromosomal and *genetic sex* are established at fertilization and depend upon whether an X-bearing sperm or a Y-bearing sperm fertilizes the ovum. *Gonadal sex* (i.e., the type of gonads that develop) is determined by the sex chromosome complex (XX or XY) that is present. Development of the male *phenotype* (appearance) requires a Y chromosome, but only the short arm of this chromosome is critical for sex determination. The gene for a *testis-determining factor* (TDF) has been localized in the "sex-determining region of the Y" (SRY) chromosome (Thompson et al., 1991). Two X chromosomes are required for the development of the female phenotype.

The Y chromosome has a strong, testis-determining effect on the medulla of the indifferent gonad. It is the presence of TDF that determines testicular differentiation. Under the influence of this determining factor, the primary sex cords differentiate into seminiferous tubules (Fig. 14–11B and D). The absence of a Y chromosome (i.e., an XX sex chromosome complement) results in formation of an ovary (Fig. 14–11C and E); thus, the type of sex chromosome complex established at fertilization determines the type of gonad that develops from the indifferent gonad.

DEVELOPMENT OF TESTES (Fig. 14–11B, D, and F). In embryos with a Y chromosome, TDF

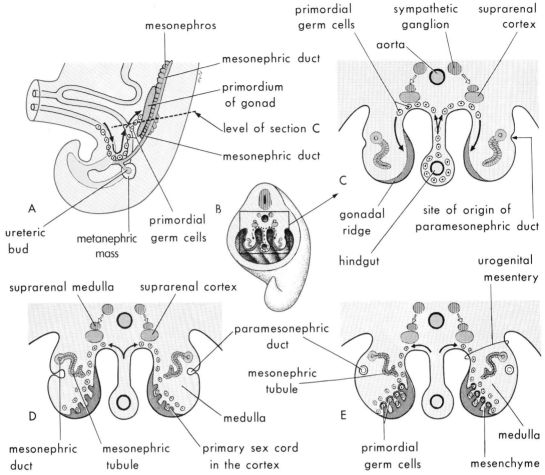

Figure 14–10. *A*, Sketch of a five-week embryo, illustrating the migration of primordial germ cells from the yolk sac. *B*, Three-dimensional sketch of the caudal region of a five-week embryo, showing the location and extent of the gonadal ridges on the medial aspect of the urogenital ridges. *C*, Transverse section showing the primordium of the suprarenal glands, the gonadal ridges, and the migration of primordial germ cells into the developing gonads (ovaries or testes). *D*, Transverse section through a six-week embryo, showing the primary sex cords and the developing paramesonephric ducts. *E*, Similar section at later stage, showing the indifferent gonads and the mesonephric and paramesonephric ducts.

Figure 14–11. Schematic sections illustrating differentiation of the indifferent gonads into testes or ovaries. *A*, Six weeks, showing the indifferent or undifferentiated gonads composed of an outer cortex and an inner medulla. *B*, Seven weeks, showing testes developing under the influence of the testis-determining factor (TDF) on the Y chromosome. Note that the primary sex cords have become seminiferous cords. *C*, 12 weeks, showing ovaries beginning to develop. Cortical cords have extended from the surface epithelium, displacing the primary sex cords centrally into the mesovarium where they form the rudimentary rete ovarii. *D*, Testis at 20 weeks, showing the rete testis and seminiferous tubules derived from the seminiferous cords. An efferent ductule has developed from a mesonephric tubule, and the mesonephric duct has become the ductus epididymis (duct of the epididymis). *E*, Ovary at 20 weeks, showing the primordial follicles formed from the cortical cords. *F*, Section of a seminiferous tubule from a 20-week fetus. Note that no lumen is present at this stage and that the seminiferous epithelium is composed of two kinds of cells. *G*, Section from the ovarian cortex of a 20-week fetus, showing three primordial follicles.

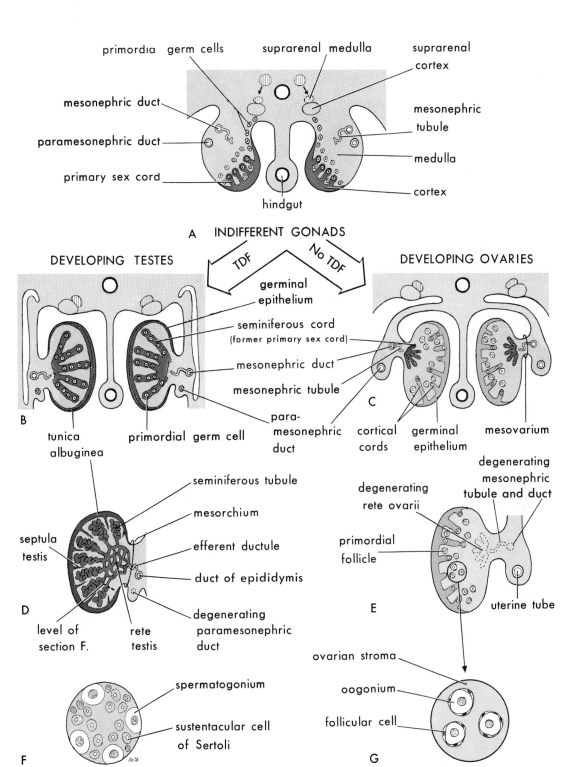

Figure 14–11. *See legend on opposite page.*

induces the primary sex cords to condense and branch. Their ends anastomose to form the *rete testis*. The sex cords, now called *seminiferous cords*, lose their connections with the germinal epithelium as a thick fibrous capsule called the *tunica albuginea* develops (Fig. 14–11*B* and *D*). The seminiferous cords develop into the seminiferous tubules, tubuli recti, and rete testis. The walls of the seminiferous tubules are composed of two kinds of cell (Fig. 14–11*F*): supporting cells or *Sertoli cells*, derived from the surface epithelium, and *spermatogonia* that differentiate from primordial germ cells.

The seminiferous tubules become separated by mesenchyme that gives rise to the *interstitial cells* (of Leydig). By about the eighth week, these cells produce the male sex hormone *testosterone*, which induces masculine differentiation of the genital ducts and external genitalia. In addition to testosterone, the testes produce a *müllerian-inhibiting factor* (MIF) that suppresses development of the paramesonephric (müllerian) ducts (Fig. 14–12).

DEVELOPMENT OF OVARIES (Fig. 14–11*C*, *E* and *G*). In female 46,XX embryos, gonadal development occurs very slowly. The X chromosomes bear genes for ovarian development, but an autosomal gene also appears to play a role in ovar-

ian organogenesis (DiGeorge, 1992). The ovary is not identifiable until about the tenth week; thereafter, the characteristic cortex begins to develop. The primary sex cords do not become prominent in the gonads of female embryos, but they extend into the medulla and form a rudimentary *rete ovarii*. The rete ovarii, comparable to the rete testis, is a transitory remnant of the cortical cords.

During the fetal period, secondary sex cords called *cortical cords* extend from the surface epithelium into the underlying mesenchyme (Fig. 14–11*C*). As these cords increase in size, *primordial germ cells* are incorporated into them. The cords break up into isolated cell clusters called *primordial follicles*, consisting of *oogonia* derived from primordial germ cells, surrounded by a layer of follicular cells (Fig. 14–11*E* and *G*). Active mitosis of oogonia occurs during fetal life, producing thousands of these primitive germ cells. *No oogonia form postnatally*. All oogonia enlarge to become *primary oocytes* before birth (see Fig. 2–5).

Development of Genital Ducts

THE INDIFFERENT STAGE (Figs. 14–10 and 14–12). Two pairs of genital ducts develop in

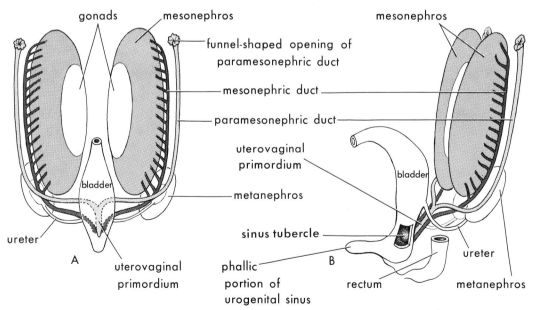

Figure 14–12. *A*, Sketch of a frontal view of the posterior abdominal wall of a seven-week embryo, showing the two pairs of genital ducts present during the indifferent stage. *B*, Lateral view of a nine-week fetus, showing the sinus tubercle (müllerian tubercle) on the posterior wall of the urogenital sinus. It becomes the hymen in females and the seminal colliculus in males. This colliculus (L., mound) is an elevated area on the posterior wall of the prostatic portion of the urethra upon which open the ejaculatory ducts (Moore, 1992).

both sexes: *mesonephric (wolffian) ducts* and *paramesonephric (müllerian) ducts.* The paramesonephric ducts come together in the median plane in both sexes and fuse into a Y-shaped *uterovaginal primordium* or canal (Fig. 14–12A). The funnel-shaped openings of the paramesonephric ducts open into the coelomic cavity (future peritoneal cavity). The uterovaginal primordium projects into the dorsal wall of the urogenital sinus and produces an elevation called the *sinus tubercle* (Fig. 14–12B).

Testosterone produced by the interstitial cells stimulates development of the mesonephric ducts into the male genital tract, and the MIF produced by the sustentacular cells suppresses development of the paramesonephric ducts, which develop into the female genital tract in female fetuses.

DEVELOPMENT OF MALE GENITAL DUCTS. As the mesonephros degenerates, some mesonephric tubules near the testis persist and are transformed into *efferent ductules* (Fig. 14–13A). These ductules open into the mesonephric duct, which becomes the *ductus epididymis* in this region. Beyond the epididymis (coiled duct of the epididymis), the mesonephric duct acquires a thick investment of smooth muscle and becomes the *ductus (vas) deferens.* A lateral outgrowth from the caudal end of each mesonephric duct gives rise to a *seminal vesicle.* The part of the mesonephric duct between the duct of this gland and the urethra becomes the *ejaculatory duct.* The remainder of the male genital duct system is formed by the urethra.

THE PROSTATE (Fig. 14–13A). Multiple endodermal outgrowths arise from the prostatic portion of the urethra and grow into the surrounding mesenchyme. The glandular epithelium of the prostate differentiates from the endodermal cells, and the associated mesenchyme differentiates into the stroma and smooth muscle fibers of the prostate.

THE BULBOURETHRAL GLANDS (Fig. 14–13A). These pea-sized structures develop from paired endodermal outgrowths from the spongy portion of the urethra. Their smooth muscle fibers and stroma differentiate from the adjacent mesenchyme. Like the prostate, the secretions of these glands contribute to the semen (Moore, 1992).

DEVELOPMENT OF FEMALE GENITAL DUCTS. In embryos with ovaries, the mesonephric ducts regress, and the paramesonephric ducts develop into the female genital tract. The cranial unfused portions of the paramesonephric ducts develop into the uterine tubes, and the fused portions called the *uterovaginal primordium* (canal) give rise to the epithelium and glands of the uterus (Fig. 14–13B and C). The endometrial stroma and myometrium are derived from the adjacent splanchnic mesenchyme. The *uterine (fallopian) tubes* develop from the cranial unfused portions of the paramesonephric ducts (Fig. 14–13).

DEVELOPMENT OF THE VAGINA. The vaginal epithelium is derived from the endoderm of the urogenital sinus (Fig. 14–8). The fibromuscular wall of the vagina develops from the surrounding splanchnic mesenchyme. A solid cord of endodermal cells called the *vaginal plate* forms, and then the central cells break down, forming the lumen of the vagina. The peripheral cells remain as the vaginal epithelium (Fig. 14–13C). Until late fetal life, the lumen of the vagina is separated from the cavity of the urogenital sinus by a membrane called the *hymen* (Figs. 14–13C and 14–14H). The hymen usually ruptures during the perinatal period and remains as a thin fold of mucous membrane around the entrance to the vagina (see Fig. 2–3).

VESTIGIAL STRUCTURES DERIVED FROM THE EMBRYONIC GENITAL DUCTS (Fig. 14–13). During conversion of the mesonephric and paramesonephric ducts into adult structures, some parts of them may remain as vestigial structures (e.g., the appendix of the testis and the epoophoron). These vestiges are rarely seen unless pathological changes develop in them. See Moore and Persaud (1993) for details.

AUXILIARY FEMALE GENITAL GLANDS. Buds grow out from the urethra into the surrounding mesenchyme and form the *urethral glands* and the *paraurethral glands.* These glands correspond to the prostate in the male. Similar outgrowths from the urogenital sinus form the *greater vestibular glands,* which are homologous with the bulbourethral glands in the male.

DESCENT OF THE TESTES. Inguinal canals develop and later form pathways for the testes to descend through the abdominal wall into the scrotum. Inguinal canals also develop in female embryos even though the ovaries do not descend through them. Descent of the testes through the inguinal canals usually begins during the twenty-eighth week and takes about three days. About four weeks later the testes enter the scrotum, and the inguinal canals contract.

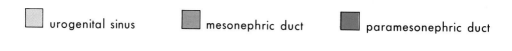

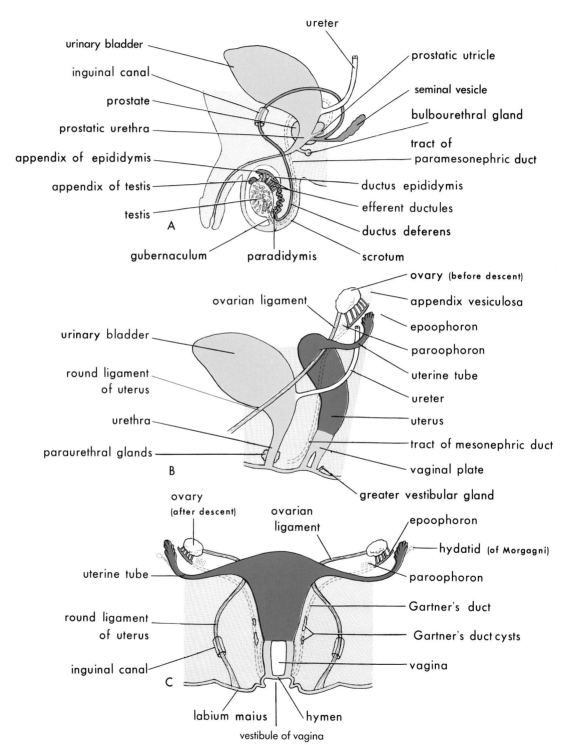

Figure 14–13. Schematic drawings illustrating development of the male and female reproductive systems from the primitive genital ducts. Vestigial structures (paradidymis, paroophoron, appendix of testis, appendix of epididymis, Gartner's duct, hydatid of Morgagni) are also shown. *A*, Reproductive system in a newborn male. *B*, Female reproductive system in a 12-week fetus. *C*, Reproductive system in a newborn female.

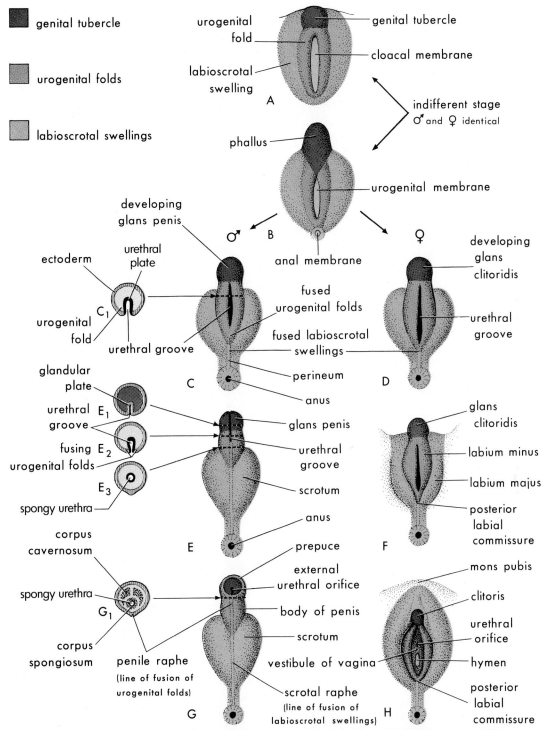

Figure 14–14. *A* and *B*, Diagrams illustrating development of the external genitalia during the indifferent or undifferentiated stage (four to seven weeks). *C, E,* and *G,* Stages in the development of male external genitalia at about 9, 11, and 12 weeks, respectively. To the left are schematic transverse sections (C_1, E_1 to E_3, and G_1) through the developing penis, illustrating formation of the spongy urethra. *D, F,* and *H,* Stages in the development of female external genitalia at 9, 11, and 12 weeks, respectively.

UNDESCENDED TESTES. This condition occurs in about three per cent of full-term male infants. A cryptorchid or undescended testis may be located in the abdominal cavity or anywhere along the usual path of descent of the testis; it usually lies in the inguinal canal. The cause of most cases of cryptorchidism is unknown, but failure of normal androgen production appears to be a factor.

Development of External Genitalia

THE INDIFFERENT OR UNDIFFERENTIATED STAGE (Fig. 14–14*A* and *B*). The external genitalia also pass through a stage that is not distinguishable as male or female. Early in the fourth week, a *genital tubercle* develops ventral to the cloacal membrane. *Labioscrotal swellings* and *urogenital folds* develop on each side of the cloacal membrane. The genital tubercle soon elongates and is called a *phallus;* initially, it is as large in females as in males. A *urethral groove* forms on the ventral surface of the phallus (Fig. 14–14*C* and *D*). Although sexual characteristics begin to appear during the early fetal period, the external genitalia of males and females appear similar until the end of the ninth week (Fig. 14–*C* and *D*). The final form is not established until the twelfth week (Fig. 14–14*G* and *H*).

DEVELOPMENT OF MALE EXTERNAL GENITALIA (Fig. 14–14*C*, *E*, and *G*). Masculinization of the external genitalia is caused by testosterone produced by the fetal testes. The *penis* develops as the phallus elongates. The *urogenital folds* fuse along the ventral surface of the penis to form the *spongy urethra* (penile urethra); as a result, the external urethral orifice moves to the *glans penis.* The *labioscrotal swellings* grow toward each other and fuse to form the *scrotum.*

DEVELOPMENT OF FEMALE EXTERNAL GENITALIA (Fig. 14–14*D*, *F*, and *H*). Feminization of the indifferent external genitalia occurs without the presence of a sex hormone. The phallus becomes the relatively small *clitoris*, which develops like the penis except that the urogenital folds do not fuse. These unfused folds form the *labia minora*, and the unfused labioscrotal folds become the *labia majora.*

Congenital Anomalies of the Genital System

Because an early embryo has the potential to develop as either a male or a female, errors in sex development may result in various degrees of intermediate sex, a condition known as *intersexuality* or hermaphroditism. A person with *ambiguous external genitalia* is called a hermaphrodite or *intersex.* Intersexual conditions are classified according to the histological appearance of the person's gonads. *True hermaphrodites* have both ovarian and testicular tissue. Some intersexes have testes and are called *male pseudohermaphrodites;* others have ovaries and are known as *female pseudohermaphrodites* (Rutgers, 1991).

TRUE HERMAPHRODITES. Persons with this rare intersexual condition usually have a 46,XX chromosome constitution. Both ovarian and testicular tissues are present, either in the same or in opposite gonads. *Ovotestes* form if both the medulla and cortex of the indifferent gonads develop (Fig. 14–11). The physical appearance (phenotype) may be male or female, but the external genitalia are usually ambiguous. This condition is the result of *an error in sex determination.*

MALE PSEUDOHERMAPHRODITISM. These persons have a 46,XY chromosome constitution. The external and internal genitalia are intersexual and variable due to varying degrees of development of the external genitalia and genital ducts. Either an inadequate amount of testosterone and MIF are produced by the fetal testes or they are formed after the period of maximum tissue sensitivity of the sexual structures has passed. Five genetic defects have been described in the enzymatic synthesis of testosterone by the fetal testes, and a defect in Leydig cell differentiation has been described (DiGeorge, 1992). These defects produce male pseudohermaphroditism through inadequate virilization of the male fetus.

ANDROGEN INSENSITIVITY SYNDROME. (Testicular Feminization [Fig. 14–15]). Persons with this uncommon condition (1 in 20,000 live births) related to intersexuality appear as normal females despite the presence of testes and XY sex chromosomes. Normal breast development occurs at puberty. The vagina usually ends blindly, and the other internal genitalia are absent or rudimentary. The testes are usually in the abdomen or the inguinal canals, but they may descend into the labia majora. The psychosexual orientation of these women is entirely female. *Medically, legally, and socially, these persons are females.*

The failure of masculinization to occur in these individuals is the result of a resistance to the action of testosterone at the cellular level in the labioscrotal and urogenital folds. Current evidence suggests that the *defect is in the*

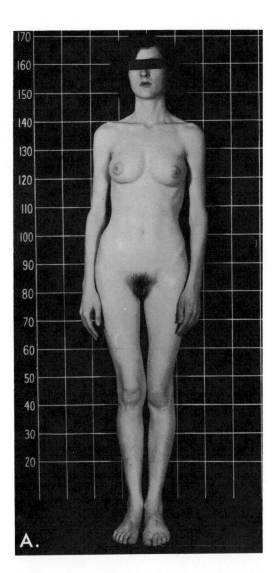

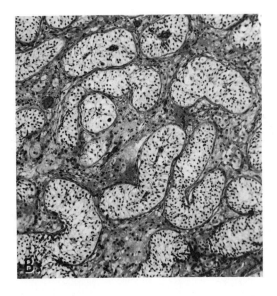

Figure 14–15. *A*, Photograph of a 17-year-old female with the androgen insensitivity syndrome (testicular feminization). The external genitalia are female, but the patient has a 46,XY karyotype and testes. *B*, Photomicrograph of a section through a testis removed from the inguinal region of this woman, showing seminiferous tubules. There are no germ cells. (From Jones HW, Scott WW: *Hermaphroditism, Genital Anomalies and Related Endocrine Disorders.* Baltimore, Williams & Wilkins, 1958.)

androgen receptor mechanism. Embryologically, these females represent an extreme form of male pseudohermaphroditism, but they are not intersexes because they have normal external genitalia.

Usually the testes are removed as soon as they are discovered because, in about one third of these women, malignant tumors develop by 50 years of age (Behrman, 1992). The androgen insensitivity syndrome follows X-linked recessive inheritance, and the gene encoding the androgen receptor has been localized (DiGeorge, 1992). For details on the genetics of this condition, see Thompson et al., 1991.

FEMALE PSEUDOHERMAPHRODITISM. These persons have a 46,XX chromosome constitution.

The most common cause of female pseudohermaphroditism is the *congenital adrenal hyperplasia* (CAH) (Fig. 14–16). There is no ovarian abnormality, but the excessive production of androgens by the hyperplastic fetal suprarenal glands causes masculinization of the external genitalia, varying from enlargement of the clitoris to almost masculine external genitalia. Commonly, there is clitoral hypertrophy, partial fusion of the labia majora, and a persistent urogenital sinus.

Persons with CAH are the most frequently encountered group of intersexes, accounting for about half of all cases of ambiguous external genitalia. The administration of *androgenic agents* to a woman during pregnancy can also cause these abnormalities of the female external genitalia (see Fig. 9–14). Most cases have resulted from the use of certain progestational compounds for the treatment of threatened abortion (p. 133).

HYPOSPADIAS (Fig. 14–17A to C). Once in about every 300 male infants, the external urethral orifice is on the ventral surface of the penis instead of at the tip of the glans. Usually the penis is curved ventrally, a condition known as *chordee*. There are four types of hypospadias: *glandular, penile, penoscrotal,* and *perineal*. The glandular and penile types constitute about 80 per cent of cases. Hypospadias is the result of inadequate production of androgens by the fetal testes and/or inadequate receptor sites for these hormones. The defects result in failure of fusion of the urogenital folds; as a consequence, there is incomplete formation of the spongy urethra. Differences in the timing and degree of

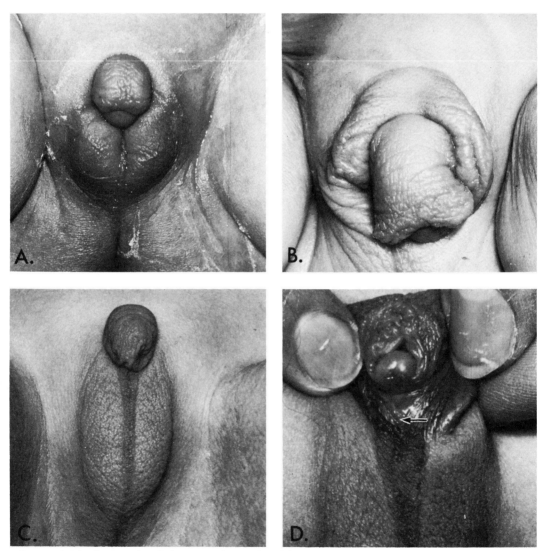

Figure 14–16. Photographs of the external genitalia of female pseudohermaphrodites resulting from congenital adrenal hyperplasia (CAH). *A,* External genitalia of a newborn female, exhibiting enlargement of the clitoris and fusion of the labia majora. *B,* External genitalia of a female infant, showing considerable enlargement of the clitoris. The labia majora have partially fused to form a scrotumlike structure. *C* and *D,* External genitalia of this six-year-old girl, showing the enlarged clitoris and fused labia majora. In *D,* note the glans clitoris and the opening of the urogenital sinus *(arrow).*

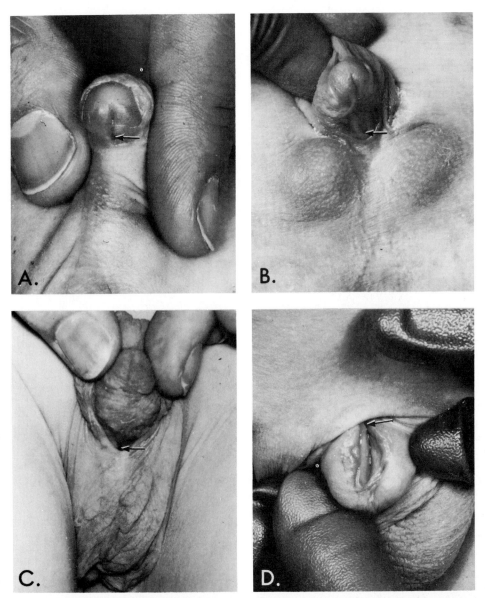

Figure 14–17. Photographs of penile malformations. *A,* Glandular hypospadias. This is the most common form of hypospadias. The external urethral orifice is indicated by the arrow. There is a shallow pit at the usual site of the orifice. Note the moderate degree of chordee causing the penis to curve ventrally. (From Jolly H: *Diseases of Children,* 2nd ed. Oxford, Blackwell Scientific Publications, 1968.) *B,* Penile hypospadias. The penis is short and curved (chordee). The external urethral orifice *(arrow)* is near the penoscrotal junction. *C,* Penoscrotal hypospadias. The external urethral orifice *(arrow)* is located at the penoscrotal junction. *D,* Epispadias. The external urethral orifice *(arrow)* is on the dorsal (upper) surface of the penis near its origin. (Courtesy of Mr. Innes Williams, Genitourinary Surgeon, The Hospital for Sick Children, Great Ormond Street, London, England.)

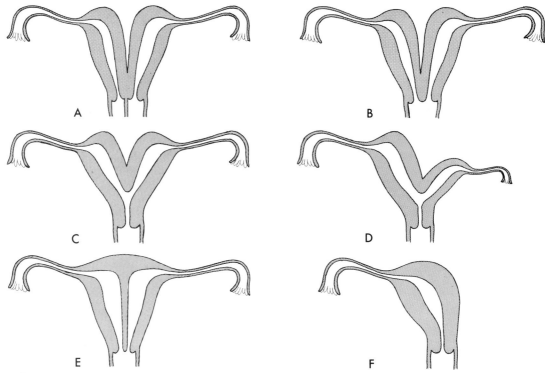

Figure 14-18. Drawings illustrating various types of congenital uterine abnormalities. *A*, Double uterus and double vagina. *B*, Double uterus with single vagina. *C*, Bicornuate uterus. *D*, Bicornuate uterus with a rudimentary left horn. *E*, Septate uterus. *F*, Unicornuate uterus.

hormonal failure account for the various types of hypospadias.

EPISPADIAS (Fig. 14–17*D*). Once in about 30,000 male infants, the urethra opens on the dorsal surface of the penis. Although epispadias may occur as a separate entity, it is *usually associated with exstrophy of the bladder* and has a similar cause (Fig. 14–9).

ANOMALIES OF THE UTERUS AND VAGINA (Fig. 14–18). Various types of uterine duplication result from failure of the paramesonephric ducts to fuse normally. *Double uterus* results from failure of fusion of the caudal parts of the paramesonephric ducts and may be associated with a double or a single vagina (Fig. 14–18*A* and *B*). If the doubling involves only the superior por-

tion of the body of the uterus, the condition is called *bicornuate (double-horned) uterus* (Fig. 14–18*C* and *D*). In some cases, the uterus is divided internally by a thin septum (Fig. 14–18*E*). Uncommonly, one paramesonephric duct degenerates or fails to form; this results in a *unicornuate (single-horned) uterus* (Fig. 14–18*F*).

Once in about every 4000 females *absence of the vagina occurs*. This results from failure of the vaginal plate to develop (Fig. 14–13*B*). When the vagina is absent, the uterus is usually also absent. Failure of canalization of the vaginal plate results in *vaginal atresia*. Failure of the hymen to rupture results in a condition known as *imperforate hymen*.

SUMMARY

The urogenital system develops from the intermediate mesoderm, the mesothelium lining the peritoneal cavity, and the endoderm of the urogenital sinus. Three successive sets of kidneys develop: (1) the transitory and nonfunctional *pronephroi,* (2) the *mesoneph-*

roi, which serve as a temporary excretory organ, and (3) the functional *metanephroi* or permanent kidneys.

The metanephroi develop from two sources: (1) the *metanephric diverticulum* or ureteric bud, which gives rise to the ureter, renal pelvis, calices, and collecting tubules, and (2) the *metanephric mesoderm*, which gives rise to the nephrons. At first the kidneys are located in the pelvis, but they gradually "ascend" to the abdomen. This apparent migration results from disproportionate growth of the lumbar and sacral regions of the embryo. The *urinary bladder* develops from the urogenital sinus and the surrounding splanchnic mesenchyme. The female urethra and almost all of the male urethra have a similar origin.

Developmental abnormalities of the kidney and ureters are common. Incomplete division of the metanephric diverticulum or ureteric bud results in bifid or double ureter and a supernumerary kidney. Failure of the kidney to "ascend" from its embryonic position in the pelvis results in an *ectopic kidney*.

The reproductive system develops in close association with the urinary or excretory system. *Genetic sex* is established at fertilization, but the gonads do not acquire sexual characteristics until the seventh week. The external genitalia do not become distinctly masculine or feminine until the twelfth week. The genital or reproductive organs in both sexes develop from primordia, which appear identical at first. During this *indifferent or undifferentiated stage,* an embryo has the potential to develop into a male or female.

Gonadal sex is determined by the *testis-determining factor* (TDF). This factor is located in the "sex-determining region of the Y" (SRY) of the short arm of the Y chromosome. *TDF directs testicular differentiation.* The Leydig cells produce testosterone that stimulates development of the mesonephric ducts into male genital ducts. These androgens also stimulate development of the indifferent external genitalia into the penis and scrotum. A *müllerian inhibiting factor* (MIF), produced by the Sertoli cells of the testes, inhibits development of the paramesonephric ducts.

In the absence of a Y chromosome and in the presence of two X chromosomes, ovaries develop, the mesonephric ducts regress, the paramesonephric ducts develop into the uterus and uterine tubes, the vagina develops from vaginal plate derived from the urogenital sinus, and the external genitalia develop into the clitoris and labia (minora and majora).

Errors of the sex-determining mechanism produce *true hermaphroditism,* an uncommon intersexual condition. These persons have both ovarian and testicular tissue and variable internal and external genitalia. Errors in sexual differentiation cause *pseudohermaphroditism.* In the male this is the result of failure of the fetal testes to produce adequate amounts of masculinizing hormones or from tissue insensitivity of the sexual structures. In the female, pseudohermaphroditism usually results from congenital adrenal hyperplasia (CAH), a disorder of the fetal suprarenal glands that causes excessive production of androgens and masculinization of the external genitalia.

Commonly Asked Questions

1. Does a horseshoe kidney usually function normally? What sort of problems may occur with this anomaly, and how can they be corrected?
2. My uncle has been told that he has two kidneys on one side and none on the other. How did this abnormality probably happen? Are there likely to be any problems associated with this condition?
3. Do true hermaphrodites ever marry? Are they ever fertile?
4. When a baby is born with ambiguous external genitalia, how long does it take to assign the appropriate sex? What does the physician tell the parents? How is the appropriate sex determined?
5. What is the most common type of disorder producing ambiguity of the external genitalia? Will masculinizing or androgenic hormones given during the fetal period of development cause ambiguity of external genitalia in female fetuses?

The answers to these questions are given on page 333.

REFERENCES

Barr ML: Correlations between sex chromatin patterns and sex chromosome complexes in man. *In* Moore KL (ed): *The Sex Chromatin.* Philadelphia, WB Saunders, 1966.

Behrman RE (ed): *Nelson Textbook of Pediatrics,* 14th ed. Philadelphia, WB Saunders, 1992.

DiGeorge AM: Hermaphroditism. *In* Behrman RE (ed): *Nelson Textbook of Pediatrics,* 14th ed. Philadelphia, WB Saunders, 1992.

Federman DD: *Abnormal Sexual Development: A Genetic and Endocrine Approach to Differential Diagnosis.* Philadelphia, WB Saunders, 1967.

Mittwoch U: Sex determination and sex reversal: Genotype, phenotype, dogma and semantics. *Human Genet 89:*467, 1992.

Moffatt DB: Developmental abnormalities of the urogenital system. *In* Chisholm GD, Williams DI (eds): *Scientific Foundations of Urology,* 2nd ed. London, Heinemann Medical, 1982.

Moore KL: The development of clinical sex chromatin tests. *In* Moore KL (ed): *The Sex Chromatin.* Philadelphia, WB Saunders, 1966.

Moore KL: Sex determination, sexual differentiation and intersex development. *Can Med Assoc J 7:*292, 1967.

Moore KL: *Clinically Oriented Anatomy,* 3rd ed. Baltimore, Williams & Wilkins, 1992.

Moore KL and Persaud TVN: *The Developing Human. Clinically Oriented Embryology,* 5th ed. Philadelphia, WB Saunders, 1993.

O'Rahilly R: The development of the vagina in the human. *In* Blandau RJ, Bergsma D (eds): *Morphogenesis and Malformations of the Genital Systems.* Original Article Series. New York, Alan R Liss, 1977.

Persaud TVN: Embryology of the female genital tract and gonads. *In* Copeland LJ, Jarrell J, McGregor J (eds): *Textbook of Gynecology.* Philadelphia, WB Saunders, 1993.

Rutgers JL: Advances in the pathology of intersex conditions. *Hum Path 22:*884, 1991.

Simpson JL: *Disorders of Sexual Differentiation: Etiology and Clinical Delineation.* New York, Academic Press, 1976.

Thompson MW, McInnes RR, Willard HF: *Thompson & Thompson Genetics in Medicine,* 5th ed. Philadelphia, WB Saunders, 1991.

15

THE CARDIOVASCULAR SYSTEM

The cardiovascular system is the first system to function in the embryo; blood begins to circulate by the end of the third week. This early development of the heart and vascular system is necessary because the rapidly growing embryo needs an efficient method of acquiring oxygen and nutrients and disposing of carbon dioxide and waste products.

EARLY HEART DEVELOPMENT

Heart development is first indicated toward the end of the third week in the *cardiogenic area* (Fig. 15–1A). A pair of endothelial strands called *angioblastic cords* appears and soon becomes canalized to form *endothelial heart tubes* (Fig. 15–2B). These tubes approach each other

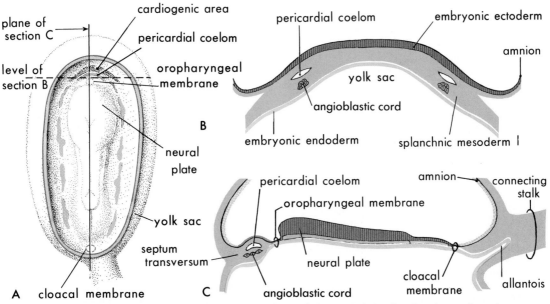

Figure 15–1. *A,* Diagrammatic dorsal view of an embryo of about 18 days, showing the cardiogenic area. *B,* Transverse section of an embryo, demonstrating the angioblastic cords. *C,* Longitudinal section of the embryo, illustrating the relationship of the angioblastic cords (developing heart) to the oropharyngeal membrane, pericardial coelom, and septum transversum (future part of diaphragm).

227

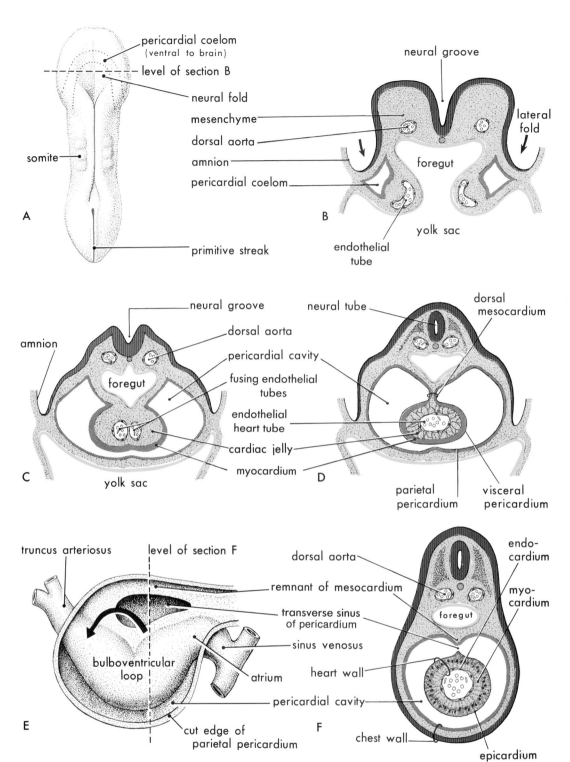

Figure 15–2. *A,* Dorsal view of an embryo of about 20 days. *B,* Transverse section through the heart region of the embryo, showing the widely separated endothelial heart tubes and the lateral folds (*arrows*). *C,* Transverse section of an embryo of about 21 days, showing the formation of the pericardial cavity and the endothelial heart tubes about to fuse. Note they are surrounded by a primitive myocardium. *D,* Similar section at 22 days, showing the single heart tube suspended by the dorsal mesocardium. *E,* Schematic drawing of the heart at about 28 days, showing degeneration of the dorsal mesocardium and formation of the transverse pericardial sinus. *F,* Transverse section through this embryo after disappearance of the dorsal mesocardium. Observe that the three layers of the heart wall are now formed.

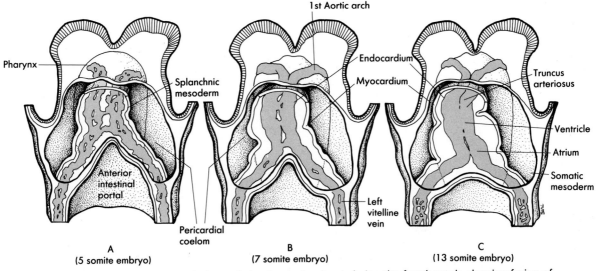

Figure 15–3. Sketches of ventral views of the developing heart during the fourth week, showing fusion of the endothelial heart tubes and bending of the single heart tube. The ventral pericardial wall has been removed.

and fuse to form a single heart tube (Figs. 15–2C and 15–3).

Three paired veins drain into the tubular heart of four-week-old embryos (Figs. 14–2 and 14–3): (1) the *vitelline veins* return blood from the yolk sac, (2) the *umbilical veins* bring oxygenated blood from the chorion (embryonic part of the placenta), and (3) the *common cardinal veins* return blood from the body of the embryo.

During development of the *head fold*, the en-dothelial heart tube and pericardial cavity come to lie ventral to the foregut and caudal to the oropharyngeal membrane (Fig. 15–4). Concurrently, the tubular heart elongates and develops alternate dilations and constrictions: truncus arteriosus, bulbus cordis, ventricle, atrium, and sinus venosus (Fig. 15–3C).

The *truncus arteriosus* is continuous cranially with the *aortic sac*, from which the *aortic arches* arise (Fig. 15–5). The large sinus venosus

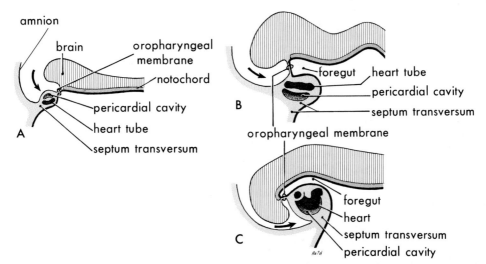

Figure 15–4. Schematic drawings of longitudinal sections through the cranial half of human embryos during the fourth week, showing the effect of the head fold (*arrow*) on the endothelial heart tube and other structures. As the head fold develops, the primitive heart and pericardial cavity come to lie ventral to the foregut and caudal to the oropharyngeal membrane.

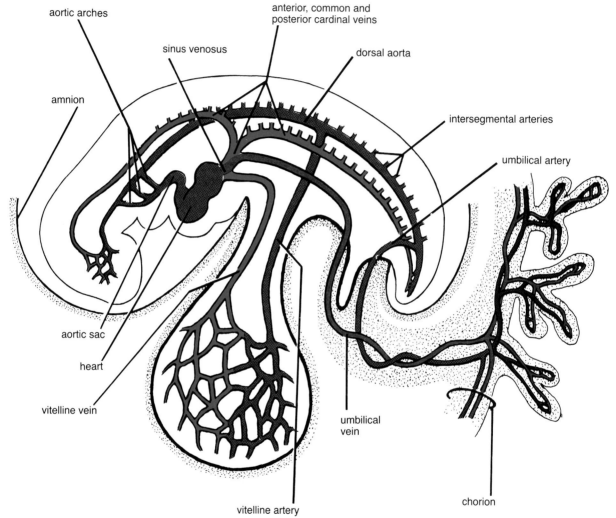

Figure 15–5. Sketch of the cardiovascular system in a 26-day embryo, showing vessels of the left side. Although blood circulates to and from the yolk sac, nourishment and oxygen for the embryo come from the chorion (part of the primitive placenta; see Fig. 5–8). The umbilical vein is colored red because it carries well-oxygenated blood. The umbilical arteries are colored medium red to indicate that they are carrying poorly oxygenated blood.

receives the umbilical, vitelline, and common cardinal veins from the chorion, yolk sac, and embryo, respectively. The **sinus venosus** is a large venous sinus, which receives blood from the umbilical, vitelline, and common cardinal veins (Figs. 15–3D and 15–5). Initially, the heart is a fairly straight tube, but it soon bends upon itself, forming a U-shaped *bulboventricular loop* (Figs. 15–2E and 15–3).

As the endothelial heart tubes fuse, an external layer of the embryonic heart is formed by splanchnic mesoderm surrounding the pericardial coelom. This layer represents the *primitive myocardium* (Fig. 15–2D). At this stage the developing heart is composed of an endothelial tube separated from another tube, the primitive myocardium, by gelatinous connective tissue called *cardiac jelly*. The endothelial tube becomes the internal endothelial lining of the heart called the *endocardium*, and the primitive myocardium becomes the muscular wall or *myocardium* of the heart. The *epicardium* or visceral pericardium (Fig. 15–2F) is derived from mesothelial cells that arise from the external surface of the sinus venosus and spread over the myocardium (Hirakow, 1992).

THE PRIMITIVE CIRCULATION

Contractions of the primitive heart begin on days 21 to 22. Movements occur in peristaltic waves that begin in the sinus venosus and force the blood through the tubular heart. The primitive blood forms in the wall of the yolk sac during the third week (see Fig. 5–7) and passes via the *vitelline veins* to the sinus venosus of the heart (Fig. 15–5). The *sinus venosus* also receives blood from the chorion via the *umbilical veins* (at first there are two). The blood from the *chorion* contains nutrients and oxygen derived from the mother's blood. Because *the yolk sac lacks yolk*, the embryo must obtain its nourishment and oxygen from its mother via the primitive placenta (Fig. 15–5; see also Fig. 5–9).

Blood from the primitive heart is distributed to the branchial or pharyngeal arches by the *aortic arches* and to the rest of the embryo's body by the *aortae* (initially there are two) and their branches (Fig. 15–5). Blood from the primitive heart also passes to the yolk sac and chorion via the vitelline and umbilical arteries, respectively.

After releasing oxygen and nutrients to the developing tissues and organs of the embryo and receiving carbon dioxide and waste products from them, the blood is returned to the heart mainly by the *cardinal veins* (Fig. 15–5). The blood that passes from the heart to the primitive placenta (chorion) and decidua releases its waste products and carbon dioxide into the *maternal blood* and receives nutrients and oxygen from it. This well-oxygenated blood is returned to the heart by the umbilical veins.

COMPLETION OF HEART DEVELOPMENT

The primitive heart has one atrium and one ventricle. Partitioning of the atrioventricular canal, atrium, and ventricle begins around the middle of the fourth week and is essentially complete by the end of the fifth week. Although described separately, these developmental processes occur concurrently.

Partitioning of the Atrioventricular Canal

Endocardial cushions develop in the dorsal and ventral walls of the heart in the region of the atrioventricular canal (Fig. 15–6B). These swellings grow toward each other and fuse (Fig. 15–6C), dividing the atrioventricular canal into right and left atrioventricular canals (Fig. 15–6D).

Partitioning of the Primitive Atrium

A thin, crescent-shaped membrane, the *septum primum*, grows from the dorsocranial wall of the primitive atrium (Figs. 15–7B and 15–8A). As this curtainlike septum grows, a large opening called the *foramen primum* forms between its free edge and the endocardial cushions. As the septum primum grows toward the *endocardial cushions*, it reduces the size of the foramen primum (Fig. 15–8B and C). Before the foramen primum is obliterated, perforations appear in the central part of the septum primum, which soon coalesce to form another opening, the *foramen secundum* (Fig. 15–8B to D). Concurrently, the septum primum fuses with the fused endocardial cushions, thereby obliterating the foramen primum.

Subsequently, another crescentic membrane, the *septum secundum*, grows from the ventrocranial wall of the atrium on the right side of the septum primum (Fig. 15–8D). This septum

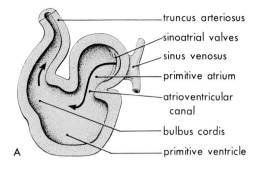

truncus arteriosus
sinoatrial valves
sinus venosus
primitive atrium
atrioventricular canal
bulbus cordis
primitive ventricle

A

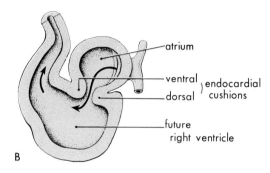

atrium
ventral ⎱ endocardial
dorsal ⎰ cushions
future right ventricle

B

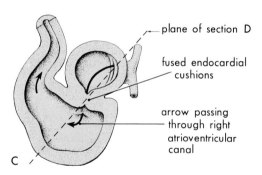

plane of section D
fused endocardial cushions
arrow passing through right atrioventricular canal

C

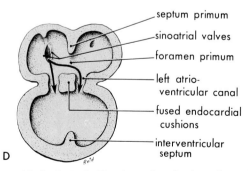

septum primum
sinoatrial valves
foramen primum
left atrio-ventricular canal
fused endocardial cushions
interventricular septum

D

Figure 15–6. *A* to *C*, Sketches of sagittal sections of the heart during the fourth and fifth weeks, illustrating division of the atrioventricular canal. *D*, Frontal section of the heart at the plane shown in *C*. The interatrial and interventricular septa have also started to develop.

gradually covers the foramen secundum (Fig. 15–8*E* to *G*). The oval opening in the septum secundum is called the *foramen ovale* (Fig. 15–8*E*). The remaining part of the septum primum forms the flap-type *valve of the foramen ovale* (Fig. 15–8*G₁* and *H₁*). *Before birth* the foramen ovale allows most of the blood entering the right atrium to pass into the left atrium (see Fig. 15–21). *After birth* the foramen ovale normally closes, and the interatrial septum becomes a complete partition (see Fig. 15–22).

FATE OF SINUS VENOSUS AND FORMATION OF ADULT RIGHT ATRIUM. Initially the sinus venosus is a separate chamber of the heart and opens into the dorsal wall of the right atrium (Figs. 15–5 and 15–6). The *left horn* of the sinus venosus forms the **coronary sinus** (Fig. 15–9*B*), and the *right horn* becomes part of the wall of the **right atrium** (Fig. 15–9*B* and *C*). The remnant of the right part of the primitive atrium is represented by the rough portion of the atrium and the *right auricle*, an appendage of the atrium (Fig. 15–9).

THE PRIMITIVE PULMONARY VEIN AND FORMATION OF THE ADULT LEFT ATRIUM. The smooth part of the wall of the left atrium is derived from the *primitive pulmonary vein*. As the atrium expands, the terminal portion of this vein and its main branches are gradually incorporated into the wall of the left atrium. The remnant of the left part of the primitive atrium is the *left auricle*, an appendage of the atrium.

Partitioning of Primitive Ventricle

Division of the primitive ventricle into right and left ventricles is indicated at the end of the fourth week by a muscular ridge, the *interventricular septum*, in the floor of the ventricle near its apex (Figs. 15–6*D* and 15–7*B*). An *interventricular foramen* between the free edge of the interventricular septum and the fused endocardial cushions permits communication between the right and left ventricles. The interventricular foramen normally closes by the end of the seventh week due to fusion of tissue from three sources (see Fig. 15–11). After closure of the interventricular foramen, the pulmonary trunk is in communication with the right ventricle and the aorta with the left ventricle.

Partitioning of the Bulbus Cordis and Truncus Arteriosus

During the fifth week elevations called *bulbar ridges* form in the walls of the bulbus cordis

Text continued on page 237

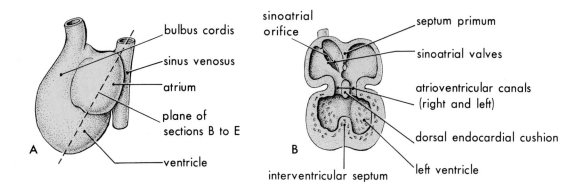

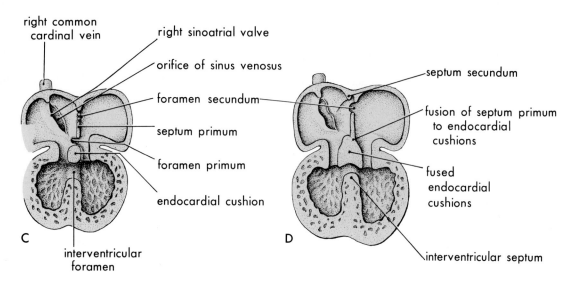

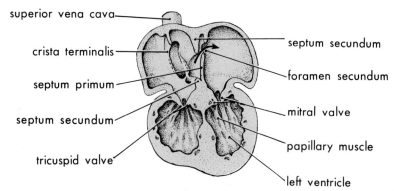

Figure 15-7. Schematic drawings of the developing heart, showing partitioning of the atrioventricular canal, primitive atrium, and ventricle. *A*, Sketch showing the plane of frontal sections *B* to *E*. *B*, About 28 days, showing the early appearance of the septum primum, interventricular septum, and dorsal endocardial cushion. *C*, About 32 days, showing perforations in the dorsal part of the septum. *D*, About 35 days, showing the foramen secundum. *E*, About eight weeks, showing the heart after partitioning of it into four chambers.

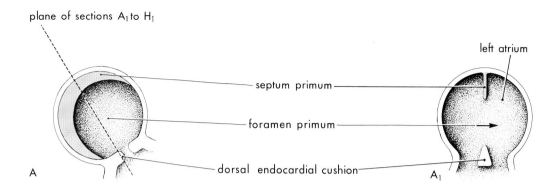

plane of sections A₁ to H₁

left atrium

septum primum

foramen primum

dorsal endocardial cushion

A   A₁

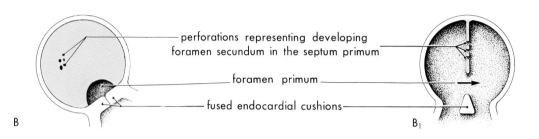

perforations representing developing
foramen secundum in the septum primum

foramen primum

fused endocardial cushions

B   B₁

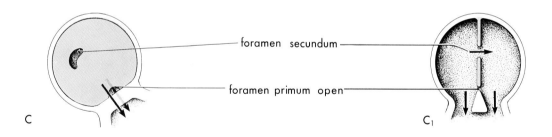

foramen secundum

foramen primum open

C   C₁

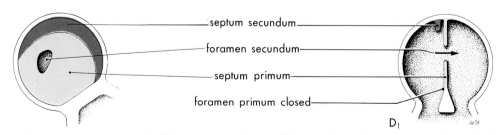

septum secundum

foramen secundum

septum primum

foramen primum closed

D   D₁

Figure 15–8. Diagrammatic sketches illustrating partitioning of the primitive atrium. *A* to *H* are views of the developing interatrial septum as viewed from the right side. *A₁* to *H₁* are frontal sections of the developing interatrial septum at the plane shown in *A*.

Illustration continued on opposite page

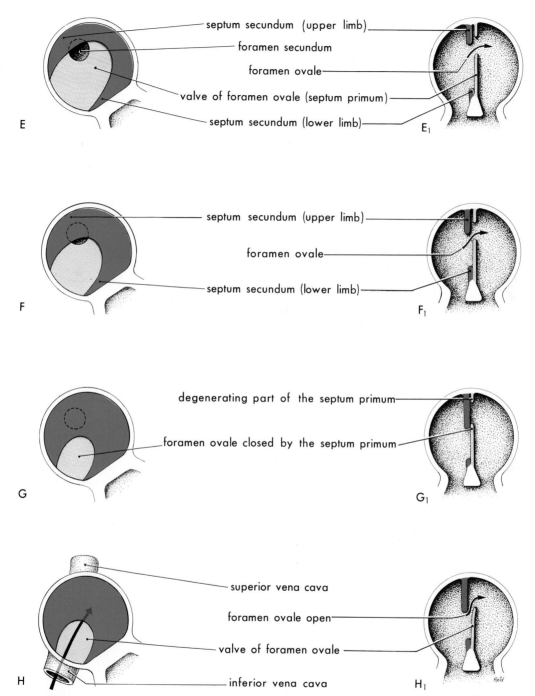

Figure 15–8. *Continued.* Note that, as the septum secundum grows, it overlaps the opening in the septum primum (foramen secundum). The valvelike nature of the foramen ovale is illustrated in G_1 and H_1. When pressure in the right atrium exceeds that in the left atrium, blood passes from the right to the left side of the heart. When the pressures are equal, the septum primum closes the foramen ovale.

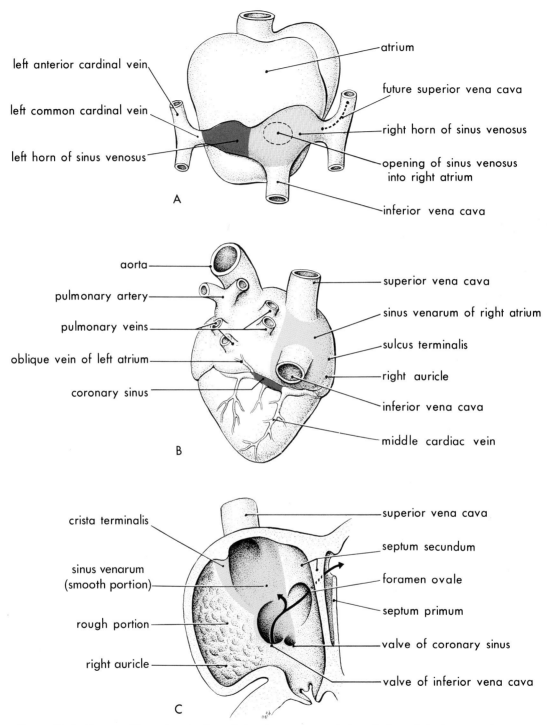

Figure 15–9. Diagrams illustrating the fate of the sinus venosus. *A,* Dorsal view of the heart at about 26 days, showing the early appearance of the sinus venosus. *B,* Dorsal view at eight weeks after incorporation of the right horn of the sinus venosus into the right atrium. The left horn of the sinus venosus has become the coronary sinus. *C,* Internal view of the fetal right atrium showing: (1) the smooth part (sinus venarum) of the wall of the right atrium derived from the right horn of the sinus venosus, and (2) the crista terminalis and the valves of the inferior vena cava and coronary sinus derived from the right sinoatrial valve. The primitive right atrium becomes the right auricle, a conical muscular pouch, which lies against the root of the aorta in the adult.

(Fig. 15–10*B* and *C*). These ridges are first filled with cardiac jelly but are later invaded by mesenchymal cells. Similar *truncal ridges* form in the truncus arteriosus, which are continuous with the bulbar ridges. The spiral orientation of the ridges, possibly caused by the streaming of blood from the ventricles, results in a spiral *aorticopulmonary septum* when these ridges fuse (Fig. 15–10*D* to *G*). This septum divides the bulbus cordis and truncus arteriosus into two channels, the *ascending aorta* and *pulmonary trunk*. Because of the spiral form of the aorticopulmonary septum, the pulmonary trunk twists around the ascending aorta (Figs. 15–10*H* and 15–11).

The **bulbus cordis** is gradually incorporated into the walls of the ventricles. In the adult right ventricle it is represented by the *conus arteriosus* (infundibulum), which gives origin to the pulmonary trunk (Moore, 1992). In the adult left ventricle the bulbus cordis forms the walls of the *aortic vestibule*, the part of the ventricular cavity just inferior to the aortic valve.

Development of the Conducting System of the Heart

Initially the muscle layers of the atrium and ventricle are continuous. The primitive atrium acts as the temporary pacemaker of the heart, but the sinus venosus soon takes over this function. The **sinoatrial node** develops during the fifth week. It is originally in the right wall of the sinus venosus, but it is incorporated into the wall of the right atrium with the sinus venosus (see Fig. 15–9).

After incorporation of the sinus venosus, cells from its left wall are found in the base of the interatrial septum just anterior to the opening of the coronary sinus. Together with cells from the atrioventricular region, they make up the **atrioventricular node** and bundle. This specialized tissue is normally the only pathway from the atria to the ventricles because, as the four chambers of the heart develop, a band of connective tissue grows in from the epicardium. This tissue subsequently separates the muscle of the atria from that of the ventricles and forms part of the adult *cardiac skeleton*. The sinoatrial node, atrioventricular node, and atrioventricular bundle soon become richly supplied with nerves.

Abnormalities of the conducting tissue may cause unexpected death during infancy. Anderson and Ashley (1974) observed conducting tissue abnormalities in the hearts of several infants who died unexpectedly from a disorder classified as "crib death" or *sudden infant death syndrome* (SIDS). There remains a lack of consensus that a single mechanism is responsible for the sudden and unexpected deaths of apparently healthy infants. Some findings in infants who later died of SIDS suggest that they have an abnormality in the autonomic nervous system (Behrman, 1992).

CONGENITAL ANOMALIES OF THE HEART AND GREAT VESSELS

Because development of the heart and great vessels is complex, congenital heart defects (CHDs) are relatively common. The overall incidence is about six to eight cases per 1000 births. The following anomalies are relatively common, and many are amenable to surgery.

Atrial Septal Defects (ASDs)

ASD is a common congenital heart defect. It occurs more frequently in females than in males. There are two main types.

SECUNDUM TYPE ASD (Fig. 15–12*A* to *D*). The defect is in the area of the foramen ovale and may include defects of the septum primum and septum secundum. *Patent foramen ovale* may result from abnormal resorption of the septum primum during the formation of the foramen secundum. If resorption occurs in abnormal locations, the septum primum is fenestrated or netlike (Fig. 15–12*A*). If excessive resorption of the septum primum occurs, the resulting short septum primum does not cover the foramen ovale (Fig. 15–12*B*).

If an abnormally large foramen ovale results from defective development of the septum secundum, a normal septum primum will not close the foramen ovale at birth (Fig. 15–12*C*). Large ASDs result from a combination of excessive resorption of the septum primum and a large foramen ovale (Fig. 15–12*D*). This heart defect is characterized by a large opening between the left and right atria. There is obviously considerable interatrial shunting of blood in these people. Females with ASDs outnumber males three to one.

ENDOCARDIAL CUSHION AND AV SEPTAL DEFECTS WITH PRIMUM TYPE ASD (Fig. 15–12*E*). The septum primum does not fuse with the endocardial cushions, leaving a *patent foramen primum*; usually there is also a cleft in the mitral valve of the heart. For a description of uncommon types of ASD, see Moore and Persaud (1993).

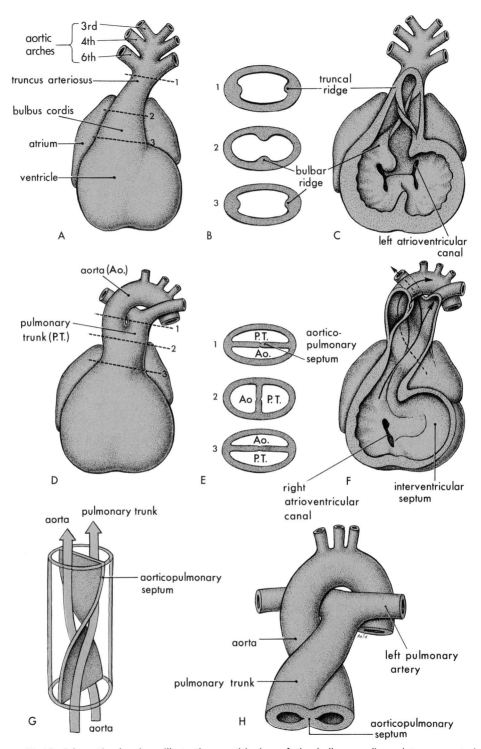

Figure 15–10. Schematic drawings illustrating partitioning of the bulbus cordis and truncus arteriosus. *A,* Ventral aspect of the heart at five weeks. *B,* Transverse sections through the truncus arteriosus and bulbus cordis, illustrating the truncal and bulbar ridges. *C,* The ventral wall of the heart has been removed to demonstrate the ridges. *D,* Ventral aspect of the heart after partitioning of the truncus arteriosus. *E,* Sections through the newly formed aorta (Ao.) and pulmonary trunk (P.T.), showing the aorticopulmonary septum. *F,* Six weeks. The ventral wall of the heart and pulmonary trunk have been removed to show the aorticopulmonary septum. *G,* Diagram illustrating the spiral form of the aorticopulmonary septum. *H,* Drawing showing the great arteries twisting around each other as they leave the heart.

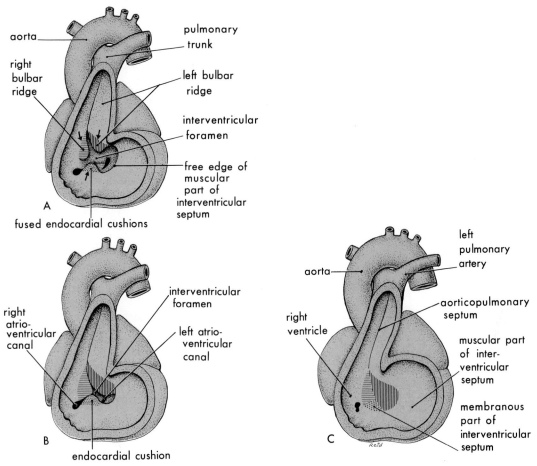

Figure 15–11. Schematic diagrams illustrating closure of the interventricular foramen and formation of the membranous part of the interventricular septum. The walls of the bulbus cordis and the right ventricle have been removed. *A*, Sagittal section at five weeks, showing the bulbar ridges and the fused endocardial cushions. *B*, Schematic coronal section at six weeks, showing how proliferation of subendocardial tissue diminishes the interventricular foramen. *C*, Seven weeks, showing the fused bulbar ridges and the membranous part of the interventricular septum, which is formed by extensions of tissue from the right side of the endocardial cushions.

Ventricular Septal Defects (VSDs)

This congenital anomaly ranks first in frequency on all lists of cardiac defects. It occurs more frequently in males than in females and accounts for about 25 per cent of congenital heart disease. *Membranous septal defect* is the commonest type of VSD (Fig. 15–13*B*). Incomplete closure of the interventricular foramen and failure of the membranous part of the interventricular septum to develop result from failure of tissue to grow from the right side of the fused endocardial cushions and fuse with the aorticopulmonary septum and the muscular part of the interventricular septum (Fig. 15–11*C*).

Abnormal Division of the Truncus Arteriosus

PERSISTENT TRUNCUS ARTERIOSUS. This anomaly is the result of failure of development of the aorticopulmonary septum. As a result, the truncus arteriosus does not divide into the aorta and pulmonary trunk. The most common type is a single arterial vessel which gives rise to the pulmonary trunk and ascending aorta (Fig. 15–14*A* and *B*). The next most common type is for the right and left pulmonary arteries to arise close together from the dorsal wall of the persistent truncus arteriosus.

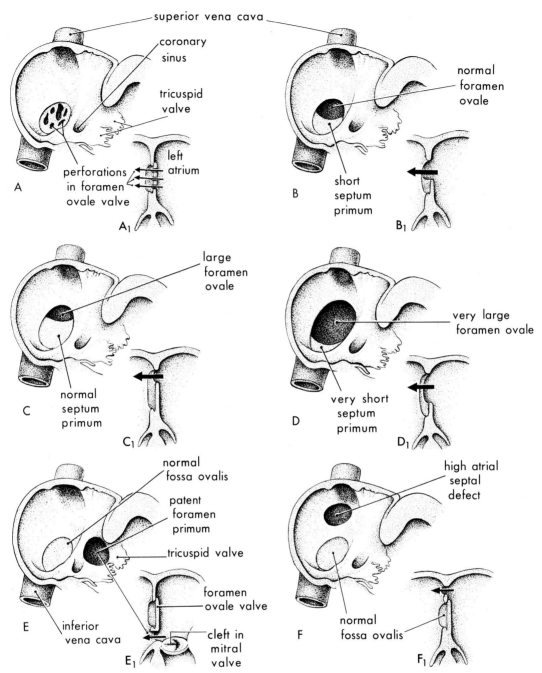

Figure 15–12. Drawings of the right aspect of the interatrial septum (*A* to *F*) and sketches of frontal sections through the septum (*A₁* to *F₁*), illustrating various types of atrial septal defects. *A*, Patent foramen ovale resulting from resorption of the septum primum in abnormal locations. *B*, Patent foramen ovale caused by excessive resorption of the septum primum, sometimes called the "short flap defect." *C*, Patent foramen ovale resulting from an abnormally large foramen ovale. *D*, Patent foramen ovale resulting from an abnormally large foramen ovale and excessive resorption of the septum primum. *E*, Endocardial cushion defect with primum type atrial septal defect. The frontal section *E₁* also shows the cleft in the septal leaflet of the mitral valve. *F*, High septal defect resulting from abnormal absorption of the sinus venosus into the right atrium. This is a very uncommon defect. Note the fossa ovalis in *E* and *F* that forms when the foramen ovale closes normally.

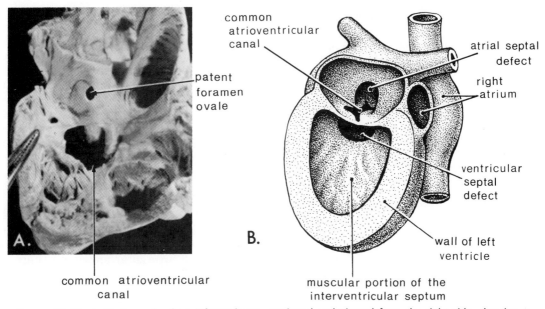

Figure 15–13. *A,* Photograph of an infant's heart, sectioned and viewed from the right side, showing a patent foramen ovale and an atrioventricular (canal) septal defect. (From Lev M: *Autopsy Diagnosis of Congenitally Malformed Hearts.* Springfield, IL, Charles C Thomas, 1953.) *B,* Schematic drawing of a heart, illustrating various defects of the cardiac septa.

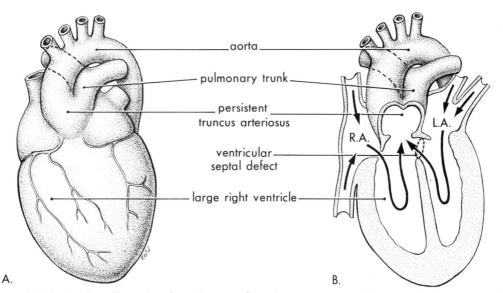

Figure 15–14. Drawings illustrating the main type of persistent truncus arteriosus. *A,* The common trunk divides into an aorta and short pulmonary trunk. *B,* Sketch to show the circulation in this heart and a ventricular septal defect.

TRANSPOSITION OF THE GREAT ARTERIES (TGA). In typical cases of TGA, the aorta lies anterior to the pulmonary trunk and arises from the right ventricle, and the pulmonary trunk arises from the left ventricle. For survival there must be a septal defect (ASD or VSD) or a patent ductus arteriosus (see Fig. 15–19B) to permit some interchange of blood between the pulmonary and systemic circulations. During partitioning of the truncus arteriosus, the aorticopulmonary septum fails to pursue a spiral course. As a result, the origins of the great arteries are reversed. According to the *conal growth hypothesis*, the conus arteriosus fails to grow normally as the bulbus cordis is incorporated into the right ventricle.

Tetralogy of Fallot

This is a combination of four cardiac defects (Fig. 15–15B) consisting of: (1) pulmonary stenosis (narrowing of the region of the right ventricular outflow), (2) ventricular septal defect (VSD), (3) overriding aorta, and (4) hypertrophy of the right ventricle. This condition causes *cyanosis* (blueness) of the lips and fingernails; consequently, these infants are sometimes referred to as "blue babies."

THE AORTIC ARCHES

As the branchial or pharyngeal arches develop during the fourth week (Fig. 15–16), they receive arteries from the heart. These aortic arches (arteries) arise from the aortic sac and terminate in the dorsal aorta of the corresponding side (Fig. 15–16B). Although six pairs of aortic arches develop, they are not all present at the same time, e.g., by the time the sixth pair of aortic arches forms, the first two pairs have disappeared (Fig. 15–16C).

Derivatives of the Aortic Arches

During the sixth to eighth weeks, the primitive aortic arch pattern of arteries is transformed into the adult arterial arrangement (Figs. 15–16 and 15–17).

The first and second pairs of aortic arches largely disappear. The proximal parts of the *third pair of aortic arches* form the *common carotid arteries*, and distal portions join with the dorsal aortae to form the *internal carotid arteries*.

The left *fourth aortic arch* forms part of the *arch of the aorta*. The right fourth aortic arch

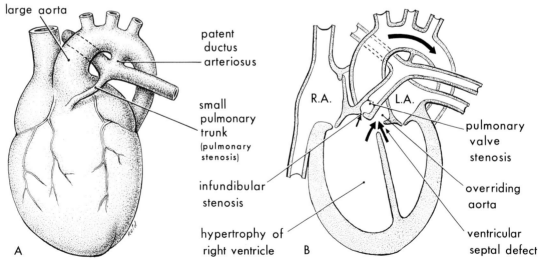

Figure 15–15. *A,* Drawing of an infant's heart, showing a small pulmonary trunk (pulmonary stenosis) and a large aorta resulting from unequal partitioning of the truncus arteriosus. There is also hypertrophy of the right ventricle and a patent ductus arteriosus. *B,* Frontal section of a defective heart, illustrating the tetralogy of Fallot. Note that the large aorta lies over the VSD and receives blood from both ventricles. There are two types of pulmonary stenosis. In *pulmonary valve stenosis,* the pulmonary valve cusps are fused, and a narrow opening remains. In *infundibular pulmonary stenosis,* the conus arteriosus (infundibulum) of the right ventricle is underdeveloped.

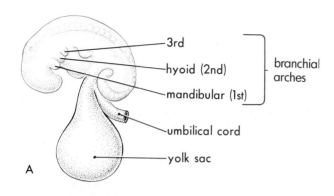

A

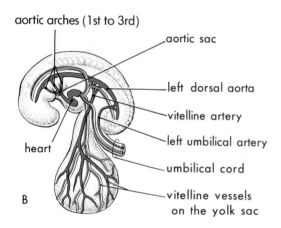

B

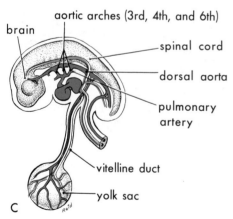

C

Figure 15–16. Drawings illustrating the aortic arches and the primitive cardiovascular system. *A,* Left side of a 26-day embryo. *B,* Schematic drawing of this embryo, showing the left aortic arches arising from the aortic sac of the truncus arteriosus, running through the branchial or pharyngeal arches, and terminating in the left dorsal aorta. *C,* 37-day embryo, showing the single dorsal aorta and that the first two pairs of aortic arches have largely degenerated.

becomes the proximal portion of the *right subclavian artery.* The distal part of this artery forms from the right dorsal aorta and the right seventh intersegmental artery (Fig. 15–17*B*). The fifth pair of aortic arches has no derivatives.

The *left sixth aortic arch* develops as follows: the proximal part persists as the proximal part of the *left pulmonary artery,* and the distal part persists as a shunt or passageway between the pulmonary artery and the aorta called the **ductus arteriosus** (Figs. 15–17*C* and 15–19). The *right sixth aortic arch* develops as follows: the proximal part persists as the proximal part of the *right pulmonary artery* and the distal part degenerates.

Anomalies of the Aortic Arches

Because of the many changes involved in transformation of the embryonic aortic arch system into the adult arterial pattern, it is understandable that variations and anomalies may occur. Abnormalities result from the persistence of parts of aortic arches that normally disappear or from disappearance of other parts that normally persist.

COARCTATION OF THE AORTA. This relatively common anomaly is characterized by a narrowing of the aorta. Most coarctations occur just distal to the origin of the left subclavian artery near the insertion of the ductus arteriosus. The embryological basis of coarctation of the aorta is unclear. One explanation is illustrated (Fig. 15–18*E* to *G*). There is abnormal involution of a small segment of the left dorsal aorta. Later, this constricted segment (area of coarctation) moves cranially with the left subclavian artery to the region of the ductus arteriosus. In the common type of coarctation, the constriction is inferior to the level of the ductus arteriosus (Fig. 15–18*A*). A collateral circulation develops during the fetal period, assisting with passage of blood to inferior parts of the body (Fig. 15–18*B*).

PATENT DUCTUS ARTERIOSUS (PDA) (Fig. 15–19*B*). This anomaly is two to three times more common in females than in males. The embryological basis of PDA is failure of the ductus arteriosus to involute after birth and form the ligamentum arteriosum. Failure of contraction of the muscular wall of the ductus arteriosus after birth is the primary cause of patency.

PDA is the most common cardiac anomaly associated with maternal rubella infection during early pregnancy (see Chapter 9). PDA may occur as an isolated anomaly or in association with cardiac defects. There is some evidence that the low oxygen content of the blood in

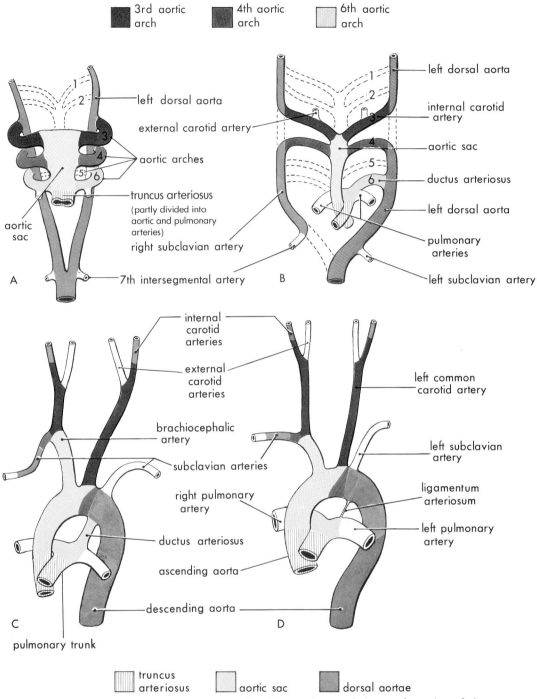

Figure 15–17. Schematic drawings illustrating the changes that result in transformation of the truncus arteriosus, aortic sac, aortic arches, and dorsal aortae into the adult arterial pattern. The vessels which are not shaded or colored are not derived from these structures. *A,* Aortic arches at six weeks; by this stage the first two pairs of aortic arches have largely disappeared. *B,* Aortic arches at seven weeks; the parts of the dorsal aortae and aortic arches that normally disappear are indicated with broken lines. *C,* Arterial arrangement at eight weeks. *D,* Sketch of the arterial vessels of a six-month infant.

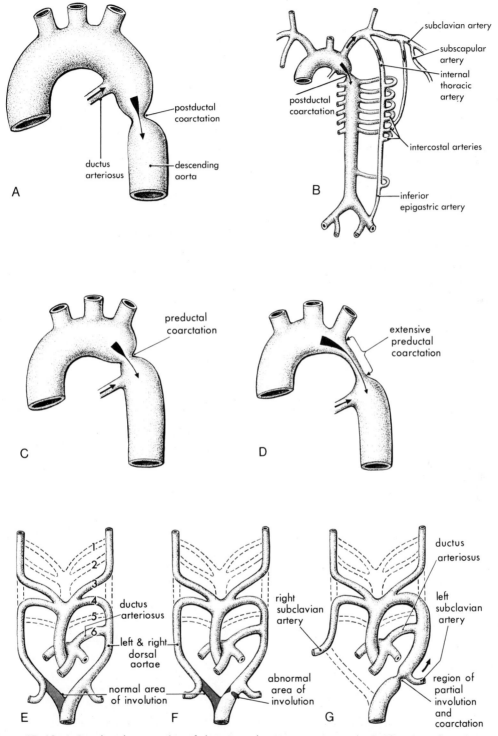

Figure 15–18. *A,* Postductal coarctation of the aorta, the most common type. *B,* Diagrammatic representation of the common routes of collateral circulation that develop with postductal coarctation of the aorta. *C* and *D,* Preductal coarctation. *E,* Sketch of the aortic arch pattern in a seven-week-old embryo, showing the areas that normally involute. *F,* Localized abnormal involution of a small distal segment of the left dorsal aorta. *G,* Later stage, showing the abnormally involuted segment appearing as a coarctation of the aorta. This moves (*arrow*) to the region of the ductus arteriosus with the left subclavian artery.

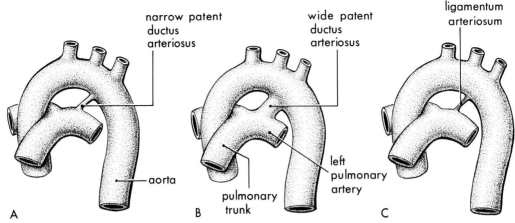

Figure 15–19. *A,* The ductus arteriosus (DA) of a newborn infant. The ductus is normally patent for about two weeks after birth. *B,* Large patent ductus arteriosus (PDA) in a six-month-old infant. In this anomaly some of the blood that should go through the aorta to the inferior part of the body goes back to the lungs via the ductus arteriosus and the pulmonary arteries. *C,* The ligamentum arteriosum, the normal remnant of the ductus arteriosus, in a six-month-old infant.

infants with *neonatal respiratory distress* can adversely affect closure of the ductus arteriosus; for example, PDA commonly occurs in small premature infants with respiratory difficulties associated with a deficiency of surfactant. Isolated PDA is more common in infants born at high altitude.

THE FETAL CIRCULATION

The fetal cardiovascular system is designed to serve prenatal needs and to permit modifications at birth that establish the postnatal circulatory pattern. Good respiration in the newborn infant is dependent upon normal circulatory changes occurring at birth.

COURSE OF THE FETAL CIRCULATION (Figs. 15–20 and 15–21). Well-oxygenated blood returns from the placenta in the *umbilical vein.* About half of this blood bypasses the liver, going through the *ductus venosus.* After a short course in the *inferior vena cava* (IVC), the blood enters the right atrium. Because the IVC also contains poorly oxygenated blood from the lower limbs, abdomen, and pelvis, the blood entering the right atrium is not as well oxygenated as that in the umbilical vein.

The blood from the IVC is largely directed by the inferior border of the septum secundum through the *foramen ovale* into the left atrium. Here it mixes with a relatively small amount of poorly oxygenated blood returning from the lungs via the pulmonary veins. The blood passes

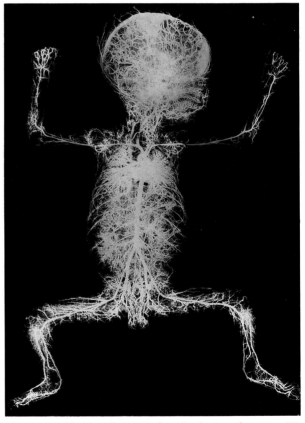

Figure 15–20. Arteriogram of male human fetus at 22 weeks' gestation, showing the entire primary arterial network. The arteries were perfused with an aqueous suspension of a radiopaque media (cinnabar or mercury sulfide) via the ascending thoracic aorta. (From Maher WP: *Am J Anat* *187*:201, 1990.)

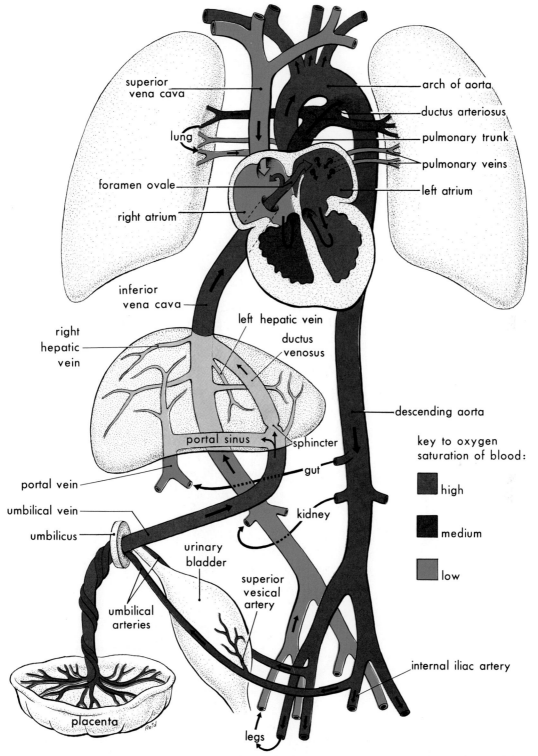

Figure 15–21. A simplified scheme of the fetal circulation. The colors indicate the oxygen saturation of the blood, and the arrows show the course of the fetal circulation. The organs are not drawn to scale. Observe that there are three shunts that permit most of the blood to bypass the liver and the lungs: (1) the *ductus venosus*, (2) the *foramen ovale*, and (3) the *ductus arteriosus*.

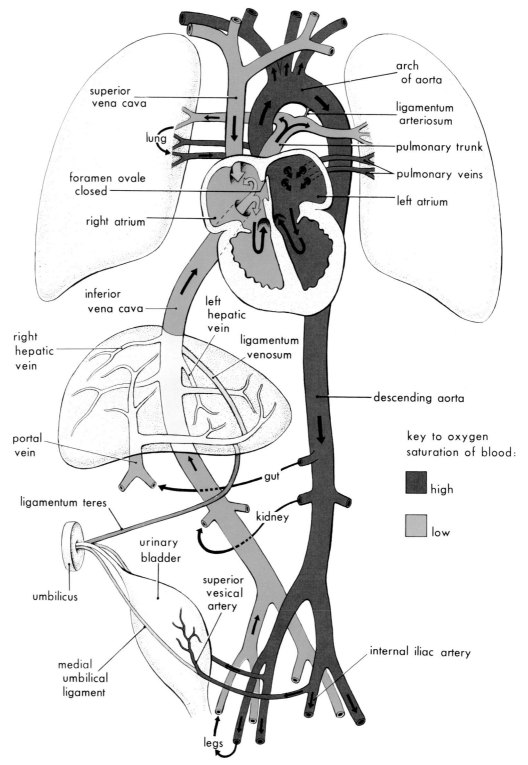

Figure 15–22. A simplified representation of the circulation after birth. The adult derivatives of the fetal vessels and structures that become nonfunctional at birth are also shown. The arrows indicate the course of the neonatal circulation. The organs are not drawn to scale. After birth the three shunts that short circuited the blood during fetal life cease to function, and the pulmonary and systemic circulations are separated.

into the left ventricle and leaves via the ascending aorta. Consequently, the arteries supplying the heart, head and neck, and upper limbs receive well-oxygenated blood.

A small amount of oxygenated blood from the IVC remains in the right atrium. This blood mixes with poorly oxygenated blood from the superior vena cava (SVC) and coronary sinus and passes into the right ventricle. The blood leaves by the pulmonary trunk, and most of it passes through the ductus arteriosus into the aorta. Very little blood goes to the lungs before birth because they are nonfunctional and so require little blood. Most of the mixed blood in the descending aorta passes into the umbilical arteries and is returned to the placenta for reoxygenation. The blood remaining in the aorta circulates through the inferior part of the body and eventually enters the IVC and passes to the right atrium.

THE POSTNATAL CIRCULATION

NEONATAL CHANGES IN THE CARDIOVASCULAR SYSTEM (Fig. 15–22). Important circulatory adjustments occur at birth when the circulation of fetal blood through the placenta ceases and the lungs begin to function. The foramen ovale, ductus arteriosus, ductus venosus, and umbilical vessels are no longer needed. Occlusion of the placental circulation causes an immediate fall of blood pressure in the IVC and right atrium.

Aeration of the lungs is associated with a dramatic fall in pulmonary vascular resistance, a marked increase in pulmonary blood flow, and a progressive thinning of the walls of the pulmonary arteries. Due to increased pulmonary blood flow, the pressure in the left atrium rises above that in the right atrium. This closes the foramen ovale by pressing its valve, the septum primum, against the septum secundum.

Because of the changes in the cardiovascular system at birth, the vessels and structures that are no longer required are transformed as follows (Fig. 15–22): the intra-abdominal portion of the *umbilical vein* becomes the *ligamentum teres*, which passes from the umbilicus to the left branch of the portal vein; the *ductus venosus* becomes the *ligamentum venosum*, which passes through the liver from the left branch of the portal vein to the IVC.

Most of the intra-abdominal portions of the *umbilical arteries* form the *medial umbilical ligaments.* The proximal parts of these vessels persist as the superior vesical arteries, which supply the superior part of the urinary bladder. The *foramen ovale* normally closes functionally at birth. Later anatomical closure results from tissue proliferation and adhesion of the septum primum (valve of foramen ovale) to the left margin of the septum secundum.

The *ductus arteriosus* eventually becomes the *ligamentum arteriosum*, which passes from the left pulmonary artery to the arch of the aorta. Anatomical closure of the ductus normally occurs by the end of the third postnatal month. The change from the fetal to the adult pattern of circulation is not sudden; it takes place over a period of days and weeks. During the transitional stage, there may be a right-to-left flow through the foramen ovale. Although the ductus arteriosus constricts at birth, it usually remains patent for two or three months.

SUMMARY

The cardiovascular system begins to develop toward the end of the third week from splanchnic mesoderm in the cardiogenic area. Paired endothelial heart tubes form and fuse into a single endothelial heart tube. The primitive myocardium soon surrounds this tube. The heart starts to beat at 21 to 22 days.

By the end of the third week a functional cardiovascular system is present. As the heart tube grows, it bends to the right and soon acquires the general external appearance of the adult heart. The heart becomes partitioned into four chambers between the fourth and seventh weeks.

The critical period of heart development is from about day 20 to day 50 after fertilization. Because partitioning of the heart is complex, defects of the cardiac septa are relatively common, particularly ventricular septal defects. Some congenital anomalies result from abnormal transformation of the aortic arches into the adult arterial pattern.

Because the lungs are nonfunctional during prenatal life, the fetal cardiovascular system is structurally designed so that blood is oxygenated in the placenta and largely bypasses the lungs. The modifications that establish the postnatal circulatory pattern at birth are not abrupt but extend into infancy. Failure of the normal changes in the circulatory system to occur at birth results in a patent foramen ovale or a patent ductus arteriosus or both.

Commonly Asked Questions

1. The pediatrician said that our newborn baby had a heart murmur. What does this mean? What causes this condition and what does it indicate?
2. Are congenital anomalies of the heart common? What is the most common congenital heart defect in children?
3. What are the causes of congenital anomalies of the cardiovascular system? Can drugs taken by the mother during pregnancy cause congenital cardiac defects? A friend of mine who drank heavily during her pregnancy had a child with a heart defect. Could her drinking have caused her infant's heart defect?
4. Can viral infections cause congenital heart disease? I have heard that if a mother has *measles during pregnancy* her baby will have an abnormality of the cardiovascular system. Is this true? I have also heard that women can be given a vaccine that will protect their babies against certain viruses. Is this true?
5. My sister's baby had its aorta arising from the right ventricle and its pulmonary artery arising from the left ventricle. The baby died during the first week. What is this anomaly called and how common is this disorder? Can the condition be corrected surgically? If so, how is this done?
6. I know a set of healthy identical twin sisters in their forties. It was found during a routine examination that one of them had a *reversed heart.* Is this a serious heart anomaly? How common is this among identical twins and what causes this condition to develop?

The answers to these questions are given on page 334.

REFERENCES

Anderson RH, Ashley GT: Growth and development of the cardiovascular system. *In* Davis JA, Dobbing J (eds): *Scientific Foundation of Paediatrics.* Philadelphia, WB Saunders, 1974.

Behrman RE (ed): *Nelson Textbook of Pediatrics,* 14th ed. Philadelphia, WB Saunders, 1992.

Butler J, Vincent RN, Reed M, Collins GF: Cardiac embryogenesis: A three-dimensional approach. *Can J Cardiol* 3:111, 1987.

Chinn A, Fitzsimmons J, Shepard TH, Fantel AG: Congenital heart disease among spontaneous abortuses and stillborn fetuses: Prevalence and associations. *Teratology 40:*475, 1989.

Clark EB: Cardiac embryology. Its relevance to congenital heart disease. *Am J Dis Child* 140:41, 1986.

Conte G, Grieco M: Closure of the interventricular foramen and morphogenesis of the membranous septum and ventricular septal defects in the human heart. *Anat Anz* 155:39, 1984.

Deanfield JE: Transposition of the great arteries: To switch or not to switch? *Curr Opin Pediatr* 1:85, 1989.

Feinberg RN, Sherer GK, Auerbach R (eds): *The Development of the Vascular System.* Basel, Karger, 1991.

Ferencz C: The etiology of congenital cardiovascular malformations: Observations on genetic risks with implications for further birth defects research. *J Med* 16:497, 1985.

Fink BW: *Congenital Heart Disease,* 2nd ed. Chicago, Year Book Medical Publishers, 1985.

Hirakow R: Development of the vertebrate heart and the extracellular matrix. *Congenital Anomalies* 26:205, 1986.

Hirakow R: Personal communication, 1992.

Kirklin JW, Colvin EV, McConnell ME, et al.: Complete transposition of the great arteries: Treatment in the current era. *Pediatr Clin North Am* 37:171, 1990.

Long WA: *Fetal and Neonatal Cardiology.* Philadelphia, WB Saunders, 1990.

Merrill WH, Bender HW: The surgical approach to congenital heart disease. *Current Problems in Surg* 22:4, 1985.

Moore KL: *Clinically Oriented Anatomy,* 2nd ed. Baltimore, Williams & Wilkins, 1992.

Moore KL, Persaud TVN: *The Developing Human. Clinically Oriented Embryology,* 5th ed. Philadelphia, WB Saunders, 1993.

Morris GK, Hampton J: Congenital heart lesions: An introduction. *Medicine International* 18:745, 1985.

O'Rahilly R: The timing and sequence of events in human cardiogenesis. *Acta Anat* 79:70, 1971.

Persaud TVN: Historical development of the concept of a pulmonary circulation. *Can J Cardiol* 5:12, 1989.

Rosenquist GC, Bergsma D (eds): *Morphogenesis and Malformation of the Cardiovascular System.* The National Foundation-March of Dimes. Birth Defects: Original Article Series, Vol. XIV, No. 7. New York, Alan R. Liss, 1978.

Schats R, Jansen CAM, Wladimiroff JW: Embryonic heart activity: Appearance and development in early pregnancy. *Brit J Obstet Gynaecol* 97:989, 1990.

Schmidt KG, Silverman WH: Evaluation of the fetal heart by ultrasound. *In* Callen PW: *Ultrasonography in Obstetrics and Gynecology,* 2nd ed. Philadelphia, WB Saunders, 1988.

Schmidt KG, Silverman NH: The fetus with a cardiac malformation. *In* Harrison MR, Golbus MS, Filly RA (eds): *The Unborn Patient: Prenatal Diagnosis and Treatment,* 2nd ed. Philadelphia, WB Saunders, 1991.

Skovránek J: Prenatal development of the heart and the blood circulatory system. *Physiol Res 40:*25, 1991.

Thompson MW, McInnes RR, Willard HF: *Thompson & Thompson Genetics in Medicine,* 5th ed. Philadelphia, WB Saunders, 1991.

Ueland K: Cardiac diseases. *In* Creasy RK, Resnik R (eds): *Maternal-Fetal Medicine: Principles and Practice.* Philadelphia, WB Saunders, 1989.

Virmani R, Atkinson JD, Fenoglio JJ: *Cardiovascular Pathology.* Philadelphia, WB Saunders, 1991.

16

THE MUSCULOSKELETAL SYSTEM

The musculoskeletal system develops from mesoderm and neural crest cells, the formation of which is described in Chapter 5. As the notochord and neural tube form, the *intraembryonic mesoderm* lateral to these structures condenses to form two longitudinal columns of *paraxial mesoderm* (Fig. 16–1A). Beginning around 20 days, the **somites** arise from the paraxial mesoderm, as the columns of paraxial mesoderm are divided into blocks of tissue. Externally, the somites appear as pairs of beadlike elevations along the dorsolateral surface of the embryo (see Figs. 6–3 to 6–5).

The development and early differentiation of the somites are illustrated in Figure 16–1. Initially, the somites are composed of compact aggregates of mesenchymal cells. Each somite soon becomes differentiated into two parts: (1) a ventromedial part called the *sclerotome* that forms the vertebrae and ribs, and (2) a dorsolateral part called the *dermomyotome* that gives rise to the dermis of the skin and the intrinsic back muscles.

Mesodermal cells give rise to *mesenchyme*, which is loosely organized embryonic connective tissue. Much of the mesenchyme in the head is derived from *neural crest cells* (p. 6). These cells migrate into the branchial or pharyngeal arches and form the bones and connective tissue of craniofacial structures (p. 152). Regardless of their source, mesenchymal cells have the ability to differentiate in many different ways (e.g., into fibroblasts, chondroblasts, or osteoblasts).

DEVELOPMENT OF BONE AND CARTILAGE

The primordia of bones first appear as condensations of mesenchymal cells that form models of the bones. Some bones develop in mesenchyme by *intramembranous bone formation*. In other cases, the mesenchymal bone models are transformed into cartilage bone models that later become ossified by *endochondral bone formation*.

HISTOGENESIS OF CARTILAGE. Cartilage develops from mesenchyme and first appears in embryos during the fifth week. In areas where cartilage is to develop, the mesenchyme condenses and the cells proliferate and become rounded. Subsequently, collagenous and/or elastic fibers are deposited in the intercellular substance or matrix. The cartilage-forming cells called *chondroblasts* secrete collagenous fibrils and the ground substance of the matrix. *Three types of cartilage* (hyaline cartilage, fibrocartilage, and elastic cartilage) are distinguished according to the type of matrix that is formed. Hyaline cartilage is the most widely distributed type.

HISTOGENESIS OF BONE. Bone develops in two types of connective tissue: mesenchyme and cartilage. Like cartilage, bone consists of cells and

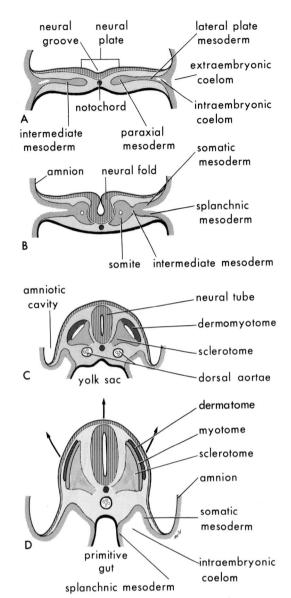

Figure 16–1. Transverse sections through embryos of various ages, illustrating the formation and early differentiation of somites. See Figure 6–3 for the external appearance of these embryos. *A*, Embryo of about 18 days, showing the paraxial mesoderm from which the somites are derived. *B*, Embryo of about 22 days. *C*, Embryo of about 26 days. The dermomyotome region of the somite gives rise to a myotome (muscle-forming body) and a skin plate (future dermis). *D*, Embryo of about 28 days. The arrows indicate directions of growth movements of somite remnants and neural tube to the notochord.

an organic intercellular substance called matrix, which comprises collagen fibrils embedded in an amorphous component. For an account of bone cells with respect to the regulation of development, structure, matrix formation, and minerali-

zation, see Marks Jr and Popoff (1988) and Dziedzic-Goclawska et al. (1988).

Intramembranous Ossification

This type of bone formation occurs in mesenchyme that has formed a membranous layer. This is why this type of ossification is called intramembranous ossification. The mesenchyme condenses and becomes highly vascular; some cells differentiate into *osteoblasts* (bone-forming cells) and begin to deposit matrix or intercellular substances called *osteoid tissue* (prebone). The osteoblasts are almost completely separated from one another, contact being maintained by a few tiny processes. Calcium phosphate is then deposited in the osteoid tissue as it is organized into bone. Bone osteoblasts are trapped in the matrix and become *osteocytes*.

At first new bone has no organized pattern. Spicules of bone soon become organized and coalesce into lamellae or layers. Concentric lamellae develop around blood vessels, forming *haversian systems*. Some osteoblasts remain at the periphery of the developing bone and continue to lay down layers, forming plates of compact bone on the surfaces. Between the surface plates, the intervening bone remains spiculated or spongy. This spongy environment is somewhat accentuated by the action of cells, called *osteoclasts*, which absorb bone. In the interstices of spongy bone, the mesenchyme differentiates into bone marrow. During fetal and postnatal life, there is continuous remodeling of bone by the simultaneous action of osteoclasts and osteoblasts. Studies of the cellular and molecular events during embryonic bone formation suggest that osteogenesis and chondrogenesis are programmed early in development and are independent events under the influence of vascular factors.

Intracartilaginous Ossification

This type of bone formation occurs in preexisting cartilaginous models (Fig. 16–2). In a long bone, for example, the **primary ossification center** appears in the *diaphysis* (the portion of a long bone between its ends). This part is later called the body or shaft. Here the cartilage cells increase in size (hypertrophy), the matrix becomes calcified, and the cells die. Concurrently a thin layer of bone is deposited under the *perichondrium* surrounding the diaphysis; thus, the perichondrium becomes the *periosteum*. Invasion

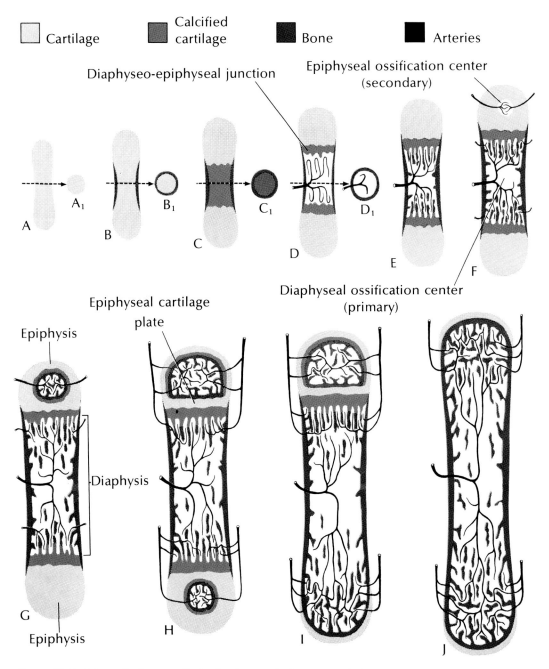

Figure 16–2. Schematic diagrams illustrating intracartilaginous or endochondral ossification and the development of a typical long bone. *A* to *J* are longitudinal sections, and *A₁* to *D₁* are cross sections at the levels indicated. *A,* Cartilage model of the bone. *B,* A subperiosteal ring of bone appears. *C,* Cartilage begins to calcify. *D,* Vascular mesenchyme enters the calcified cartilage. *E,* At each diaphyseal-epiphyseal junction there is a zone of ossification. *F,* Blood vessels and mesenchyme enter the superior epiphyseal cartilage. *G,* The epiphyseal ossification center grows. *H,* A similar center develops in the inferior epiphyseal cartilage plate. *I,* The inferior epiphyseal cartilage plate is ossified. *J,* The superior epiphyseal cartilage plate ossifies, forming a continuous bone marrow cavity. When the epiphyseal plates ossify, the bone can no longer grow in length. (Modified from Bloom W, Fawcett DW: *A Textbook of Histology,* 11th ed. Philadelphia, WB Saunders, 1986.)

of vascular connective tissue from the periosteum breaks up the cartilage. Some invading cells differentiate into the *hemopoietic (hematopoietic) cells* of the bone marrow, and others differentiate into osteoblasts that deposit bone matrix on the spicules of calcified cartilage. This process continues toward the *epiphyses* or ends of the bone. The spicules of bone are remodeled by the action of osteoclasts and osteoblasts.

Lengthening of long bones occurs at the *diaphyseal-epiphyseal junction.* Cartilage cells in this region proliferate by mitosis. Toward the diaphysis, the cartilage cells hypertrophy, and the matrix becomes calcified and broken up into spicules by vascular tissue from the bone marrow or medullary cavity. Bone is deposited on these spicules; absorption of this bone keeps the spongy bone masses relatively constant in length and enlarges the marrow cavity.

Ossification of limb bones begins at the end of the embryonic period and thereafter makes demands on the maternal supply of calcium and phosphorus. Pregnant women are therefore advised to maintain an adequate intake of these elements in order to preserve healthy bones and teeth. The region of bone formation at the center of the body (shaft) of a long bone is called the ***primary ossification center*** (Fig. 16–2F). At birth, the bodies or diaphyses are largely ossified, but most of the ends or *epiphyses* are still cartilaginous.

Most ***secondary ossification centers*** in the epiphyses *appear during the first few years after birth.* The epiphyseal cartilage cells hypertrophy, and there is invasion by vascular connective tissue. As previously described, ossification spreads in all directions, and only the articular cartilage and a transverse plate of cartilage, the *epiphyseal cartilage plate,* remain cartilaginous. Upon completion of growth, the epiphyseal plate is replaced by spongy bone; the epiphyses and diaphysis are united, and further elongation of the bone does not occur.

In most bones the epiphyses have fused with the diaphyses by the age of 20 years. Growth in the diameter of a bone results from deposition of bone at the periosteum and from absorption on the medullary surface. The rate of deposition and absorption is balanced to regulate the thickness of the compact bone and the size of the marrow cavity. The internal reorganization of bone continues throughout life. The development of irregular bones is similar to that of the epiphyses of long bones. Ossification begins centrally and spreads in all directions. In addition to membranous and endochondral ossification, *chondroid tissue,* which also differentiates from mesenchyme, is now recognized as an important factor for skeletal growth (Dhem et al., 1989).

DEVELOPMENT OF JOINTS

Most junctions between bones are constructed to allow movement of parts of the body (e.g., the knee joint). The terms *articulation* and *joint* are used synonymously to refer to the structural arrangements that join two or more bones together at their place of meeting. Joints are classified in several ways. Those with little or no movement are classified according to the type of material holding the bones together, e.g., the bones involved in *fibrous joints* are joined by fibrous tissue (Fig. 16–3D). Joints begin to develop during the sixth week; and, by the end of the eighth week, they closely resemble adult joints.

SYNOVIAL JOINTS (Fig. 16–3*B*). The mesenchyme between the developing bones known as *interzonal mesenchyme* differentiates as follows: (1) peripherally, it gives rise to the capsular and other ligaments, (2) centrally, it disappears and the resulting space becomes the joint cavity, and (3) where it lines the capsule and the articular surfaces, it forms the *synovial membrane.* Probably as a result of joint movement, the mesenchymal cells subsequently disappear from the surfaces of the articular cartilages. Examples of this type of joint are the knee and elbow joints.

CARTILAGINOUS JOINTS (Fig. 16–3*C*). The interzonal mesenchyme between the developing bones differentiates into hyaline cartilage (e.g., the costochondral joints) or fibrocartilage (e.g., the pubic symphysis). For a description of the anatomy of these joints, see Moore (1992).

FIBROUS JOINTS (Fig. 16–3*D*). The interzonal mesenchyme between the developing bones differentiates into dense fibrous connective tissue, e.g., the sutures of the skull (see Fig. 16–9).

DEVELOPMENT OF THE VERTEBRAL COLUMN

Precartilaginous Mesenchymal Stage

During the fourth week, mesenchymal cells from the somites are found in three main areas (Figs. 16–1D and 16–4A):

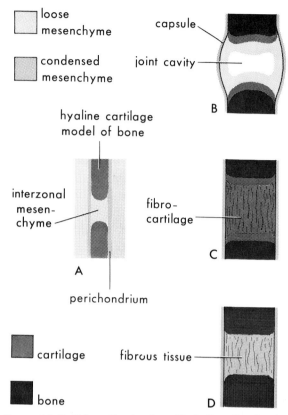

Figure 16–3. Schematic drawings illustrating the development of joints during the sixth and seventh weeks. *A,* Condensed mesenchyme continues across the gap or interzone between the developing bones, enclosing some loose mesenchyme (the interzonal mesenchyme) between them. This primitive joint may differentiate into *B,* a synovial joint, *C,* a cartilaginous joint, or *D,* a fibrous joint.

1. *Surrounding the notochord.* In a frontal section of a four-week embryo, the sclerotomes appear as paired condensations of mesenchymal cells around the notochord (Fig. 16–4*B*). Each *sclerotome* consists of loosely arranged cells cranially and densely packed cells caudally. Some of the densely packed cells move cranially opposite the center of the myotome and form the *intervertebral disc* (Fig. 16–4*D*). The remaining densely packed cells fuse with the loosely arranged cells of the immediately caudal sclerotome to form the mesenchymal *centrum,* the primordium of the body of a vertebra. Thus, each centrum develops from two adjacent sclerotomes and becomes an intersegmental structure. The nerves now lie in close relationship to the intervertebral discs, and the *intersegmental arteries* lie on each side of the vertebral bodies. In

the thorax, the dorsal intersegmental arteries become the *intercostal arteries.*

The **notochord** degenerates and disappears where it is surrounded by the developing vertebral bodies. Between the vertebrae, the notochord expands to form the gelatinous center of the intervertebral disc called the *nucleus pulposus* (Fig. 16–4*D*). This nucleus is later surrounded by the circularly arranged fibers of the *anulus fibrosus.* The nucleus pulposus and anulus (annulus) fibrosus together constitute the intervertebral disc.

> Remnants of the notochord may persist and give rise to a *chordoma.* This slow-growing neoplasm occurs most frequently in the base of the skull and in the lumbosacral region.

2. *Surrounding the neural tube.* These mesenchymal cells form the vertebral (neural) arch, which covers and protects the spinal cord (Fig. 16–5).

3. *In the body wall.* These mesenchymal cells form the costal processes, which form ribs in the thoracic region.

Chondrification of Typical Vertebrae

During the sixth week, *chondrification centers* appear in each mesenchymal vertebra (Fig. 16–5). At the end of the embryonic period, the two centers in each centrum fuse to form the cartilaginous *centrum.* Concomitantly, the centers in the vertebral arches fuse with each other and the centrum. The spinous and transverse processes develop from extensions of chondrification centers in the vertebral arch. Chondrification spreads until a cartilaginous vertebral column is formed.

Ossification of Typical Vertebrae

Ossification begins during the embryonic period and ends around the 25th year (Figs. 16–5*C* and *F* and 16–6).

PRENATAL PERIOD (Fig. 16–5*C* to *F*). At first there are two primary ossification centers, ventral and dorsal, for the centrum. The **primary ossification centers** soon fuse to form one center. Three primary centers are present by the end of the embryonic period: one in the centrum and one in each half of the vertebral arch (Fig. 16–5*C*). Ossification becomes evident in the vertebral arches in the eighth week. At birth, each vertebra consists of three bony parts connected by cartilage (Fig. 16–5*D*).

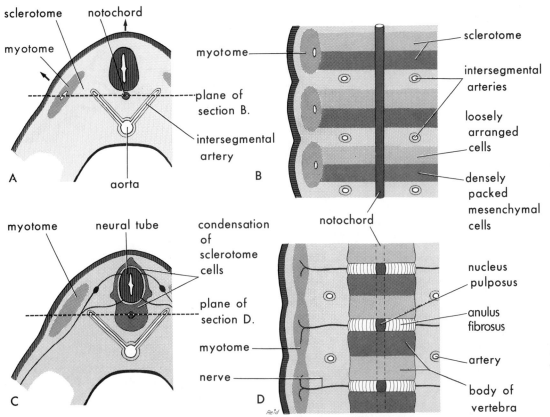

Figure 16–4. *A,* Partial transverse section through a four-week embryo. The arrows indicate the dorsal growth of the neural tube and the simultaneous dorsolateral movement of the somite remnant leaving behind a trail of sclerotomal cells. *B,* Diagrammatic frontal section of this embryo, showing that the condensation of sclerotome cells around the notochord consists of a cranial area of loosely packed cells and a caudal area of densely packed cells. *C,* Partial transverse section through a five-week embryo, showing the condensation of sclerotome cells around the notochord and the neural tube, forming a mesenchymal vertebra. *D,* Diagrammatic frontal section, illustrating that the vertebral body forms from the cranial and caudal halves of two successive sclerotome masses. The intersegmental arteries now cross the bodies of the vertebrae, and the spinal nerves lie between the vertebrae. The notochord is degenerating, except in the region of the intervertebral disc where it forms the nucleus pulposus.

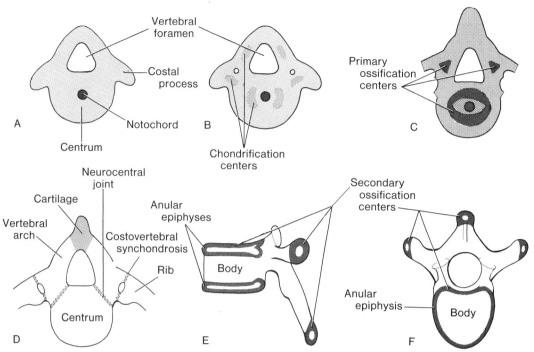

Figure 16–5. Drawings illustrating the stages of vertebral development. *A,* Mesenchymal vertebra at five weeks. *B,* Chondrification centers in a mesenchymal vertebra at six weeks. *C,* Primary ossification centers in a cartilaginous vertebra at seven weeks. *D,* A thoracic vertebra at birth, consisting of three bony parts. Note the cartilage between the halves of the vertebral arch and between the arch and the centrum (the neurocentral joint). *E* and *F,* Two views of a typical thoracic vertebra at puberty, showing the location of the secondary centers of ossification.

POSTNATAL PERIOD (Fig. 16–5*E* and *F*). The halves of the vertebral arch fuse during the first three to five years. The laminae of the arches first unite in the lumbar region, and subsequent union progresses cranially. Initially, the vertebral arch articulates with the centrum at cartilaginous *neurocentral joints*, which permit the vertebral arches to grow as the spinal cord enlarges. These joints disappear when the vertebral arch fuses with the centrum during the third to sixth years.

Five **secondary ossification centers** appear after puberty: one for the tip of the spinous process, one for the tip of each transverse process, and two rim epiphyses called *anular epiphyses*, one on the superior and one on the inferior rim of the vertebral body (Fig. 16–5*E*). The vertebral body is a composite of the superior and inferior anular epiphyses and the mass of bone between them. It includes the centrum, parts of the vertebral arch, and the facets for the heads of the ribs. All secondary centers unite with the rest of the vertebra at about 25 years.

Vertebral Anomalies

VARIATION IN THE NUMBER OF VERTEBRAE. About 95 per cent of people have seven cervical, 12 thoracic, five lumbar, and five sacral vertebrae. About three per cent of people have one or two more vertebrae, and about two per cent have one less. To determine the number of vertebrae, it is necessary to examine the entire vertebral column (e.g., in a radiograph), because an apparent extra (or absent) vertebra in one segment of the column may be compensated for by an absent (or extra) vertebra in an adjacent segment, e.g., 11 thoracic-type vertebrae with six lumbar-type vertebrae.

SPINA BIFIDA OCCULTA (see Fig. 17–10*A*). This defect of the vertebral arch results from failure of development and fusion of the halves of the vertebral arch. It is commonly observed in radiographs of the cervical, lumbar, and sacral regions and can be diagnosed *in utero* by sonography. Frequently, only one vertebra is affected. Spina bifida occulta of the first sacral vertebra occurs in about 20 per cent of people who are

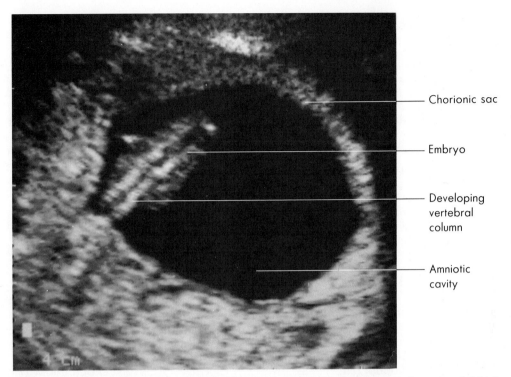

Chorionic sac

Embryo

Developing
vertebral
column

Amniotic
cavity

Figure 16–6. Ultrasound image of a 7-week-old human embryo. This coronal scan shows two bright lines, which represent lateral parts of the vertebrae surrounding the vertebral (neural) canal. (Courtesy of Dr. E.A. Lyons, Professor of Radiology and Obstetrics and Gynecology, Head of Radiology, Health Sciences Centre, University of Manitoba, Winnipeg, Manitoba, Canada).

usually unaware of the defect. The spinal cord and spinal nerves are usually normal, and neurological symptoms are commonly absent. The skin over the defect is intact, and there may be no external evidence of the abnormality. Sometimes the anomaly is indicated by a dimple or a tuft of hair (see Fig. 17–10A).

RACHISCHISIS (see Fig. 16–10). The term rachischisis (cleft vertebral column) refers to the vertebral anomalies encountered in a complex group of developmental defects that primarily affect the axial structures of the body. In these cases the neural folds fail to fuse, either due to faulty induction by the underlying notochord and its associated mesenchyme, or because of the action of teratogenic agents on the neuro-epithelial cells making up the neural folds. The neural and vertebral defects may be extensive (see Fig. 16–10C), or they may be restricted to a small area.

HEMIVERTEBRA (Fig. 16–7B). The developing vertebral bodies have two chondrification centers that normally unite (Fig. 16–5B). A hemivertebra results from failure of one of the chondrification centers to appear and subsequent failure of half of the vertebra to form.

These defective vertebrae produce *scoliosis* (lateral curvature) of the vertebral column. There are other causes of scoliosis, such as weakness of the spinal muscles (Moore, 1992).

DEVELOPMENT OF RIBS

Ribs develop from the mesenchymal *costal processes* of the thoracic vertebrae (Fig. 16–5A). They become cartilaginous during the embryonic period and later ossify. The original union of the costal processes with the vertebra is replaced by synovial joints, the *costovertebral joints* (Fig. 16–5D).

Anomalies of the Ribs

ACCESSORY RIBS (Fig. 16–7A). Accessory ribs are usually rudimentary. They result from the development of the costal processes of cervical or lumbar vertebrae. These processes usually form ribs only in the thoracic region. The most common type of accessory rib is a *lumbar rib*, but it causes no problems (Moore, 1992).

Cervical ribs are less common but are present in 0.5 to one per cent of people. A cervical rib is attached to the seventh cervical vertebra and may be unilateral or bilateral (Fig. 16–7). Pressure of a cervical rib on the *brachial plexus* of nerves or the subclavian vessels may produce neurovascular symptoms (Moore, 1992).

FUSED RIBS. Fusion of ribs occasionally occurs posteriorly when two or more ribs arise from a single vertebra. Fused ribs are often associated with a hemivertebra.

FORKED RIBS (Fig. 16–7A). Forking of a rib at its anterior end is not uncommon. Usually the anomaly is unilateral and of no clinical significance. Rib anomalies are often seen in combination with vertebral anomalies and scoliosis (Gr., crookedness) of the vertebral column.

DEVELOPMENT OF THE SKULL

The skull develops from mesenchyme around the developing brain. It consists of the *neurocranium*, a protective case for the brain, and the *viscerocranium*, the skeleton of the face.

CARTILAGINOUS NEUROCRANIUM (Fig. 16–8). Initially, the cartilaginous neurocranium or *chondrocranium* consists of the cartilaginous base of the developing skull, which forms by fusion of several cartilages (Fig. 16–8A). Later, endo-

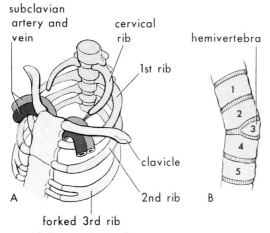

Figure 16–7. Drawings of vertebral and rib anomalies. *A,* Cervical and forked ribs. Observe that the left cervical rib has a fibrous band that passes posterior to the subclavian vessels and attaches to the sternum. This condition very likely produced neurovascular changes in the left upper limb. *B,* Anterior view of the vertebral column, showing a hemivertebra (half vertebra). The right half of the third thoracic vertebra is absent. Note the associated lateral curvature (scoliosis) of the vertebral column.

chondral ossification of this chondrocranium forms various bones in the base of the skull (Fig. 16–8D).

MEMBRANOUS NEUROCRANIUM (Figs. 16–8D and 16–9). Intramembranous ossification occurs in the mesenchyme investing the brain and forms the bones of the *calvaria* (cranial vault). During fetal life and infancy, the flat bones of the skull are separated by dense connective tissue membranes that constitute fibrous joints called *sutures* (Fig. 16–9). Six large fibrous areas ("soft spots") called *fontanelles* are present where several sutures meet.

The softness of the bones and their loose connections at the sutures enable the calvaria to undergo changes of shape during birth called *molding* (e.g., the forehead becomes flattened and the occiput [back of the head] drawn out as the bones overlap). Within a day or so after birth, the shape of the calvaria returns to normal. This construction of the skull also enables the skull to enlarge rapidly with the brain during infancy and childhood.

CARTILAGINOUS VISCEROCRANIUM (Fig. 16–8D). This consists of the cartilaginous skeleton of the first two pairs of *branchial (pharyngeal) arches* (see Fig. 11–5). During endochondral ossification, the dorsal end of the *first arch cartilage* (Meckel's cartilage) forms two middle ear bones: the malleus and incus. The dorsal end of the *second arch cartilage* (Reichert's cartilage) forms the stapes of the middle ear and the styloid process of the temporal bone. The ventral end ossifies to form the lesser cornu and superior part of the body of the hyoid bone. The ventral end of the *third arch cartilage* gives rise to the greater cornu and inferior part of the body of the hyoid bone.

MEMBRANOUS VISCEROCRANIUM (Fig. 16–8D). Intramembranous ossification occurs in the maxillary prominence of the first branchial or pharyngeal arch (see Fig. 11–5). This forms the premaxilla, maxilla, zygomatic, and squamous temporal bones. The mesenchyme of the mandibular prominence of this arch condenses around the first arch cartilage and undergoes intramembranous ossification to form the mandible.

THE FETAL AND NEWBORN SKULL (Fig. 16–9). The fetal skull is large in proportion to the rest of the skeleton, and the face is relatively small compared with the calvaria (cranial vault). The small facial region is the result of the small size of the jaws, the virtual absence of paranasal si-

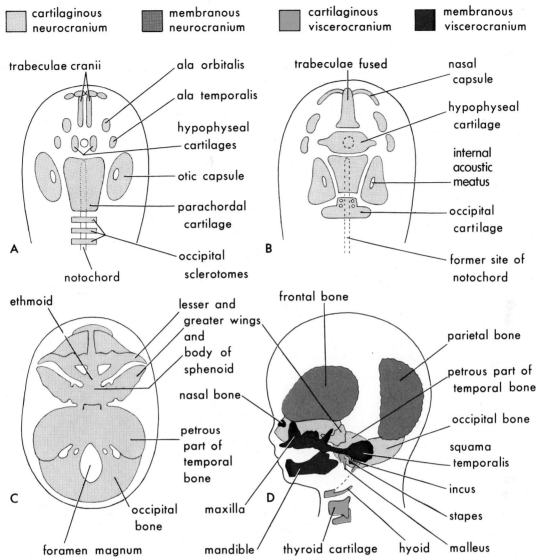

cartilaginous neurocranium

membranous neurocranium

cartilaginous viscerocranium

membranous viscerocranium

trabeculae cranii

ala orbitalis

ala temporalis

hypophyseal cartilages

otic capsule

parachordal cartilage

occipital sclerotomes

notochord

A

trabeculae fused

nasal capsule

hypophyseal cartilage

internal acoustic meatus

occipital cartilage

former site of notochord

B

ethmoid

lesser and greater wings and body of sphenoid

nasal bone

petrous part of temporal bone

foramen magnum

occipital bone

C

frontal bone

parietal bone

petrous part of temporal bone

occipital bone

squama temporalis

incus

stapes

maxilla

mandible   thyroid cartilage   hyoid   malleus

D

Figure 16–8. Diagrams illustrating development of the skull. *A* to *C* show the base of the developing skull as viewed superiorly; *D* is a lateral view. *A,* Six weeks, showing the various cartilages that will fuse to form the chondrocranium. *B,* Seven weeks after fusion of some of the paired cartilages. *C,* 12 weeks, showing the cartilaginous base of the skull or chondrocranium formed by the fusion of various cartilages. *D,* 20 weeks, indicating the derivation of the bones of the fetal skull. The sides and roof of the skull (calvaria) develop from the mesenchyme investing the brain that undergoes intramembranous ossification.

nuses, and the general underdevelopment of the facial bones.

POSTNATAL GROWTH OF THE SKULL. The fibrous sutures of the newborn calvaria permit it and the brain to enlarge during infancy and childhood. The increase in the size of the calvaria is greatest during the first two years, the period of most rapid postnatal growth of the brain. A person's calvaria normally increases in capacity until 15 to 16 years of age. This growth is also related to growth and development of the brain.

There is also rapid growth of the face and jaws, coinciding with the eruption of the primary or deciduous teeth; these changes are still more marked after the permanent teeth erupt (see Chapter 19). There is concurrent enlargement of the frontal and facial regions associated with the increase in the size of the paranasal sinuses. Most of the paranasal sinuses are

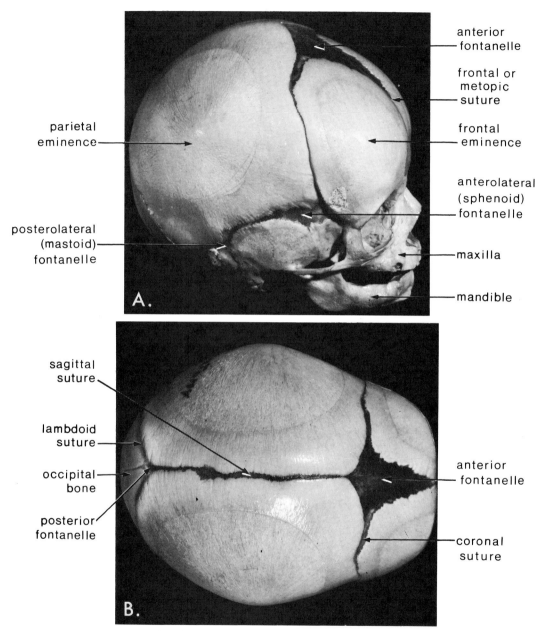

Figure 16–9. Photographs of a fetal skull, showing the bones, fontanelles, and connecting sutures. *A,* Lateral view. *B,* Superior view. The posterior and anterolateral fontanelles close within two to three months after birth by growth of the surrounding bones. The posterolateral fontanelles close similarly by the end of the first year, and the anterior fontanelle closes about the middle of the second year. The two halves of the frontal bone normally begin to fuse during the second year, and the metopic (frontal) suture is usually obliterated by the eighth year. The other sutures begin to disappear during adult life, but the times when the sutures close are subject to wide variations.

rudimentary or absent at birth. Growth of these sinuses is important in altering the shape of the face and in adding resonance to the voice.

Anomalies of the Skull

ACRANIA (Fig. 16–10). The calvaria is absent and a large defect of the vertebral column is usually present. Acrania is associated with *anencephaly* or *meroanencephaly* (absence of most of the brain); this severe brain anomaly is discussed in Chapter 17.

CRANIOSYNOSTOSIS. Several rare skull anomalies result from premature closure of the skull sutures. Prenatal closure results in the most severe abnormalities. The cause of craniosynostosis is unknown, but genetic factors appear to be important. These abnormalities are much more common in males than in females, and they are often associated with other skeletal defects. The type of deformed skull produced depends upon which sutures close prematurely. If the sagittal suture closes early, the skull becomes long, narrow, and wedge-shaped (*scaphocephaly*); this

type constitutes about half the cases of craniosynostosis. Another 30 per cent of cases involve premature closure of the coronal suture. This results in high, towerlike skull (*oxycephaly* or *turricephaly*, Fig. 16–11A). If the coronal or the lambdoid suture closes prematurely on one side only, the skull is twisted and asymmetrical (*plagiocephaly*; Fig. 16–11B).

The *appendicular skeleton* consists of the pectoral (shoulder) and pelvic girdles and the limb bones.

LIMB DEVELOPMENT

The general features of early limb development are described and illustrated in Chapter 6. The **limb buds** first appear as small elevations of the ventrolateral body wall toward the end of the fourth week (Fig. 16–12A). The early stages of limb development are alike for the upper and lower limbs (Figs. 16–13 and 16–14) except that development of the upper limb buds

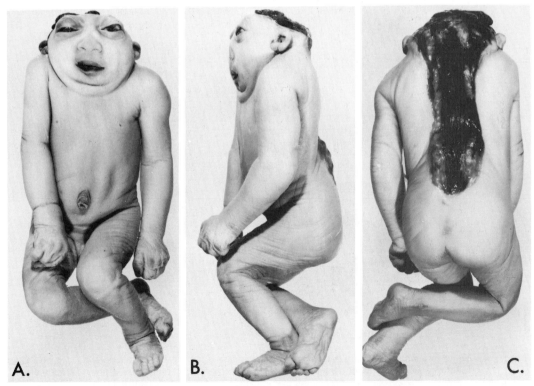

Figure 16–10. Photographs of anterior, lateral, and posterior views of a newborn infant with acrania (absence of cranial vault), meroanencephaly (partial absence of the brain), rachischisis (extensive cleft in vertebral column), and myeloschisis (severe type of spina bifida [see Fig. 17–10D]). Infants with these extensive craniovertebral defects usually die within a few days after birth.

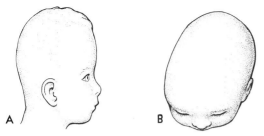

Figure 16–11. Drawing illustrating two types of skull anomaly. *A*, Oxycephaly (turricephaly), showing the towerlike skull resulting from premature closure of the coronal suture. *B*, Plagiocephaly, a type of asymmetrical skull resulting from premature closure of the coronal and lambdoid sutures on the left side.

precedes that of the lower limb buds by two days. The *upper limb buds* develop opposite the caudal cervical segments, and the *lower limb buds* form opposite the lumbar and upper sacral segments. Each limb bud consists of a mass of mesenchyme that is covered by a layer of ectoderm. The mesenchyme is derived from the somatic layer of lateral mesoderm.

The *apical ectodermal ridge* (Fig. 16–12*B*), a thickening of the ectoderm at the apex of the limb, exerts an inductive influence on the mesenchymal cells in the limb bud, which promotes growth and development of the bones and muscles. *Retinoic acid* is believed to play a modulating role in pattern formation and limb morphogenesis. The ends of the flipperlike limb buds flatten into paddlelike hand or foot plates; the digits differentiate at the margins of these plates (Fig. 16–14).

By the end of the sixth week, the mesenchymal tissue in the **hand plates** has condensed to form *digital (finger) rays*. These mesenchymal condensations outline the pattern of the future digits (fingers). During the seventh week, similar condensations of mesenchyme form *digital (toe) rays* in the **foot plates**. At the tip of each digital

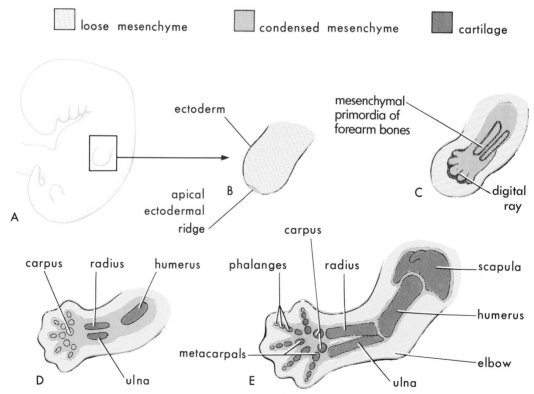

Figure 16–12. *A*, An embryo of about 28 days, showing the early appearance of the limb buds (see also Fig. 6–7). *B*, Schematic drawing of a longitudinal section through an early upper limb bud. The apical ectodermal ridge, a thickening of the ectoderm, has an inductive influence on the loose mesenchyme in the limb bud; it promotes growth of the mesenchyme and appears to give it the ability to form specific cartilaginous elements. *C*, Similar sketch of an upper limb bud at 33 days, showing the mesenchymal primordium of the limb bones. *D*, Upper limb at six weeks, showing the hyaline cartilage models of the various bones. *E*, Later in the sixth week, showing the completed cartilaginous models of the bones of the upper limb.

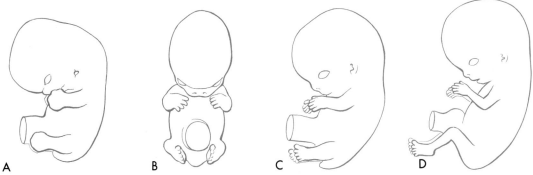

Figure 16–13. Drawing illustrating positional changes of the developing limbs. *A,* About 48 days, showing the limbs extending ventrally and the hand and foot plates facing each other. *B,* About 51 days, showing the upper limbs bent at the elbows and the hands curved over the thorax. *C,* About 54 days, showing the soles of the feet facing each other. *D,* About 56 days. Note that the elbows now point caudally and the knees cranially.

ray is a portion of the apical ectodermal ridge. It induces development of the mesenchyme into the primordia of the bones (phalanges) in the digits. The intervals between the digital rays are occupied by loose mesenchyme. The intervening regions of mesenchymal tissue soon break down, forming notches between the digital rays (Fig. 16–14*D* and *J*). As this tissue breakdown progresses, separate digits are produced by the end of the eighth week. If this process is incomplete or is arrested, varying degrees of webbing (*syndactyly*) result (see Fig. 16-19).

As the limbs elongate and the bones form, *myoblasts* (muscle-forming cells) aggregate and develop into a large muscle mass in each limb. In general, this muscle mass separates into dorsal (extensor) and ventral (flexor) components. Initially, the limbs are directed caudally; later,

they extend ventrally as the developing upper and lower limbs rotate in opposite directions and to different degrees (see Fig. 16–13). Originally the flexor aspect of the limbs is ventral and the extensor aspect dorsal. The preaxial and postaxial borders are cranial and caudal, respectively (Fig. 16–15).

The upper limb buds rotate laterally through 90 degrees on their longitudinal axes; thus, the future elbows point backward or dorsally, and the extensor muscles come to lie on the lateral and dorsal aspects of the upper limb. *The lower limb buds rotate medially* through almost 90 degrees; thus, the future knees point forward or ventrolaterally, and the extensor muscles lie on the ventral aspect of the lower limb. It should also be clear that the radius and tibia and the ulna and fibula are homologous bones, just as

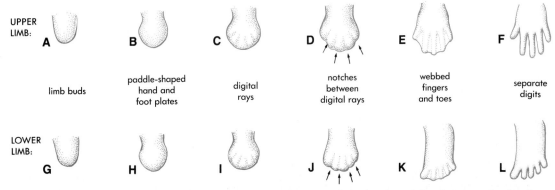

Figure 16–14. Drawings illustrating stages in the development of the hands and feet between the fourth and eighth weeks. The early stages of limb development are alike, except that development of the hands precedes that of the feet by a day or so. *A,* 27 days. *B,* 32 days. *C,* 41 days. *D,* 46 days. *E,* 50 days. *F,* 54 days. *G,* 28 days. *H,* 36 days. *I,* 46 days. *J,* 49 days. *K,* 52 days. *L,* 56 days.

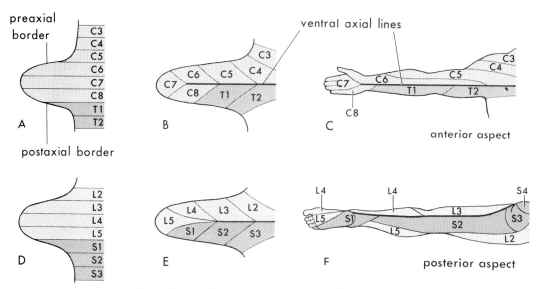

Figure 16–15. Diagrams illustrating development of the dermatomal patterns of the limbs. The *axial lines* indicate where there is no sensory overlap. *A* and *D*, Ventral aspect of the limb buds early in the fifth week. At this stage the dermatomal patterns show the primitive segmental arrangement. *B* and *E*, Similar views later in the fifth week, showing the modified arrangement of dermatomes. *C* and *F*, The dermatomal patterns in the adult upper and lower limbs. The primitive dermatomal pattern has disappeared, but an orderly sequence of dermatomes can still be recognized. In *F*, note that most of the original ventral surface of the lower limb lies on the posterior aspect of the adult limb. This results from the medial rotation of the lower limb that occurs toward the end of the embryonic period. In the upper limb, the ventral axial line extends along the anterior surface of the arm and forearm. In the lower limb, the ventral axial line extends along the medial side of the thigh and knee to the posteromedial aspect of the leg to the heel.

the thumb and the big toe are homologous digits.

During the sixth week, the mesenchymal primordia of bones in the limb buds undergo chondrification to form hyaline cartilage models of the future appendicular skeleton (Fig. 16–12D and E). The models of the pectoral girdle and the upper limb bones appear slightly before those of the pelvic girdle and lower limb bones. The bone models in each limb appear in a proximodistal sequence. By the end of the embryonic period, all the cartilage bones of the limbs are present. Ossification begins in the long bones by the end of the embryonic period. By 12 weeks, primary ossification centers have appeared in nearly all bones of the limbs. Secondary ossification centers usually appear after birth.

DERMATOMES AND CUTANEOUS INNERVATION OF THE LIMBS (Fig. 16–15). Because of its relationship to the growth and rotation of the limbs, the cutaneous segmental nerve supply of the limbs is considered in this chapter rather than in the chapter dealing with the nervous system or the integumentary system.

A dermatome is defined as the *area of skin supplied by a single spinal nerve and its spinal ganglion.* During the fifth week, the peripheral nerves grow from the limb plexuses (brachial and lumbosacral) into the mesenchyme of the limb buds. The spinal nerves are distributed in segmental bands and supply both dorsal and ventral surfaces of the limb buds. As the limbs elongate, the cutaneous distribution of the spinal nerves migrates along the limbs and no longer reaches the surface in the distal part of the limbs. Although the original dermatomal pattern changes during growth of the limbs, an orderly sequence of distribution can still be recognized in the adult (Fig. 16–15C and F).

A cutaneous nerve area is the *area of skin supplied by a peripheral nerve.* Both cutaneous nerve areas and dermatomes show considerable overlapping. The dermatomal patterns indicate that, if the dorsal root of that segment is cut, there may be a slight deficit in the area indicated. Because there is overlapping of dermatomes, however, a particular area is not exclusively innervated by a single segmental nerve. The limb dermatomes may be traced progressively down the lateral aspect of the upper limb and back up its medial aspect.

A comparable distribution of dermatomes occurs in the lower limbs, which may be traced down the ventral and up the dorsal aspect of the lower limb. When the limbs descend they carry their nerves with them; this explains the oblique course of the nerves of the brachial and lumbosacral plexuses.

LIMB DEFECTS

Minor limb anomalies or structural defects are relatively common but they can usually be corrected surgically. Major limb anomalies are relatively uncommon. An "epidemic" of limb anomalies occurred from 1957 to 1962 as a result of maternal ingestion of *thalidomide* (Fig. 16–16; see also Chapter 9, p. 136).

The terminology used to describe limb deficiencies in this text follows the international nomenclature in which only two basic descriptive terms are used: (1) *amelia*, complete absence of a limb or limbs (Fig. 16–16A), and (2) *meromelia* (Gr. *meros*, part, + *melos*, extremity), partial absence of a limb or limbs (Fig. 16–16B and C). Descriptive terms such as hemimelia, peromelia,

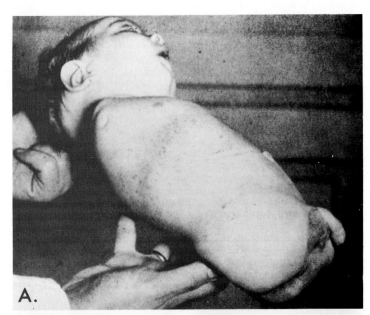

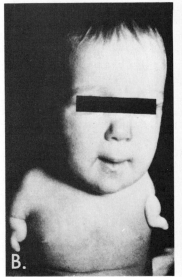
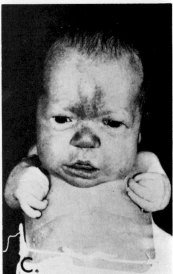

Figure 16–16. Limb defects caused by thalidomide. *A,* Quadruple amelia. The upper and lower limbs are absent. *B,* Meromelia of the upper limbs. The upper limbs are represented by rudimentary stumps. *C,* Meromelia of the upper limbs with the rudimentary upper limbs attached directly to the trunk. (From Lenz W, Knapp K: *German Med Monthly* 7:253, 1962.)

ectromelia, and phocomelia are not used in current nomenclature because of their imprecision.

The most *critical period of limb development* is from 24 to 36 days after fertilization (Newman, 1986). Hence, a drug or agent that could cause absence of the limbs or of parts of them would have to act before the end of this period. Major limb defects are now found about twice in 1000 newborns; most of them are caused by genetic factors (Connor and Ferguson-Smith, 1988; Thompson et al.,1991).

ABSENCE OF THE HANDS AND PHALANGES (Fig. 16–17*A* to *D*). Absence of the digits and often part of the hand is not common. Genetic factors cause these abnormalities (Chapter 9).

CLEFT HAND AND CLEFT FOOT (Fig. 16–17*E* and *F*). In these uncommon anomalies, often called *lobster-claw deformities*, there is absence of one or more central digits. This results from failure of development of one or more digital rays (Fig. 16–14). The hand or foot is thus divided into two parts that oppose each other like lobster claws. The remaining digits are partially or completely fused (syndactyly).

BRACHYDACTYLY (Fig. 16–18*A*). Abnormal shortness of the digits (fingers or toes) is uncommon. This anomaly is the result of reduction in the length of the phalanges. It is usually inherited as a dominant trait and is often associated with shortness of stature (see Fig. 9–11).

POLYDACTYLY (Fig. 16–18*C* and *D*). Supernumerary (extra) fingers or toes are common. Often the extra digit is incompletely formed and rudimentary. If the hand is affected, the extra digit is most commonly medial or lateral in position rather than central. In the foot, the extra toe is usually in the lateral position. Polydactyly is inherited as a dominant trait.

SYNDACTYLY (Fig. 16–19). Fusion of the fingers or toes (webbed digits) is a fairly common limb defect (occurs in one to 2000 births). Webbing of the skin between fingers or toes (cutaneous syndactyly) is due to failure of the tissue to break down between the digits during development (Fig. 16–14*E* and *K*). Syndactyly is most frequently observed between the third and fourth fingers and the second and third toes. It is inherited as a simple dominant or simple recessive trait. In unusual cases there is also fusion of the bones *(osseous syndactyly)*.

CONGENITAL CLUBFOOT (Fig. 16–19*C*). Any deformity of the foot involving the talus (ankle bone) is called a clubfoot or talipes (L. *talus*, ankle + *pes*, foot). *Talipes equinovarus* is the common type of clubfoot, occurring about once in 1000 births. It is about twice as frequent in males. The sole of the foot is turned medially and the foot is inverted. This abnormal position of the foot prevents normal weight-bearing.

Flexible types of clubfoot appear to be due to abnormal positioning or restricted movement of the lower limbs *in utero*. The feet in these deformities are structurally normal, and the abnormalities usually correct themselves spontaneously. *Rigid types of clubfoot* result from abnormal development of the ankle and foot joints during the sixth and seventh weeks. In these cases, there are bony deformities, particularly of the talus. Hereditary and environmental factors appear to be involved in most cases of clubfoot (i.e., *multifactorial inheritance*, p. 139).

CONGENITAL DISLOCATION OF THE HIP. This deformity occurs in about one of every 1500 newborn infants and is more common in females than in males. The capsule of the hip joint is very relaxed at birth, and there is underdevelopment of the acetabulum of the hip bone and the head of the femur. The actual dislocation almost always occurs after birth. Two causative factors commonly suggested are:

1. *Abnormal development of the acetabulum.* About 15 per cent of infants with congenital dislocation of the hip are breech deliveries, suggesting that breech posture during the terminal months may result in abnormal development of the acetabulum and the head of the femur.

2. *Generalized joint laxity* appears to be associated with congenital dislocation of the hip. Joint laxity is often a dominantly inherited condition; hence, congenital dislocation of the hip appears to have a multifactorial pattern of inheritance (Thompson et al., 1991).

ACHONDROPLASIA (see Fig. 9–11). This condition is the most common cause of *dwarfism* (shortness of stature). It occurs about once in 10,000 births. The limbs are short because of disturbance of endochondral ossification at the epiphyseal cartilage plates, particularly of long bones, during fetal life. The trunk is normal length, but the head may be slightly enlarged, with a bulging forehead and "scooped-out" nose. Achondroplasia is an *autosomal dominant disorder*, and about 80 per cent of cases arise from new mutations; the rate increases with paternal age (Strewler, 1985). For details of the inheritance of achondroplasia, see Thompson et al. (1991).

Causes of Limb Defects

Anomalies of the limbs originate at different stages of development. Suppression of limb development during the early part of the fourth week results in absence of the limbs, which is known as *amelia* (see Fig. 16–16A). Arrest or disturbance of differentiation or growth of the limbs during the fifth week results in various types of *meromelia* (see Figs. 16–16*B* and *C* and

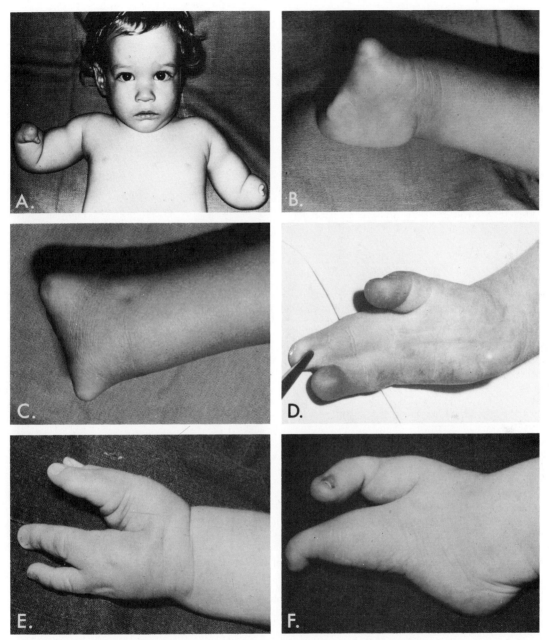

Figure 16–17. Photographs illustrating various types of meromelia (partial absence of the limbs). *A,* Absence of the hands and most of the forearms. *B,* Absence of the digits. *C,* Absence of the hand. *D,* Absence of the fourth and fifth digits and metacarpal bones. There is also syndactyly. *E,* Absence of the third digit, resulting in a cleft hand (lobster claw). *F,* Absence of the second and third toes, resulting in a cleft foot. (*D* from Swenson O: *Pediatric Surgery*, 1958. Courtesy of Appleton-Century-Crofts, Publishing Division of Prentice-Hall, Englewood Cliffs, NJ.)

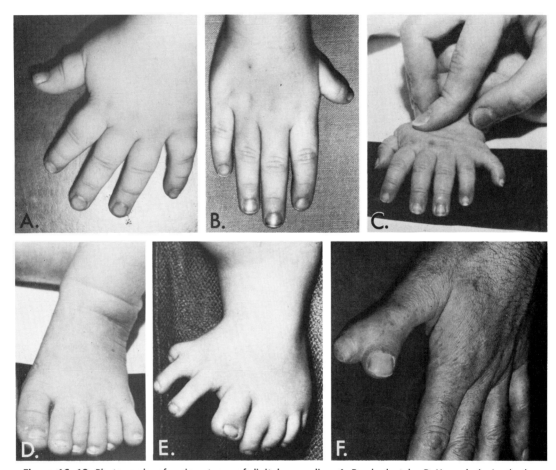

Figure 16–18. Photographs of various types of digital anomalies. *A,* Brachydactyly. *B,* Hypoplasia (underdevelopment) of the thumb. *C,* Polydactyly, showing a supernumerary finger. *D,* Polydactyly, showing a supernumerary toe. *E,* Partial duplication of the foot. *F,* Partial duplication of the thumb. (*C* and *D* from Swenson O: *Pediatric Surgery*, 1958. Courtesy of Appleton-Century-Crofts, Publishing Division of Prentice-Hall, Englewood Cliffs, NJ.)

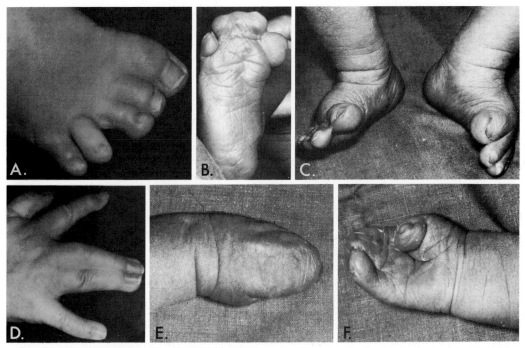

Figure 16–19. Photographs of various types of limb defects of the hands and feet. *A,* Syndactyly, showing skin webs between the first and second and second and third toes. *B,* Syndactyly involving fusion of all the toes except the fifth. *C,* Syndactyly associated with clubfoot. *D,* Syndactyly involving webbing of the third and fourth digits. *E* and *F,* Dorsal and palmar views of a child's right hand, showing syndactyly of the second to fifth digits. (*A* and *D* from Swenson O: *Pediatric Surgery*, 1958. Courtesy of Appleton-Century-Crofts, Publishing Division of Prentice-Hall, Englewood Cliffs, NJ.)

16–17). Meromelia denotes the partial absence of a limb; this may be terminal, e.g., absence of the hand or the digits (see Fig. 16–17*C*).

Like other anomalies, some limb defects are caused by: (1) genetic factors, e.g., chromosomal abnormalities as in trisomy 18 (see Fig. 9–5) or mutant genes as in brachydactyly (Fig. 16–18*A*) or osteogenesis imperfecta (Cole and Cohen Jr., 1991); (2) environmental factors, e.g., thalidomide (Fig. 16–16*A*); and (3) combination of genetic and environmental factors *(multifactorial inheritance)*, e.g., congenital dislocation of the hip (Thompson et al., 1991). Vascular disruption may also lead to limb reduction defects (Van Allen, 1992).

THE MUSCULAR SYSTEM

The muscular system develops from mesoderm except for the muscles of the iris (see Chapter 18). Muscle tissue develops from primitive cells called *myoblasts,* which are derived from *mesenchyme* (embryonic connective tissue).

Skeletal Muscles

The myoblasts that form the skeletal musculature are derived from the myotome regions of the *somites* (Figs. 16–1*D* and 16–20*A*), the *branchial (pharyngeal) arches,* and the *somatic mesoderm.* The **myoblasts** elongate, aggregate to form parallel bundles, and then fuse to form multinucleated cells. During early fetal life, *myofibrils* appear in the cytoplasm and show the characteristic cross-striations by the twelfth week.

The migration of myoblasts from the branchial (pharyngeal) arches to form the *muscles of facial expression,* mastication, and of the pharynx and larynx is described in Chapter 11 and is illustrated in Figures 11–6 and 16–20. Myoblasts from the *occipital myotomes* form the tongue muscles. *Limb muscles* develop from mesenchyme in the limb buds (Fig. 16–12). The mesenchyme that gives rise to these muscles is derived from the somatic layer of lateral mesoderm (Fig. 16–1).

Most skeletal muscle develops before birth, and almost all the remaining ones are formed by the end of the first year. The increase in the size of a muscle occurs due to an increase in the diameter of the fibers through the formation of more myofilaments. After birth, muscles increase in length and width in order to grow with the skeleton. Their ultimate size depends on the amount of exercise that is performed. Not all embryonic muscle fibers persist; many of them fail to establish themselves as necessary units of the muscle and soon degenerate.

Visceral Muscles

SMOOTH MUSCLE. Smooth muscle fibers differentiate from *splanchnic mesoderm* surrounding the primordium of the gut and its derivatives (see Fig. 13-1D). Elsewhere, smooth muscle develops from mesenchyme in the area concerned. The myoblasts elongate and develop contractile elements. The *muscles of the iris* and the myoepithelial cells of mammary and sweat glands appear to be derived from mesenchymal cells that *originate from ectoderm.*

CARDIAC MUSCLE. Cardiac muscle develops from *splanchnic mesoderm* surrounding the endothelial heart tube (see Figs. 15–2 and 15–3). Cardiac myoblasts differentiate from the primordial myocardium. They adhere to each other, as in developing skeletal muscle, but the intervening cell membranes do not disintegrate. These areas of adhesion become the *intercalated discs.* There is usually a single central nucleus, and myofibrils develop as in skeletal muscle cells. Heart muscle is recognizable in the fourth week. Late in the embryonic period, special bundles of muscle cells develop with relatively few myofibrils and relatively larger diameters than typical cardiac muscle cells. These atypical cardiac muscle cells called *Purkinje fibers* form the conducting system of the heart (Moore, 1992; Moore and Persaud, 1993).

Anomalies of Muscles

Absence of one or more muscles is more common than is generally recognized. Usually only a single muscle is absent on one side of the body or only a portion of the muscle fails to develop.

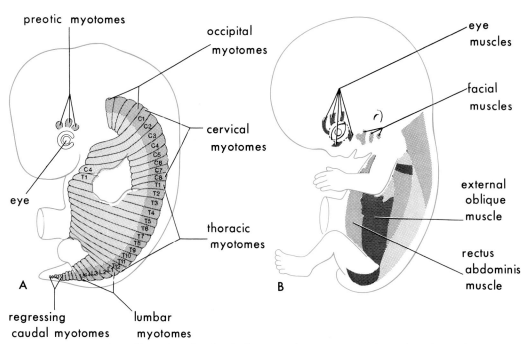

Figure 16–20. Drawings illustrating the developing muscular system. *A,* Six-week embryo, showing the myotome regions of the somites that give rise to most skeletal muscles. *B,* Eight-week embryo, showing the developing superficial trunk musculature. The limb muscles are not shown here because they are not derived from the somites; they differentiate from somatic mesoderm. Mesenchyme from this layer migrates into the limb buds early in the fourth week and gives rise to myoblasts (primordial muscle cells).

Occasionally, the same muscle or muscles may be absent on both sides of the body. Any muscle in the body may occasionally be absent; common examples are the sternocostal head of the pectoralis major, the palmaris longus, the trapezius, the serratus anterior, and the quadratus femoris (Moore, 1992).

Absence of the pectoralis major muscle, usually its sternal portion, is often associated with syndactyly (fusion of the digits). These anomalies are part of the *Poland syndrome*. Absence of this muscle is occasionally associated with absence of the mammary gland and/or hypoplasia of the nipple. In rare instances, failure of normal muscle development may be widespread, leading to immobility of multiple joints, a condition known as *arthrogryposis multiplex congen-*

ita (Behrman, 1992). Persons with this disorder have congenital stiffness of one or more joints, associated with hypoplasia of the associated muscles.

Variations in Muscles

All muscles are subject to a certain amount of variation, but some are affected more often than others. Certain muscles are functionally vestigial (e.g., those of the external ear and scalp). Some muscles present in other primates appear in only some humans (e.g., the sternalis muscle). Variations in the form, position, and attachments of muscles are common and are usually functionally insignificant.

SUMMARY

Most of the articular, skeletal, and muscular systems are derived from mesoderm. The skeleton mainly develops from condensed mesenchyme, which undergoes chondrification to form hyaline cartilage models of the bones. Ossification centers appear in these models by the end of the embryonic period, and the bones ossify by *endochondral ossification* during the fetal period. Some bones (e.g., the flat bones of the skull) develop by *intramembranous ossification.*

The vertebral column and ribs develop from sclerotomal cells that arise from the somites. The developing skull consists of a neurocranium and a viscerocranium, each of which has membranous and cartilaginous components.

The limb buds appear toward the end of the fourth week as slight elevations of the ventrolateral body wall. The *apical ectodermal ridge* (AER) exerts an inductive influence on the mesenchyme in the limb buds that pro-

motes growth and development of the limbs. The upper limb buds develop slightly before the lower limb buds. The tissues of the limb buds are derived from two main sources, the somatic layer of the lateral mesoderm and the surface ectoderm. The nerves grow into the limb buds during the fifth week. The upper and lower limbs rotate in opposite directions and to different degrees.

Most skeletal muscle is derived from the myotome regions of the somites, but some head and neck muscles are derived from branchial or pharyngeal arch mesoderm. The limb musculature develops from mesenchyme derived from the somatic layer of lateral mesoderm. Cardiac muscle and smooth muscle are derived from splanchnic mesoderm.

Most defects of the skeletal and muscular systems are caused by genetic factors; however, many congenital defects probably result from an interaction of genetic and environmental factors (multifactorial inheritance).

Commonly Asked Questions

1. An acquaintance of ours had a baby with very short limbs. His trunk is normally proportioned, but his head is slightly larger than normal. Both parents have normal limbs, and these problems have never occurred in either of their families. Could her ingestion of drugs during pregnancy have caused these abnor-

malities? If not, what is the probable cause of these skeletal disorders? Could they occur again if they have more children?

2. My sister is interested in marrying a man with very short fingers *(brachydactyly)*. He says that two of his relatives have exhibited short fingers, but none of his brothers or sisters has them. My sister has normal digits and so has everyone else in our family. She asked

me what the chances are that her children would have brachydactyly if she were to marry him. I know that heredity is involved, but I could not give her a helpful answer. Can you?

3. About a year ago I read in the paper about a woman who had a child with no right hand. She started to take a drug called *Bendectin* to alleviate nausea during the tenth week of her pregnancy (eight weeks after fertilization) and is instituting legal proceedings against the drug company that makes the drug. Does this drug cause limb defects; and, if it does, could it have caused failure of the child's hand to develop?

4. When I was a nurse I saw a baby with *syndactyly* (fused digits) of the left hand and absence of the left sternal head of the pectoralis major muscle. The baby seemed normal except that the nipple on the left side was

about two inches lower than the other one. What is the cause of these anomalies? Can they be corrected?

5. Following a routine x-ray examination of my young sister's chest, my parents were told that she had a rib in her neck. Is this possible? They were told that it might cause some pain and tingling in her upper limb after puberty. What is the embryological basis of cervical ribs? How common are they? Why may pain and tingling develop in her upper limb as she matures?

6. I know a fellow who has a long, narrow head. When he was a boy, he was called "peanut head" because of the cranial anomaly. He had normal intelligence and no apparent disability. What would cause such an abnormally shaped skull? Was it a birth injury?

The answers to these questions are given on page 334.

REFERENCES

Behrman RE (ed): *Nelson Textbook of Pediatrics*, 14th ed. Philadelphia, WB Saunders, 1992.

Blechschmidt E, Gasser RF: *Biokinetics and Biodynamics of Human Differentiation.* Springfield, Ill, Charles C Thomas, 1978.

Bruder SP, Caplan AL: Cellular and molecular events during embryonic bone development. *Connect Tissue Res 20*:65, 1989.

Cole DEC, Cohen Jr MM: Osteogenesis imperfecta: an update. *J Pediatr 119*:73, 1991.

Connor JM, Ferguson-Smith MA: *Essential Medical Genetics*, 2nd ed. Oxford, Blackwell Scientific Publications, 1988.

Daniels K, Solursh M: Modulation of chondrogenesis by the cytoskeleton and extracellular matrix. *J Cell Sci 100 (Pt. 2)*:249, 1991.

Dhem A, Goret-Nicaise M, Dambrain R, Nyssen-Behets C, Lengele B, Manzanares MC: Skeletal growth and chondroid tissue. *Arch Ital Anat Embriol 94*:237, 1989.

Dziedzic-Goclawska A, Emerich J, Grzesik W, Stachowicz W, Michalik J, Ostrowski K: Differences in the kinetics of the mineralization process in endochondral and intramembranous osteogenesis in human fetal development. *J Bone Miner Res 3*:533, 1988.

Filly RA, Golbus MS: Ultrasonography of the normal and pathologic fetal skeleton. *Radiol Clin North Am 20*:311, 1982.

Gasser RF: Evidence that sclerotomal cells do not migrate medially during normal embryonic development of the rat. *Am J Anat 154*:509, 1979.

Marin-Padilla M: Cephalic axial skeletal-neural dysraphic disorders: embryology and pathology. *Can J Neurol Sci 18*:153, 1991.

Marks Jr, SC, Popoff SN: Bone cell biology: The regulation of development, structure, and function in the skeleton. *Am J Anat 183*:1, 1988.

Moore KL: *Clinically Oriented Anatomy*, 3rd ed. Baltimore, Williams & Wilkins, 1992.

Moore KL, Persaud TVN: *The Developing Human: Clinically Oriented Embryology*, 5th ed. Philadelphia, WB Saunders, 1993.

Newman CGH: Clinical aspects of thalidomide embryopathy —a continuing preoccupation. *Teratogen Update. Environmentally Induced Birth Risks.* New York, Alan R. Liss, 1986.

O'Rahilly R, Müller F, Meyer DB: The human vertebral column at the end of the embryonic period proper. 3. The thoracolumbar region. *J Anat 168*:81, 1990a.

O'Rahilly R, Müller F, Meyer DB: The human vertebral column at the end of the embryonic period proper. 4. The sacrococcygeal region. *J Anat 168*:95, 1990b.

Smith MM, Hall BK: Development and evolutionary origins of vertebrate skeletogenic and odontogenic tissue. *Biol Rev Camb Philos Soc 65*:277, 1990.

Sperber GH: *Craniofacial Embryology*, 4th ed. London, Butterworth, 1989.

Stedman H, Sarkar S: Molecular genetics in basic myology: a rapidly evolving perspective. *Muscle Nerve 11*:668, 1991.

Strewler GJ: Osteonecrosis, osteosclerosis and other disorders of bone. *In* Wyngaarden JB, Smith Jr, LH (eds): *Cecil Textbook of Medicine*, 17th ed. Philadelphia, WB Saunders, 1985.

Thompson MW, McInnes RR, Willard HF: *Thompson & Thompson Genetics in Medicine*, 5th ed. Philadelphia, WB Saunders, 1991.

Uhthoff HK: *The Embryology of the Human Locomotor System.* New York, Springer-Verlag, 1990.

Van Allen MI: Structural anomalies resulting from vascular disruption. *Pediatr Clin NA 39*:255, 1992.

van der Harten HJ, Brons JT, Schipper NW, Dijkstra PF, Meijer CJ, van Geijin HP: The prenatal development of the normal human skeleton: a combined ultrasonographic and post-mortem radiographic study. *Pediatr Radiol 21*:52, 1990.

17

THE NERVOUS SYSTEM

The nervous system develops from the **neural plate,** a thickened, slipper-shaped area of embryonic ectoderm that appears around the middle of the third week (Fig. 17–1). Formation of the neural tube and neural crest from the neural plate is described and illustrated in Chapter 5. For more details, see Schoenwolf and Smith (1990). The **neural tube** differentiates into the *central nervous system* (CNS), consisting of the brain and spinal cord, and the **neural crest** gives rise to most of the *peripheral nervous system.* Neural crest cells also differentiate into other structures (see Fig. 17–8).

The neural tube begins to form 22 to 23 days after fertilization and is temporarily open both cranially and caudally (Figs. 17–1C and 17–2). These openings called *neuropores* normally close during the fourth week. The walls of the neural tube thicken and differentiate to form the brain and spinal cord (Fig. 17–3). The *neural canal* becomes the ventricular system of the brain and the central canal of the spinal cord.

DEVELOPMENT OF THE SPINAL CORD

The neural tube caudal to the fourth pair of somites develops into the spinal cord. The lateral walls of the neural tube thicken until only a minute central canal remains at nine weeks (Fig. 17–4C). The wall of the neural tube is composed of a thick neuroepithelium, which gives rise to all neurons and macroglial cells of the spinal cord (Fig. 17–5). The marginal zone of the neuroepithelium gradually becomes the white matter of the cord as axons grow into it and over it from nerve cell bodies in the spinal cord, spinal ganglia, and brain.

Some neuroepithelial cells differentiate into primordial neurons called *neuroblasts.* These embryonic nerve cells form an *intermediate zone* between the ventricular and marginal zones (Fig. 17–4E). When the neuroepithelial cells cease producing neuroblasts and glioblasts, they differentiate into ependymal cells, which form the ependyma (ependymal epithelium) lining the central canal of the spinal cord. Neuroblasts become *neurons* as they develop cytoplasmic processes (Fig. 17–5). The *microglial cells* (microglia), a smaller type of neuroglial cell, differentiate from mesenchymal cells surrounding the central nervous system (Fig. 17–5). They enter the spinal cord late in the fetal period with developing blood vessels.

Differential thickening of the lateral walls of the spinal cord soon produces a shallow longitudinal groove called the *sulcus limitans* (Figs. 17–4B and 17–6). This groove demarcates the dorsal part or *alar plate* (lamina) from the ventral part or *basal plate* (lamina). The alar and basal plates are later associated with afferent and efferent functions, respectively.

Text continued on page 282

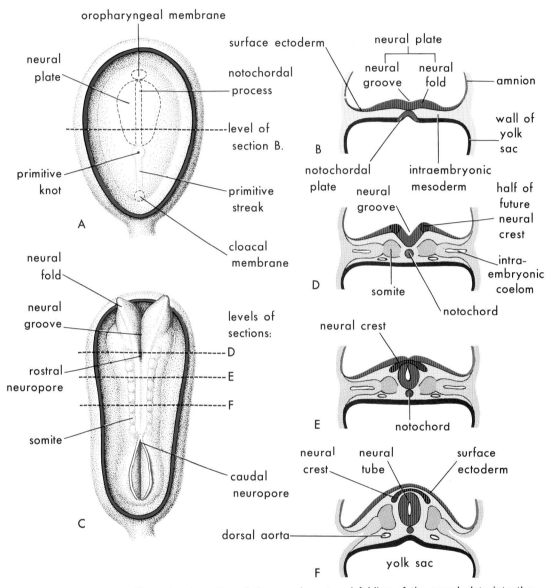

Figure 17–1. Diagrams illustrating formation of the neural crest and folding of the neural plate into the neural tube. *A,* Dorsal view of an embryo of about 18 days, exposed by removing the amnion. *B,* Transverse section of this embryo, showing the neural plate and early development of the neural groove. *C,* Dorsal view of an embryo of about 22 days. The neural folds have fused opposite the somites but are widely spread out at both ends of the embryo. Closure of the neural tube occurs initially in the region corresponding to the future junction of the brain and spinal cord. *D, E,* and *F,* Transverse sections of this embryo at the levels shown in *C,* illustrating formation of the neural tube and its detachment from the surface ectoderm. Note that some neuroectodermal cells are not included in the neural tube but remain between it and the surface ectoderm as the neural crest. (See Figure 17–8 for the derivatives of the neural crest.)

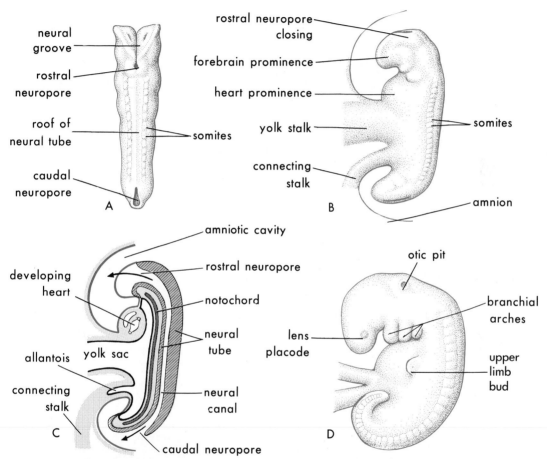

Figure 17–2. *A,* Dorsal view of an embryo of about 23 days, showing advanced fusion of the neural folds. *B,* Lateral view of an embryo of about 24 days, showing the forebrain prominence and closing of the rostral neuropore. *C,* Sagittal section of this embryo, showing the transitory communication of the neural canal with the amniotic cavity *(arrows). D,* Lateral view of an embryo of 27 days after closure of the neuropores.

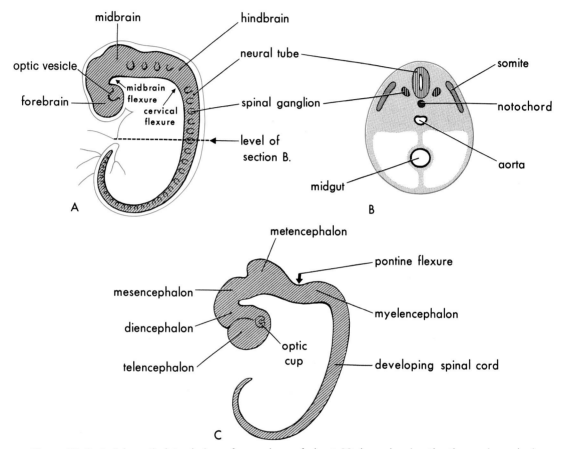

Figure 17–3. *A,* Schematic lateral view of an embryo of about 28 days, showing the three primary brain vesicles (forebrain, midbrain, and hindbrain). The two flexures demarcate the primary divisions of the brain. *B,* Transverse section of this embryo, showing the neural tube which, in this region, will develop into the spinal cord. The spinal ganglia derived from the neural crest are also shown. *C,* Schematic lateral view of the central nervous system of a six-week embryo, showing the secondary brain vesicles and the pontine flexure. The flexures occur as the brain grows rapidly. They are important in determining the final shape of the brain.

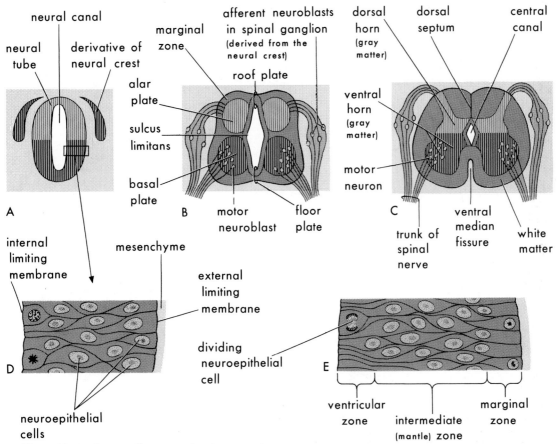

Figure 17–4. Diagrams illustrating development of the spinal cord. *A,* Transverse section through the neural tube of an embryo of about 23 days. *B* and *C,* Similar sections at six and nine weeks, respectively. *D,* Section through the wall of the early neural tube shown in *A. E,* Section through the wall of the developing spinal cord, showing the three different zones. Note that the neural canal of the neural tube becomes the central canal of the spinal cord.

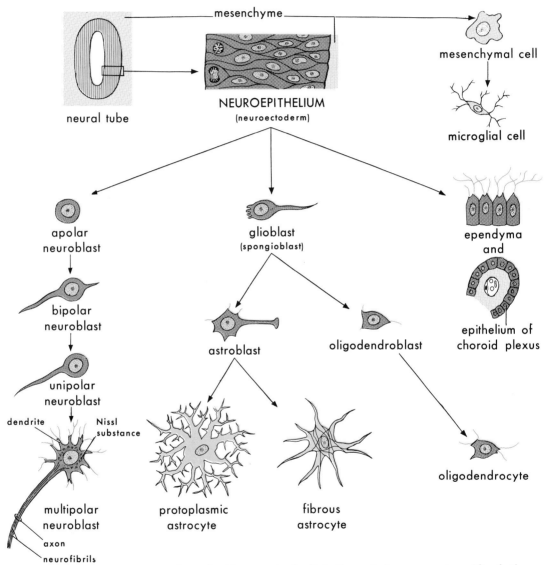

Figure 17–5. Schematic diagram illustrating histogenesis of cells in the central nervous system. After further development, the multipolar neuroblast (lower left) becomes a nerve cell (neuron). Neuroepithelial cells give rise to all neurons and macroglial cells. Microglial cells are derived from mesenchymal cells, which invade the developing nervous system with the developing blood vessels. There is substantial evidence that they are derived postnatally from blood monocytes.

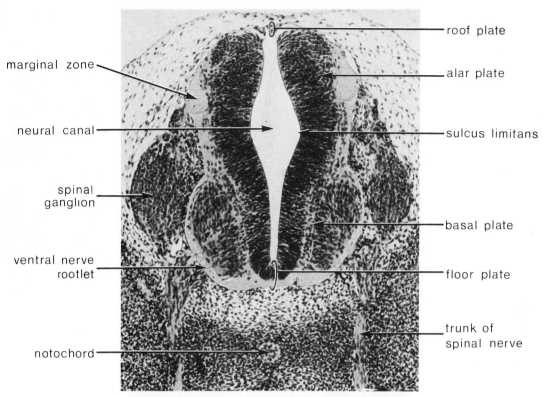

roof plate

alar plate

marginal zone

neural canal

sulcus limitans

spinal ganglion

basal plate

ventral nerve rootlet

floor plate

trunk of spinal nerve

notochord

Figure 17–6. Photomicrograph of a transverse section of the developing spinal cord in a 14-mm human embryo of about 44 days (×75). The dorsal wall (roof plate) and the ventral wall (floor plate) contain no neuroblasts and are relatively thin. Observe the notochord inside the developing vertebra. (Courtesy of Dr. J. W. A. Duckworth, Professor Emeritus of Anatomy and Cell Biology, University of Toronto.)

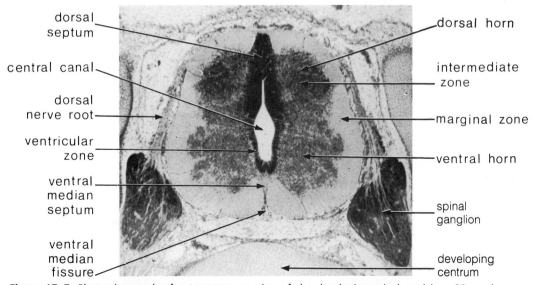

dorsal septum

dorsal horn

central canal

intermediate zone

dorsal nerve root

marginal zone

ventricular zone

ventral horn

ventral median septum

spinal ganglion

ventral median fissure

developing centrum

Figure 17–7. Photomicrograph of a transverse section of the developing spinal cord in a 20-mm human embryo of about 50 days (×60). (Courtesy of Professor Jean Hay, Department of Anatomy, Faculty of Medicine, University of Manitoba, Winnipeg, Canada.)

The Alar Plates

Cell bodies in the alar plates form the *dorsal gray matter* in columns that extend the length of the spinal cord. These columns are called *dorsal gray horns* (Fig. 17–7). As the alar plates enlarge, the *dorsal septum* forms, and the central canal is reduced in size (Figs. 17–4C and 17–7).

The Basal Plates

Cell bodies in the basal plates form the ventral and lateral gray columns, which are called *ventral gray horns* and *lateral gray horns*, respectively. Axons of ventral horn cells grow out of the spinal cord and form large bundles of nerves called the *ventral roots* of the spinal nerves (Fig. 17–6). As the basal plates enlarge, they produce the *ventral median septum*, and a deep longitudinal groove known as the *ventral median fissure* develops on the ventral surface of the spinal cord (Figs. 17–4C and 17–7).

SPINAL GANGLIA (Figs. 17–6 to 17–8). The unipolar neurons in the spinal ganglia (dorsal root ganglia) are derived from *neural crest cells*. The axons of cells in the ganglia are at first bipolar, but the two processes soon unite in a T-shaped

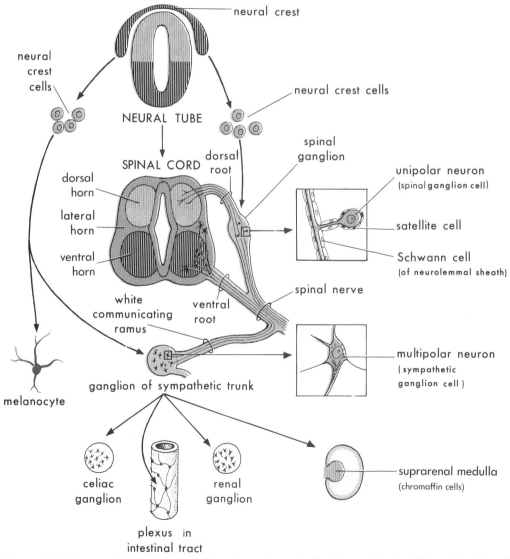

Figure 17–8. Diagram showing the derivatives of neural crest cells. These cells also differentiate into cells of the afferent ganglia of cranial nerves. Formation of a spinal nerve is also illustrated.

fashion into central and peripheral processes. The central processes enter the spinal cord and constitute the *dorsal roots of the spinal nerves.* The peripheral processes pass in the spinal nerves to special sensory endings in somatic or visceral structures.

Positional Changes of the Developing Spinal Cord

The spinal cord initially extends the entire length of the vertebral canal, and the spinal nerves pass through the intervertebral foramina at their levels of origin (Fig. 17–9A). This relationship does not persist because the vertebral column and the dura mater (outer covering of the spinal cord) grow more rapidly than the spinal cord. The caudal end of the spinal cord gradually comes to lie at relatively higher levels. As a result, the spinal roots, especially those of the lumbar and sacral segments, run obliquely from the spinal cord to the corresponding level of the vertebral column (Fig. 17–9B to D). These nerve roots form the *cauda equina.*

In the newborn infant the spinal cord terminates at the level of the second or *third lumbar vertebra* (Fig. 17–9C). *In the adult* the spinal cord usually terminates at the inferior border of the *first lumbar vertebra* (Fig. 17–9D). The dorsal and ventral nerve roots inferior to the end of the spinal cord form a sheaf of nerve roots called the *cauda equina* (L., horse's tail).

Although the dura extends the length of the vertebral column in the adult, the other layers of the meninges do not. The pia mater inferior to the caudal end of the spinal cord forms a long fibrous thread, the *filum terminale* (Fig. 17–9D). It extends from the *conus medullaris* (conical extremity of the spinal cord) to the periosteum of the first coccygeal vertebra in the adult. The filum terminale also indicates the line of regression of the embryonic spinal cord.

A portion of the subarachnoid space extends inferior to the spinal cord from which cerebrospinal fluid (CSF) may be removed without damaging the cord. CSF is obtained by inserting a needle between the vertebral arches of the lumbar vertebrae (usually between L3 and L4 or

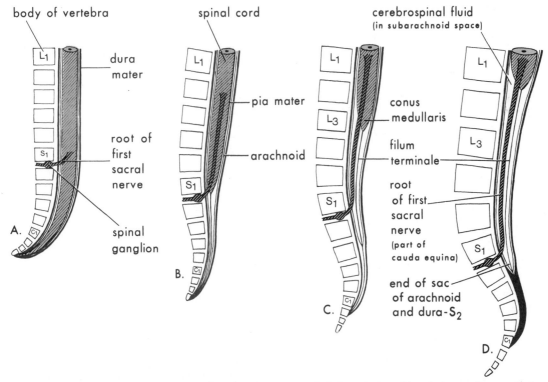

Figure 17–9. Diagram showing the position of the caudal end of the spinal cord in relation to the vertebral column and the meninges at various stages of development. The increasing inclination of the root of the first sacral nerve is also illustrated. *A,* Eight weeks. *B,* 24 weeks. *C,* Newborn. *D,* Adult.

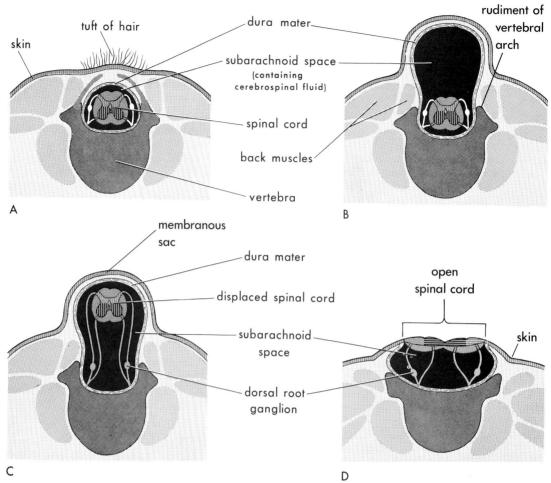

Figure 17–10. Diagrammatic sketches illustrating various types of spina bifida and the commonly associated anomalies of the nervous system. *A,* Spina bifida occulta. The halves of the vertebral arch are not fully developed; as a result, they are unfused, and the spinous process has not formed. About ten per cent of people have this defect in L5 or S1 vertebra or in both locations. It usually causes no back problems. *B,* Spina bifida with meningocele. *C,* Spina bifida with meningomyelocele. *D,* Spina bifida with myeloschisis. The types illustrated in *B* through *D* are often referred to collectively as *spina bifida cystica* because of the cystlike sac associated with them. Of these defects, 75 per cent are meningomyeloceles, and 25 per cent are meningoceles.

L4 and L5). This procedure is known as *lumbar puncture* (Moore, 1992).

MYELINATION OF NERVES. The myelin sheaths around the axons of peripheral nerve fibers begin to form in the spinal cord during the late fetal period and continue during the first post-natal year. The myelin sheath is formed around axons or axis cylinders by the plasma membranes of *Schwann cells.* The myelin sheaths of axons in the spinal cord are formed in a somewhat similar manner by *oligodendrocytes.* Fiber tracts generally become myelinated at about the time they become functional.

Congenital Anomalies of the Spinal Cord

Most congenital anomalies of the spinal cord are the result of defective closure of the caudal neuropore toward the end of the fourth week of development. The resulting *neural tube defects* (NTDs) also involve the tissues overlying the spinal cord: meninges, vertebral arches, dorsal muscles, and skin (Fig. 17–10). Defects involving the neural tube, meninges, and vertebral arches are referred to as *spina bifida cystica* (Figs. 17–10 and 17–11). "Spina bifida" de-

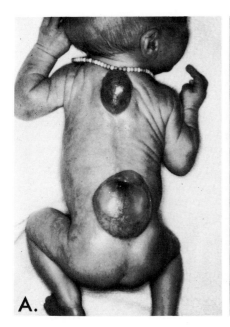
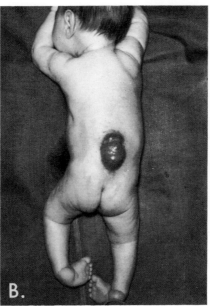

Figure 17–11. Photographs of infants with spina bifida cystica, showing the common locations of these defects. *A,* Spina bifida with meningomyelocele in the thoracic and lumbar regions. *B,* Spina bifida with myeloschisis in the lumbar region (see Fig. 17–10*D*). Note the nerve involvement affecting the lower limbs. (Courtesy of Dr. Dwight Parkinson, Children's Centre, Winnipeg.)

notes nonfusion of the halves of the vertebral (neural) arches, which is common to all types of spina bifida.

SPINA BIFIDA OCCULTA (Fig. 17–10*A*). This *vertebral defect* is due to failure of the embryonic halves of the vertebral arch to develop fully and fuse, usually in the sacral, lumbar, and cervical regions. Spina bifida occulta occurs in L5 or S1 vertebrae in about ten per cent of people. In its most minor form, there is no defect in the skin, and the only evidence of its presence may be a small dimple with a tuft of hair. *Spina bifida occulta usually produces no symptoms;* however, a small percentage of affected infants have associated developmental defects of the spinal cord and spinal roots which may produce symptoms (Behrman, 1992).

SPINA BIFIDA CYSTICA (Figs. 17–10*B* and C and 17–11). Severe types of spina bifida, involving protrusion of the spinal cord and/or the meninges through defects in several vertebral arches, are referred to as *spina bifida cystica* because of the cystlike protrusion (sac) that is associated with these anomalies. Spina bifida cystica occurs about once in every 1000 births. When the sac contains meninges and cerebrospinal fluid, the anomaly is called *spina bifida with meningocele* (Fig. 17–10*B*). The spinal cord and spinal roots are in their normal positions, but there may be spinal cord abnormalities. When the spinal cord and/or nerve roots are included in the sac, the condition is known as *spina bifida with meningomyelocele* (Fig. 17–10*C*).

Of the defects known collectively as *spina bifida cystica,* 75 per cent are meningomyeloceles. Most infants with this defect also have *hydrocephalus* (see Fig. 17–25). Often, nervous tissue is incorporated in the wall of the sac, which impairs development of nerve fibers. *Meningomyeloceles are often associated with a marked neurological deficit* inferior to the level of the protruding sac. This deficit occurs because the spinal cord is herniated into the sac and either ends there or continues in an abnormal way farther caudally. *Meningomyeloceles* may be covered by skin or a thin, easily ruptured membrane. About 15 to 20 per cent of defects have a covering of intact skin (closed lesions). These tend to cause less neurological disability than open lesions.

The most severe type of spina bifida is called *spina bifida with myeloschisis.* It is also known as spina bifida with *myelocele* (Figs. 17–10*D* and 17–11*B*). In these cases the spinal cord is open because the neural folds failed to meet and fuse during the fourth week (Gr. *schisis,* a cleaving). As a result, the spinal cord in the affected area is represented by a flattened mass of nervous tissue. Extensive *myeloschisis is associated with rachischisis* (see Fig. 16–10). It is much more usual for a short segment of the neural tube to fail to close (Fig. 17–11*B*).

Spina bifida with myeloschisis in the lumbosacral region is probably due to failure of the caudal neuropore to close during the fourth week. Another hypothesis, not as well supported, is that the neural tube ruptures after closure secondary to increased pressure within the neural canal. *Sphincter paralysis* (bladder and/or anal sphincters) is common with severe types of spina bifida.

Spina bifida cystica and/or meroanencephaly (see Fig. 17–23) is strongly suspected in utero when there is a high level of alpha-fetoprotein (AFP) in the amniotic fluid (p. 90). In these cases, AFP may also be elevated in the maternal blood serum. *Amniocentesis* (p. 89) is usually performed on pregnant women with high levels of AFP for the determination of the AFP level in the amniotic fluid. An ultrasound scan would also be requested to try to confirm the presence of a neural tube defect that has resulted in spina bifida cystica. The fetal vertebral column can be detected by ultrasound at nine weeks' gestation (see Fig. 16–6); and, if present, *spina bifida cystica* is sometimes visible as a cystic mass adjacent to the affected area of the vertebral column (Fig. 17–12).

Nutritional and environmental factors undoubtedly play a role in the production of neural tube defects (NTDs). Studies have sug-gested that vitamins and folic acid supplements taken prior to conception reduce the incidence of NTDs (Cockroft, 1991). Certain drugs are known to increase the risk of myelomeningocele (e.g., *valproic acid*, p. 135). This anticonvulsant causes NTDs in one to two per cent of pregnancies if given during early pregnancy (fourth week of development) when the neural folds are fusing (Holmes, 1992).

Pregnant animals exposed to hypothermia or vitamin A produce offspring with NTDs (Behrman, 1992). Studies have suggested that NTDs might result from specific biochemical abnormalities of the basement membrane, particularly hyaluronate, which plays a role in cell division and the shape of the primitive neuroepithelium (Copp and Bernfield, 1988).

DEVELOPMENT OF THE BRAIN

The neural tube cranial to the fourth pair of somites develops into the brain (Figs. 17–1 and 17–3). The adult brain consists of several regions; the relationship of these to each other will be understood better after the development of the brain has been considered. Fusion of the neural folds in the cranial region and closure of the rostral neuropore result in the formation of *three primary brain vesicles* from which the brain develops (Fig. 17–13).

The Brain Vesicles

During the fourth week the neural folds expand and fuse to form three primary brain vesicles: the **forebrain** or prosencephalon (Gr. *enkephalos*, brain), the *midbrain* or mesencephalon, and the *hindbrain* or rhombencephalon (Figs. 17–3 and 17–13). During the fifth week the **forebrain** partly divides into two vesicles, the *telencephalon* and the *diencephalon*, and the hindbrain partly divides into the *metencephalon* and the *myelencephalon*. As a result, there are five secondary brain vesicles.

The Brain Flexures

During the fourth week the brain grows rapidly and bends ventrally with the *head fold* (Figs. 17–3 and 17–14; see also Fig. 15–4). This produces the *midbrain flexure* in the midbrain region and the *cervical flexure* at the junction of the hindbrain and spinal cord in the cervical (neck) region. Later, unequal growth in the hindbrain between these flexures produces the

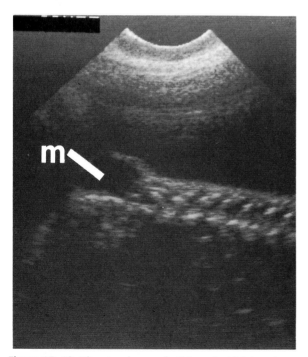

Figure 17–12. Ultrasound scan of a 14-week-old fetus, showing a cystlike protrusion representing a *meningomyelocele (m)* in the sacral region of the vertebral column. The well-formed vertebral arches of the vertebrae superior to the neural tube defect are clearly visible. (Courtesy of Dr. Lyndon M. Hill, Magee-Women's Hospital, Pittsburgh, Pennsylvania.)

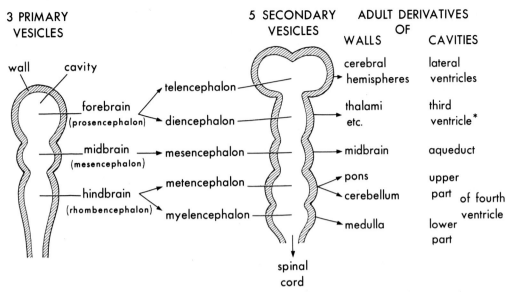

Figure 17–13. Diagrammatic sketches of the brain vesicles, indicating the adult derivatives of their walls and cavities. The cerebrum comprises all the derivatives of the forebrain. *The rostral or anterior part of the third ventricle forms from the cavity of the telencephalon.

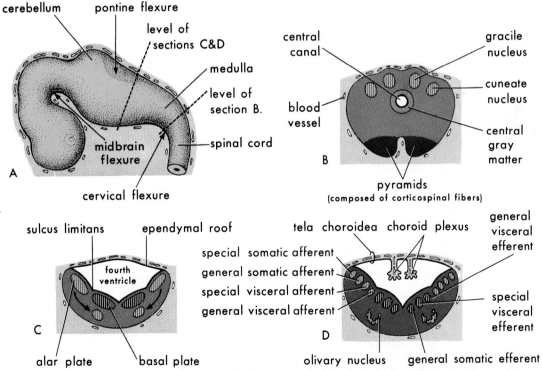

Figure 17–14. *A,* Sketch of the developing brain at the end of the fifth week, showing the three primary divisions of the brain and the brain flexures. *B,* Transverse section through the caudal part of the myelencephalon (developing closed part of the medulla). *C* and *D,* Similar sections through the rostral part of the myelencephalon (developing "open" part of the medulla), showing the position and successive stages of differentiation of the alar and basal plates. The arrows show the pathway taken by neuroblasts from the alar plates to form the olivary nuclei.

pontine flexure. This flexure causes thinning of the roof of the hindbrain (Fig. 17–14). Initially, the developing brain has the same basic structure as the developing spinal cord; however, the brain flexures produce considerable variation in the outline of transverse sections at different levels of the brain and in the position of the gray and white matter.

The Hindbrain

The *cervical flexure* demarcates the hindbrain (rhombencephalon) from the developing spinal cord (Fig. 17–14A). The pontine flexure appears in the future pontine region. The bend of this flexure divides the hindbrain into caudal (myelencephalon) and rostral (metencephalon) parts. The myelencephalon becomes the *medulla oblongata,* and the metencephalon gives rise to the *pons* and *cerebellum.* The cavity of the hindbrain becomes the **fourth ventricle** of the brain and the central canal in the caudal part of the medulla.

THE MYELENCEPHALON (Fig. 17–14). The caudal part of the myelencephalon (closed portion of the medulla) resembles the spinal cord both developmentally and structurally. The lumen of the neural tube becomes the small *central canal.* Unlike those of the spinal cord, neuroblasts from the alar plates in the myelencephalon migrate into the marginal zone and form the *gracile nucleus* medially and the *cuneate nucleus* laterally (Fig. 17–14B). The ventral area contains a pair of fiber bundles called the *pyramids,* which consist of nerve fibers from the developing cerebral cortex.

The rostral part of the myelencephalon ("open" portion of the medulla) is wide and rather flat, especially opposite the pontine flexure (Fig. 17–14A and C). The pontine flexure causes the lateral walls of the medulla to move laterally like the pages of an opening book and the roof plate to become stretched and greatly thinned. The cavity of this part of the myelencephalon becomes the caudal half of the fourth ventricle.

THE METENCEPHALON (Fig. 17–15). The walls of the metencephalon form the pons and cerebellum, and its cavity forms the superior part of the fourth ventricle. As in the rostral part of the myelencephalon, the pontine flexure causes divergence of the lateral walls of the medulla and spreading of the gray matter in the floor of the fourth ventricle.

The **cerebellum** develops from thickenings of dorsal parts of the alar plates, which enlarge and

fuse in the median plane. These cerebellar primordia soon overgrow the rostral half of the fourth ventricle and overlap the pons and medulla (Fig. 17–15D). Nerve fibers connecting the cerebral and cerebellar cortices with the spinal cord pass through the marginal layer of the ventral region of the metencephalon. This region of the *brain stem* is called the **pons** (L., bridge) because of this large band of nerve fibers.

Choroid Plexuses and Cerebrospinal Fluid (CSF)

The thin ependymal roof of the fourth ventricle is covered externally by *pia mater* derived from the mesenchyme associated with the hindbrain. This internal layer of the **meninges** (covering of the brain) together with the ependymal roof forms the *tela choroidea,* which invaginates the fourth ventricle. These tufts of capillaries differentiate into the *choroid plexuses,* which secrete CSF. Similar choroid plexuses develop in the roof of the third ventricle and in the medial walls of the lateral ventricles.

The thin roof of the fourth ventricle bulges outward in three locations. These small evaginations rupture to form foramina. The *median and lateral apertures* (foramen of Magendie and foramina of Luschka, respectively) permit the CSF from the fourth ventricle to enter the *subarachnoid space* (Fig. 17–9D).

The main site of absorption of CSF into the venous system is through the *arachnoid villi* (protrusions of the arachnoid layer of meninges) into the *dural venous sinuses* (Moore, 1992). These villi consist of a thin, cellular layer derived from the epithelium of the arachnoid and the endothelium of the venous sinus.

The Midbrain

The midbrain (mesencephalon) undergoes less change than any other part of the developing brain except the caudal part of the hindbrain. The neural canal narrows to form the *cerebral aqueduct* (Figs. 17–15D and 17–16D), which joins the third and fourth ventricles. Neuroblasts migrate from the alar plates of the midbrain into the roof or *tectum* and aggregate to form four large groups of neurons, the paired *superior* and *inferior colliculi.* They are concerned with visual and auditory reflexes, respectively.

The basal plates give rise to the neurons in the intermediate region of the brain stem called

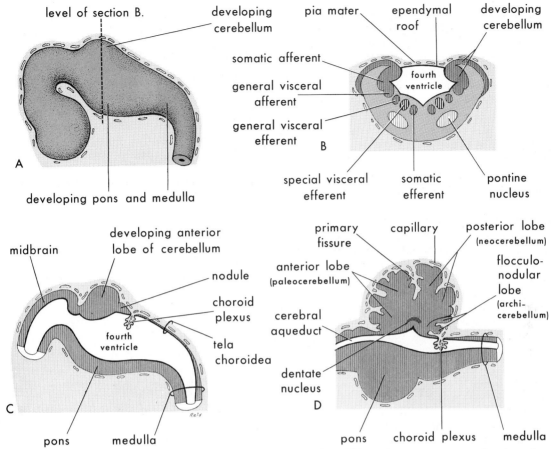

Figure 17–15. *A,* Sketch of the developing brain at the end of the fifth week. *B,* Transverse section through the metencephalon (developing pons and cerebellum), showing the derivatives of the alar and basal plates. *C* and *D,* Sagittal sections of the hindbrain at six and 17 weeks, respectively, showing successive stages in the development of the pons and cerebellum.

the *tegmentum.* It contains the red nuclei, the nuclei of the third and fourth cranial nerves, and neurons in the reticular nuclei. Fibers growing from the cerebrum form the massive crura cerebri or *cerebral peduncles,* which are features of the ventral surface of the midbrain. The *substantia nigra* (black nucleus), a broad layer of gray matter adjacent to the *cerebral peduncle* (Fig. 17–16C), may also differentiate from the basal plate; however, some authorities believe that this nucleus is formed by cells from the alar plate.

The Forebrain

As closure of the rostral neuropore occurs, two lateral outgrowths (diverticula) called *optic vesicles* appear on each side of the forebrain (Fig. 17–3A). The optic vesicles are the primor-

dia of the *retinae* and *optic nerves* (see Chapter 18). A second pair of larger diverticula arise more dorsally and rostrally; these are called the *cerebral (telencephalic) vesicles* (Fig. 17–16C). They are the primordia of the **cerebral hemispheres,** and their cavities become the *lateral ventricles.*

The rostral or anterior part of the forebrain, including the primordia of the cerebral hemispheres, is known as the *telencephalon,* and the caudal or posterior part of the forebrain is called the *diencephalon.* The cavities of the telencephalon and diencephalon both contribute to the formation of the *third ventricle* (Fig. 17–12), although the cavity of the diencephalon contributes more.

THE DIENCEPHALON (Fig. 17–17). Three swellings develop in the lateral walls of the third ventricle; later, they differentiate into the epithalamus, thalamus, and hypothalamus. The epithalamus is separated from the thalamus by the *epithalamic sulcus*. The *thalamus* on each side develops rapidly and bulges into the cavity of the third ventricle, reducing it to a narrow cleft.

The *hypothalamus* arises by proliferation of neuroblasts in the intermediate zone of the diencephalic walls inferior to the hypothalamic sulcus (Fig. 17–17E). The *pineal body* (gland) develops as a median diverticulum of the caudal part of the diencephalic roof (Fig. 17–17D). Proliferation of cells in its walls soon convert it into a solid, cone-shaped gland. The pineal body secretes *melatonin*.

The Pituitary Gland (Hypophysis Cerebri)

The pituitary gland develops from ectoderm, but the cells are derived from two sources: oral ectoderm of the *stomodeum* (primitive mouth cavity) and neuroectoderm of the *diencephalon* called the neurohypophyseal bud (Fig. 17–20; Table 17–1). This double origin explains why the pituitary gland is composed of two completely different types of tissue. The **adenohypophysis** (glandular portion) arises from the oral ectoderm (ectoderm of the oral cavity), and the **neurohypophysis** (nervous portion) originates from neuroectoderm of the diencephalon.

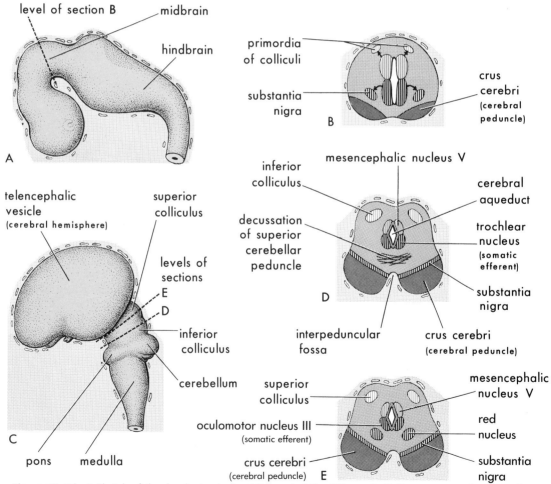

Figure 17–16. *A,* Sketch of the developing brain at the end of the fifth week. *B,* Transverse section through the developing midbrain, showing the early migration of cells from the basal and alar plates. *C,* Sketch of the developing brain at 11 weeks. *D* and *E,* Transverse sections of the developing midbrain at the level of the inferior and superior colliculi, respectively.

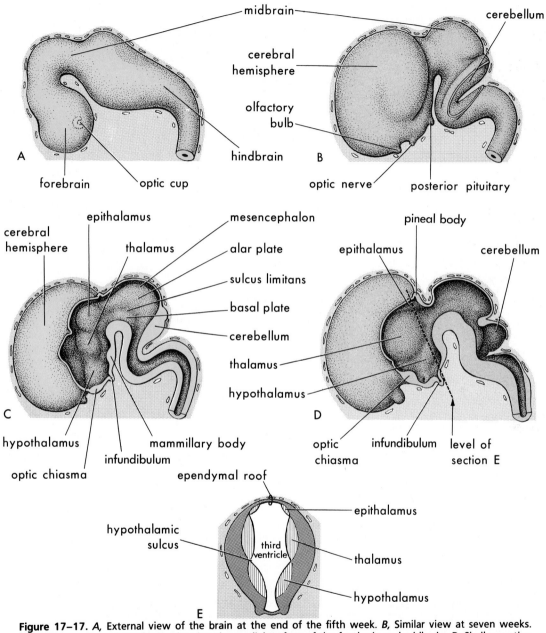

Figure 17–17. *A,* External view of the brain at the end of the fifth week. *B,* Similar view at seven weeks. *C,* Median section of this brain, showing the medial surface of the forebrain and midbrain. *D,* Similar section at eight weeks. *E,* Transverse section through the diencephalon, showing the epithalamus dorsally, the thalamus laterally, and the hypothalamus ventrally.

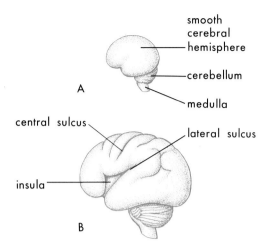

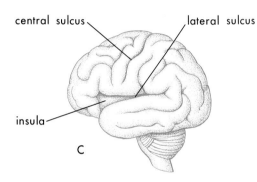

Figure 17–18. Sketches of lateral views of the left cerebral hemisphere, showing successive stages in the development of the sulci and gyri. Half actual size. Note the gradual narrowing of the lateral sulcus and formation of the insula (L., island), an area of cerebral cortex that is concealed from surface view. A, 13 weeks. B, 26 weeks. C, 35 weeks. D, Newborn.

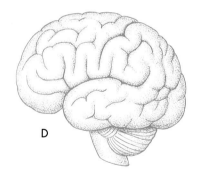

Table 17–1. DERIVATION AND TERMINOLOGY OF THE PITUITARY GLAND

| **Oral Ectoderm** (From roof of stomodeum) | → | Adenohypophysis (glandular portion) | Pars distalis / Pars tuberalis / Pars intermedia | } Anterior lobe |
| **Neuroectoderm** (From floor of diencephalon) | → | Neurohypophysis (nervous portion) | Pars nervosa / Infundibular stem / Median eminence | } Posterior lobe |

During the fourth week a diverticulum called the hypophyseal *(Rathke's) pouch* arises from the roof of the *stomodeum* and grows toward the brain. By the fifth week this pouch has elongated and come into contact with the *infundibulum,* a ventral diverticulum of the floor of the diencephalon (Figs. 17–19A and 17–20B).

Adenohypophysis. During the sixth week the connection of the hypophyseal pouch with the oral cavity degenerates and disappears (Fig. 17–18D and E). Cells of the anterior wall of the pouch proliferate actively and give rise to the *pars distalis* of the pituitary gland. Later, a small extension, the *pars tuberalis,* extends around the *infundibular stem.*

Proliferation of the anterior wall of the hypophyseal (Rathke's) pouch reduces its lumen to a narrow cleft (Fig. 17–20E). This cleft is usually not recognizable in the adult gland, but it may be represented by a few cysts. The posterior wall does not proliferate; it remains as the thin, poorly defined *pars intermedia.*

Neurohypophysis. This part of the pituitary gland is derived from the neuroectoderm of the diencephalon (Fig. 17–20; Table 17–1). The small infundibulum gives rise to the *median eminence,* the *infundibular stem,* and the *pars nervosa* (Fig. 17–20F). Nerve fibers grow into the pars nervosa from the hypothalamic area to which the infundibular stem is attached.

THE TELENCEPHALON (Fig. 17–19). The telencephalon consists of a median part and two cerebral vesicles (primordia of the *cerebral hemispheres*). The cavity of the median portion forms

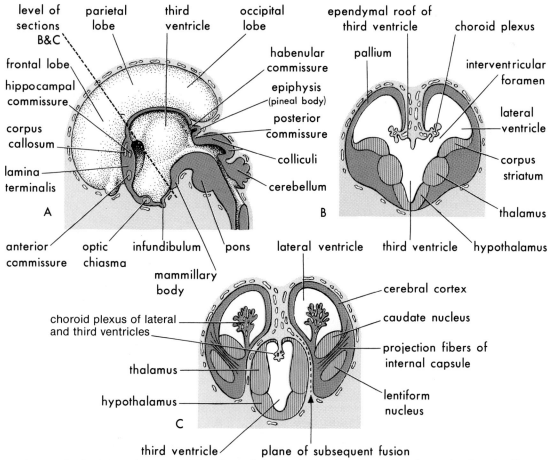

Figure 17–19. *A,* Drawing of medial surface of the forebrain of a ten-week embryo, showing the diencephalic derivatives, the main commissures, and the expanding cerebral vesicle. *B,* Transverse section through the forebrain at the level of the interventricular foramen, showing the corpus striatum and the choroid plexuses of the lateral ventricle. *C,* Similar section at about 11 weeks, showing division of the corpus striatum into caudate and lentiform nuclei by the internal capsule. The developing relationship of the cerebral hemispheres to the diencephalon is also illustrated.

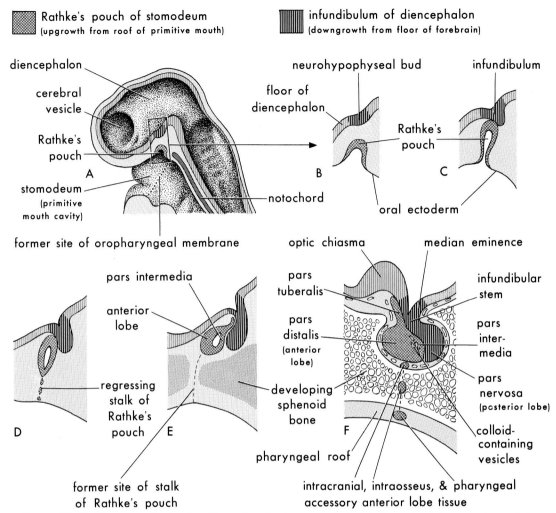

Figure 17-20. Diagrammatic sketches illustrating development of the pituitary gland (hypophysis cerebri). *A,* Sagittal section of the cranial end of an embryo of about 36 days showing the hypophyseal (Rathke's) pouch, an upgrowth from the roof of the primitive mouth cavity, and the neurohypophyseal bud from the floor of the diencephalon. *B* to *D,* Successive stages of the developing pituitary gland. By eight weeks, the hypophyseal (Rathke's) pouch loses its connection with the oral cavity. *E* and *F,* Later stages, showing proliferation of the anterior wall of the pouch and obliteration of its lumen.

the anterior part of the *third ventricle,* and the cavities of the cerebral vesicles become the *lateral ventricles.* At first the cerebral vesicles are in wide communication with the cavity of the third ventricle through the *interventricular foramina* (Fig. 17–19*B*). As the hemispheres expand they cover the diencephalon, midbrain, and hindbrain. The hemispheres eventually meet each other in the midline, flattening their medial surfaces (Fig. 17–19*A* and *C*).

The **corpus striatum** appears during the sixth week as a prominent swelling in the floor of each hemisphere (Fig. 17–20*B*). The floor of the hemisphere expands more slowly than the thin cortical wall because it contains the rather large corpus striatum; consequently, the cerebral hemispheres become C-shaped (Fig. 17–18). Posterior extension of the hemispheres is limited; thus, their caudal ends turn ventrally and rostrally, forming the temporal lobes of the brain. As the cerebral cortex differentiates, fibers passing to and from it go through the corpus striatum and divide it into *caudate* and *lentiform nuclei.* This important fiber pathway is called the *internal capsule* (Fig. 17–19*C*).

THE CEREBRAL CORTEX. The walls of the developing cerebral hemispheres initially show the typical zones of the neural tube. Cells of the intermediate zone migrate into the marginal zone and give rise to the cortical layers. The gray matter is thus located marginally, and axons from its cell bodies pass centrally and not peripherally, as in the spinal cord. These fibers form the large volume of white matter known as the *medullary center.*

Initially, the surface of the cerebral hemispheres is smooth (Fig. 17–18A); but, as growth proceeds, sulci (grooves) and gyri (convolutions) develop. These permit an increase in the surface area of the cerebral cortex without requiring an extensive increase in cranial size. As each hemisphere grows, the cortex covering the external surface of the corpus striatum grows relatively slowly and is soon overgrown (Fig. 17–18C and D). This buried cortex, hidden from view in the depths of the lateral sulcus of the cerebral hemisphere, is known as the *insula* (L., island).

Congenital Anomalies of the Brain

Due to the complexity of its embryological history, abnormal development of the brain is common (about three per 1000 births). Most major congenital anomalies are the result of defective closure of the rostral neuropore during the fourth week and involve the overlying tissues (future meninges and calvaria). The factors causing the **neural tube defects** (NTDs) are genetic and/or environmental in nature. Congenital anomalies of the brain can result from alterations in the morphogenesis or the histogenesis of the nervous tissue or they can result from developmental failures occurring in associated structures (notochord, somites, mesenchyme, and skull).

Abnormal histogenesis of the cerebral cortex can result in various types of congenital **mental retardation.** Severe mental retardation may result from exposure of the embryo or fetus to viruses and *high levels of radiation* during the eight- to 16-week period of development (see Fig. 9–12). *Maternal alcohol abuse* during pregnancy can also produce mental retardation of the fetus (p. 133).

Defects in the formation of the calvaria (e.g., cranium bifidum) are often associated with congenital anomalies of the brain and/or meninges, or both. These defects are usually in the median

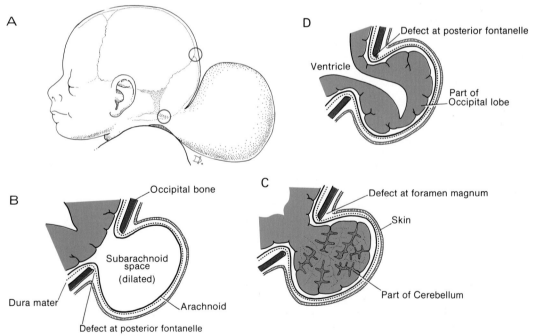

Figure 17–21. Schematic drawings illustrating cranium bifidum (bony defect in the cranium) and the various types of herniation of the brain and/or meninges. *A,* Sketch of the head of a newborn infant with a large protrusion from the occipital region of the skull, similar to that shown in Figure 17–22. The *upper red circle* indicates a cranial defect at the posterior fontanelle, and the *lower red circle* indicates a cranial defect near the foramen magnum. *B,* Meningocele consisting of a protrusion of the cranial meninges that is filled with cerebrospinal fluid. *C,* Meningoencephalocele consisting of a protrusion of part of the cerebellum that is covered by meninges and skin. *D,* Meningohydroencephalocele consisting of a protrusion of part of the occipital lobe that contains part of the posterior horn of a lateral ventricle.

plane of the calvaria (cranial vault), often in the squamous part of the occipital bone. They may include the posterior part of the foramen magnum (Fig. 17–21). When the defect in the cranium is small, usually only the meninges herniate, and this condition is called a cranial meningocele or *cranium bifidum with meningocele* (Fig. 17–21*B*).

When the cranial defect is large, the meninges and part of the brain herniate, forming a *meningoencephalocele* (Fig. 17–21*C*). If the protruding part of the brain contains part of the ventricular system, the defect is called a *meningohydroencephalocele* (Figs. 17–21*D* and 17–22). The part of the brain that is in the meningeal sac is dependent on the location of the cranial defect. Cranium bifidum associated with herniation of the brain and/or its meninges occurs about once in every 2000 births.

Exencephaly, Meroanencephaly, and Anencephaly (see Figs. 16–10 and 17–23). These severe defects of the brain are the result of failure of the rostral neuropore to close properly during the fourth week. As a result, the forebrain primordium is abnormal or absent, and the calvaria is defective or absent. Most of the embryo's brain is exposed or extruding from the skull, a condition known as *exencephaly.*

Due to the abnormal structure and vascularization of the embryonic exencephalic brain, the nervous tissue undergoes degeneration. The remains of the brain appear as a spongy, vascular mass mostly consisting of hindbrain structures

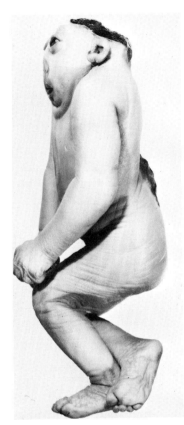

Figure 17–23. Photograph of an infant with acrania (absence of the cranial vault), meroanencephaly (partial absence of the brain, often called anencephaly [absence of the brain]); rachischisis (failure of fusion of several vertebral arches), and spina bifida with myeloschisis (failure of closure of the neural folds).

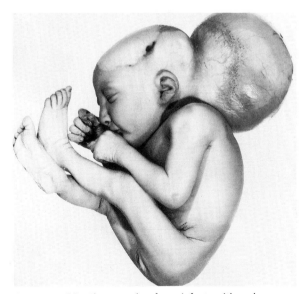

Figure 17–22. Photograph of an infant with a large meningoencephalocele in the occipital area. (Courtesy of Dr. Dwight Parkinson, Children's Centre, Winnipeg, Canada.)

(Fig. 17–23). Although this condition is usually called *anencephaly* (Gr., without a brain), a rudimentary brain stem and traces of the basal ganglia are present; for this reason, the term *meroanencephaly* (Gr. *meros*, part brain) is a better name for this anomaly.

Meroanencephaly (anencephaly) is a common *lethal anomaly* occurring about once in every 1000 births. It is two to four times more common in females than in males. It is always associated with *acrania* (absence of the calvaria) and may be associated with *rachischisis* when defective closure of the neural tube is extensive (see Fig. 16–10). Sustained extrauterine life is impossible in infants born with meroanencephaly. Infants afflicted with this defect survive for a few hours after birth at most. Prenatal diagnosis of meroanencephaly is possible by a combination of ultrasonography and measurement of alpha-fetoprotein in amniotic fluid (p. 90).

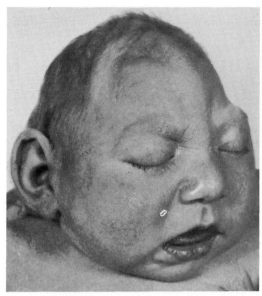

Figure 17–24. Photograph of an infant with microcephaly, showing the typical, normal-sized face and small calvaria (cranial vault) covered with loose, wrinkled skin. (From Laurence KM, Weeks R: Abnormalities of the central nervous system. *In* Norman AP (ed): *Congenital Abnormalities in Infancy*, 2nd ed. Oxford, Blackwell Scientific Publications, 1971.)

sorption of CSF; as a result, there is an excess of CSF. In obstructive or noncommunicating hydrocephalus there is interference with the circulation of CSF inside the brain. Obstructive hydrocephalus is often the result of *congenital aqueductal stenosis* in which the cerebral aqueduct is narrow or consists of several minute channels. Blockage of CSF circulation results in dilation of the ventricles superior to the obstruction and in pressure on the cerebral hemispheres. This squeezes the brain between the ventricular fluid and the bones of the calvaria. In infants, the internal pressure results in expansion of the brain and calvaria because the sutures and fontanelles are still open (see Fig. 16–9).

Hydrocephalus usually refers to obstructive hydrocephalus in which all or part of the ventricular system is enlarged. All ventricles are enlarged if the apertures of the fourth ventricle or the subarachnoid space and/or cisterns are blocked; whereas, the lateral and third ventricles are dilated when only the cerebral aqueduct is obstructed. In *nonobstructive or communicating hydrocephalus*, there is an accumulation

MICROCEPHALY (Fig. 17–24). In this uncommon condition the calvaria and brain are small, but the face is of normal size. These infants are *grossly mentally retarded* because the brain is underdeveloped, a condition known as microencephaly. Microcephaly (Gr. *mikros*, small, + *kephale*, head) results from *microencephaly* (Gr. *mikros*, small, + *enkephalos*, brain) because growth of the calvaria is largely due to pressure from the growing brain. The cause of microcephaly is often uncertain. Some cases appear to be genetic in origin, and others seem to be associated with environmental factors. Exposure to large amounts of ionizing radiation during the eight- to 16-week period and to infectious agents (e.g., cytomegalovirus, rubella, *Toxoplasma gondii*) during this period is a possible contributing factor (see Chapter 9). Microcephaly can be detected in utero by ultrasound (see Chapter 7).

HYDROCEPHALUS (Fig. 17–25). This term describes any condition in which there is enlargement of the ventricular system of the brain[1] due to an imbalance between production and ab-

---

[1] Persons unfamiliar with the production, circulation, and absorption of CSF would benefit from the clinically oriented account of the ventricular system in the brain described by Moore (1992).

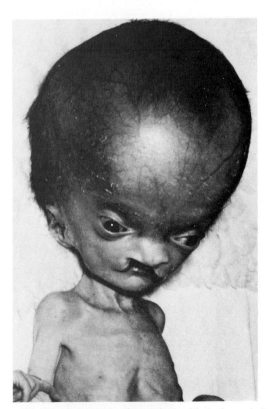

Figure 17–25. Photograph of an infant with **hydrocephalus**, bilateral cleft lip, and deformed limbs.

of CSF outside the brain, i.e., in the subarachnoid space between the brain and dura mater. The CSF pathways inside the brain are open. This condition results from interference with the absorption of CSF.

Hydrocephalus may be associated with spina bifida cystica (Figs. 17–10 and 17–11), although the hydrocephalus may not be obvious at birth. Hydrocephalus often produces thinning of the bones of the calvaria, prominence of the forehead, atrophy of the cerebral cortex and white matter, and compression of the basal ganglia and diencephalon.

Mental Retardation

Congenital impairment of intelligence may be due to various genetically determined conditions (e.g., Down syndrome). The relation of chromosomal abnormalities to mental retardation is briefly discussed in Chapter 9. *Maternal alcohol abuse* is thought to be the most common cause of environmentally-induced mental retardation. Disorders of protein, carbohydrate, or fat metabolism may also cause mental retardation. *Fetal infections* (syphilis, German measles, toxoplasmosis, and cytomegalic inclusion disease), high levels of ionizing radiation, and cretinism are commonly associated with mental retardation (Holmes, 1992; Greenough et al., 1992).

The period of eight to 16 weeks of human development appears to be the period of greatest sensitivity for fetal brain damage resulting from high doses of radiation (see Chapter 9). Cell depletion of sufficient degree in the cerebral cortex results in mental retardation. By the end of the sixteenth week, most neuronal proliferation and cell migration to form the cerebral cortex are complete.

THE PERIPHERAL NERVOUS SYSTEM

The peripheral nervous system (PNS) consists of the cranial, spinal, and visceral nerves and the cranial, spinal, and autonomic ganglia. It develops from various sources. Afferent neurons in the spinal ganglia and ganglia of cranial nerves develop from *neural crest cells* (Figs. 17–1 and 17–8). Cells of the neural crest also differentiate into multipolar neurons of the *autonomic ganglia*, including ganglia of the sympathetic trunks along the sides of the vertebral bodies, collateral or prevertebral ganglia in plexuses of the thorax and abdomen (e.g., the cardiac, celiac, and mesenteric plexuses), and parasympathetic or terminal ganglia in or near the viscera, e.g., the submucosal plexus (Meissner plexus).

Chromaffin cells of paraganglia are also derived from the neural crests. The carotid and aortic bodies also have small islands of chromaffin cells associated with them. These widely scattered groups of chromaffin cells constitute the *chromaffin system*. Formation of the spinal ganglia and nerves has been discussed previously (p. 282). The development of cranial nerves is described in Chapter 11. For a further discussion of these nerves and the autonomic nervous system, see Moore and Persaud (1993).

SUMMARY

The central nervous system (CNS) develops from a dorsal thickening of ectoderm known as the *neural plate*. This plate appears around the middle of the third week and soon infolds to form a neural groove with neural folds on each side. When the neural folds fuse to form the neural tube during the fourth week, some neuroectodermal cells are not included in it, but remain between the neural tube and the surface ectoderm as the *neural crest*. The spinal ganglia and ganglia of the autonomic nervous system are derived from *neural crest cells*, as are the sheaths of peripheral nerves (Schwann cells), cells of the suprarenal medulla, melanocytes, and cartilages in the branchial or pharyngeal arches.

The cranial end of the neural tube forms the brain, consisting of the forebrain, midbrain, and hindbrain. The *forebrain* gives rise to the cerebral hemispheres and the diencephalon; the *midbrain* becomes the adult midbrain; and the *hindbrain* gives rise to the pons, cerebellum, and medulla oblongata. The remainder and longest part of the neural tube becomes the *spinal cord*.

The lumen of the neural tube becomes the ventricles of the brain and the central canal of the spinal cord. The walls of the neural tube become thickened by proliferation of its neuroepithelial cells, which give rise to all nerve and macroglial cells in the central nervous system. The *microglia* are believed to differentiate from mesenchymal cells, which enter the central nervous system with the blood vessels.

The *pituitary gland* (hypophysis cerebri) develops from two completely different parts: (1) an ectodermal upgrowth from the stomodeum known as the hypophyseal *(Rathke's) pouch,* and (2) a neuroectodermal downgrowth from the diencephalon called the neurohypophyseal bud. The *adenohypophysis* arises from the oral ectoderm, and the *neurohypophysis* develops from the neuroectoderm (see Table 17–1).

Congenital anomalies of the CNS are common (about three per 1000 birth). Defects of closure of the neural tube *(neural tube defects)* account for most abnormalities (e.g., spina bifida cystica). The defects may be limited to the nervous system or they may include overlying tissues (bone, muscle, and connective tissue). Some defects are caused by genetic abnormalities; others result from such environmental factors as infectious agents, drugs, and metabolic disease. Most anomalies, however, are probably caused by an interaction of genetic and environmental factors.

Most gross anomalies (e.g., meroanencephaly [anencephaly]) are usually incompatible with life. Other severe defects (e.g., spina bifida cystica) often cause functional disability (e.g., muscle paralysis).

There are two main types of *hydrocephalus*: obstructive or noncommunicating hydrocephalus (blockage of CSF flow in the ventricular system) and nonobstructive or communicating hydrocephalus (blockage of CSF in the subarachnoid space).

Mental retardation may result from chromosomal abnormalities, metabolic disorders, maternal and fetal infections, maternal alcohol abuse, and exposure to high levels of radiation during the period of eight to 16 weeks of prenatal life.

Commonly Asked Questions

1. Are neural tube defects (NTDs) hereditary? The reason I ask is because my mother had a baby with spina bifida cystica and my sister had one with meroanencephaly. Is my sister likely to have another child with a NTD? Can meroanencephaly and spina bifida be detected early in fetal life?

2. I recently read in the paper about a baby born with no cerebral hemispheres and yet its head appeared normal; however, the baby exhibited excessive sleepiness, continuous crying when awake, and feeding problems. What is this condition called? What is its embryological basis? Do these children usually survive?

3. I have heard that pregnant women who are heavy drinkers may have babies who exhibit mental and growth retardation. Is this true? I have seen women get drunk during pregnancy and their babies seem to be normal. Is there a safe threshold for alcohol consumption during pregnancy?

4. My aunt told me that my cigarette smoking during pregnancy probably caused the slight mental retardation in my baby. I am not a heavy smoker. Is my aunt's accusation correct?

5. Do all types of spina bifida cause loss of motor function in the lower limbs? Which type of spina bifida cystica is more common and serious? How are infants with spina bifida cystica treated?

The answers to these questions are given on page 335.

REFERENCES

Adams J: Prenatal exposure to teratogenic agents and neurodevelopmental outcome. *Research in Infant Assessment (BD:OAS)* 25:63, 1989.

Alvarez IS, Schoenwolf GC: Expansion of surface epithelium provides the major extrinsic force for bending of the neural plate. *J Exp Zool* 26:340, 1992.

Behrman RE: *Nelson Textbook of Pediatrics,* 14th ed. Philadelphia, WB Saunders, 1992.

Bell JE: The pathology of central nervous system defects in human fetuses of different gestational ages. *In* Persaud TVN (ed): *Advances in the Study of Birth Defects, Vol. 7. Central Nervous System and Craniofacial Malformations.* New York, Alan R Liss, 1982.

Bruni JE, Del Bigio MR, Cardoso ER, Persaud TVN: Hereditary hydrocephalus in laboratory animals and humans. *Exp Pathol* 35:239, 1988.

Chuong CM: Adhesion molecules (N-CAM and tenascin) in embryonic development and tissue regeneration. *J Craniofac Genet Dev Biol* 10:147, 1990.

Cockroft DL: Vitamin deficiencies and neural tube defects: human and animal studies. *Hum Reprod* 6:148, 1991.

Copp AJ, Bernfield M: Accumulation of basement membrane-associated hyaluronate is reduced in the posterior neuropore region of mutant (curly tail) mouse embryo developing spinal neural tube defects. *Devel Biol* 130:583, 1988.

Crelin ES: Development of the Nervous System. A Logical Approach to Neuroanatomy. *Clin Symp, Vol. 26(2),* 1974.

DeVellis J, Ciment G, Lauder J (eds): *Neuroembryology. Cellular and Molecular Approaches.* New York, Alan R Liss, 1988.

Flint G: Embryology of the nervous system. *Br J Neurosurg* 3:131, 1989.

Greenough A, Osborne J, Sutherland S (eds): *Congenital, Perinatal and Neonatal Infections.* Edinburgh, Churchill Livingstone, 1992.

Holmes LB: Teratogens. *In* Behrman RD (ed): *Nelson Textbook of Pediatrics,* 14th ed. Philadelphia, WB Saunders, 1992.

Jacobson M: *Developmental Neurobiology,* 3rd ed. New York, Plenum Publishing, 1992.

Lemire RJ, Loeser JD, Leech RW, Alvord Jr EC: *Normal and Abnormal Development of the Human Nervous System.* Hagerstown, Harper & Row, 1975.

Mann RA, Persaud TVN: Histogenesis of experimental open neural defects in the chick embryo. *Anat Anz* 146:171, 1979.

Mole RH: Consequences of pre-natal radiation exposure for post-natal development. *Int J Radiat Biol* 42:1, 1982.

Moore KL: *Clinically Oriented Anatomy,* 3rd ed. Baltimore, Williams & Wilkins, 1992.

Moore KL, Persaud TVN: *The Developing Human. Clinically Oriented Embryology,* 5th ed. Philadelphia, WB Saunders, 1993.

Müller F, O'Rahilly R: The development of the human brain from a closed neural tube at stage 13. *Anat Embryol (Berl)* 177:55, 1988.

Müller F, O'Rahilly R: The development of the human brain, including the longitudinal zoning in the diencephalon at stage 15. *Anat Embryol (Berl)* 177:55, 1988.

Müller F, O'Rahilly R: Development of anencephaly and its variants. *Am J Anat* 190:193, 1991.

O'Rahilly R, Müller F: *Developmental Stages in Human Embryos.* Washington, Carnegie Institution of Washington, 1987.

Otake M, Schull WJ: *In utero* exposure to A-bomb radiation and mental retardation: A reassessment. *Brit J Radiol* 52:409, 1984.

Persaud TVN: Abnormal development of the central nervous system. *Anat Anz* 150:44, 1981.

Persaud TVN: *Environmental Causes of Human Birth Defects.* Springfield, Charles C Thomas, 1990.

Prechtl HF: Developmental neurology of the fetus. *Baillieres Clin Obstet Gynaecol* 2:21, 1988.

Rutishauser U, Jessell TM: Cell adhesion molecules in vertebrate neural development. *Physiol Rev* 68:819, 1988.

Sanes JR: Extracellular matrix molecules that influence neural development. *Annu Rev Neurosci* 12:491, 1989.

Schoenwolf GG, Smith JL: Mechanisms of neurulation: Traditional viewpoint and recent advances. *Development* 109:243, 1990.

Taeusch HW, Ballard RA, Avery ME (eds): *Schaffer and Avery's Diseases of the Newborn,* 6th ed. Philadelphia, WB Saunders, 1991.

Thompson MW, McInnes RR, Willard HF: *Thompson & Thompson Genetics in Medicine,* 5th ed. Philadelphia, WB Saunders, 1991.

Wald NJ, Cuckle HS: AFP screening in early pregnancy. *In* Spencer JAD (ed): *Fetal Monitoring.* Oxford, Oxford University Press, 1991.

Williams PL, Warwick R, Dyson M, Bannister LH: *Gray's Anatomy,* 37th ed. Edinburgh, Churchill Livingstone, 1989.

18

THE EYE
AND
EAR

THE EYE

The visual organs or eyes develop from three sources: (1) neuroectoderm of the forebrain, (2) surface ectoderm of the head, and (3) mesoderm between these layers. The ectodermal outgrowth from the brain becomes the retina, iris, and optic nerve. The surface ectoderm forms the lens, and the surrounding mesoderm gives rise to the vascular and fibrous coats of the eye.

Eye development is first evident early in the fourth week when a pair of grooves called *optic sulci* appear in the neural folds at the cranial end of the embryo (Fig. 18–1A and B). As the neural folds fuse to form the forebrain vesicle, the optic sulci evaginate to form a pair of hollow diverticula called *optic vesicles.* These vesicles project from the sides of the forebrain into the adjacent mesenchyme (see Figs. 17–3A and 18–1C). The cavities of the optic vesicles are continuous with the lumen of the forebrain vesicle. It is the mesenchyme adjacent to the forebrain that induces the optic vesicles to form, probably through a chemical mediator. As the bulblike optic vesicles grow laterally, their distal ends expand, and their connections with the forebrain become constricted to form hollow *optic stalks* (Fig. 18–1D).

As the optic vesicles contact the surface ectoderm, their lateral surfaces become flattened. At the site of contact the surface ectoderm thickens to form *lens placodes,* which are the primordia

of the *lenses* (Fig. 18–1C). The formation of lens placodes is induced by a signal produced by the optic vesicles. The inducing agent is probably a chemical substance produced by the optic vesicles (see Chapter 6, p. 63). The central region of each lens placode rapidly invaginates and sinks deep to the surface, forming a *lens pit* (Fig. 18–1D). The edges of the pit gradually approach each other and fuse to form a *lens vesicle* (Fig. 18–1F), which is soon pinched off from the surface ectoderm (Fig. 18–1H).

As the lens vesicles are developing, the optic vesicles invaginate and become double-walled structures called *optic cups* (see Figs. 17–3C and 18–1H). The opening of each optic cup is large at first, but the rim of the optic cup infolds and converges around the lens (Figs. 18–2 to 18–4). By this stage, the lens vesicles have separated from the surface ectoderm, and grooves called *optic fissures* have developed on the ventral surfaces of the optic cups and along the optic stalks (Fig. 18–1E to H). Hyaloid blood vessels develop from the mesenchyme in these fissures. The *hyaloid artery* supplies the inner layer of the optic cup, the lens vesicle, and the mesenchyme within the optic cup. The hyaloid vein returns blood from these structures. As the edges of the optic fissure come together and fuse, the hyaloid vessels are enclosed within the optic nerve (Fig. 18–2E and F). The distal

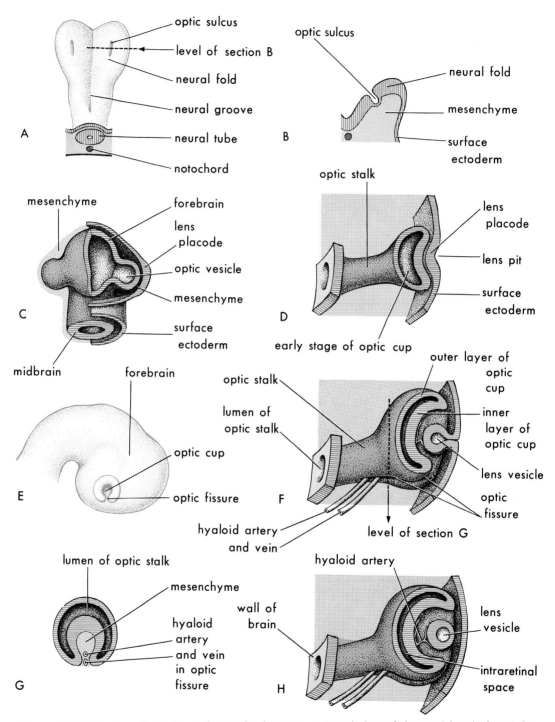

Figure 18–1. Drawings illustrating early eye development. *A*, Dorsal view of the cranial end of a 22-day embryo, showing the first indication of eye development. *B*, Transverse section through a neural fold, showing an optic sulcus. *C*, Schematic drawing of the forebrain and its covering layers of mesenchyme and surface ectoderm from an embryo of about 28 days. *D*, *F*, and *H*, Schematic sections of the developing eye, illustrating successive stages in the development of the optic cup and the lens vesicle. *E*, Lateral view of the brain of an embryo of about 32 days, showing the external appearance of the optic cup. *G*, Transverse section through the optic stalk, showing the optic fissure and its contents.

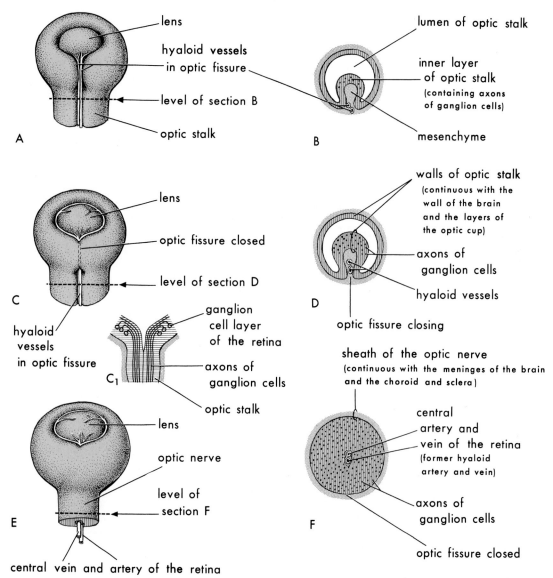

Figure 18–2. Diagrams illustrating closure of the optic fissure and formation of the optic nerve. *A, C,* and *E,* Views of the inferior surface of the optic cup and stalk, showing progressive stages in the closure of the optic fissure. *C₁,* Schematic sketch of a longitudinal section of a portion of the optic cup and optic stalk, showing axons of ganglion cells of the retina growing through the optic stalk to the brain. *B, D,* and *F,* Transverse sections through the optic stalk, showing successive stages in the closure of the optic fissure and in formation of the optic nerve. The optic fissure normally closes during the sixth week. Note that the lumen of the optic stalk is gradually obliterated as axons of ganglion cells accumulate in the inner layer of the optic stalk as the optic nerve forms.

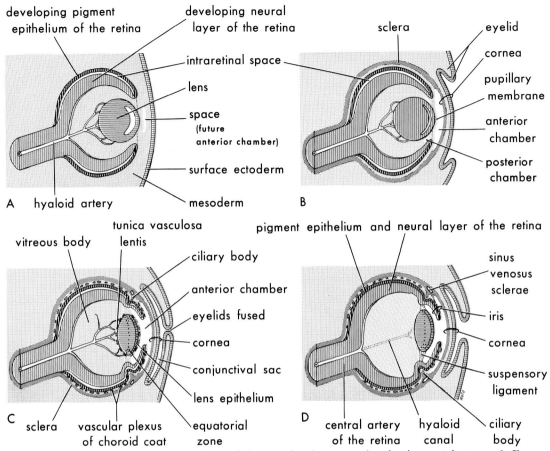

Figure 18–3. Drawings of sagittal sections of the eye showing successive developmental stages. *A,* Five weeks. *B,* Six weeks. *C,* 20 weeks. *D,* Newborn. Note that the layers of the optic cup are fused and form the retinal pigment epithelium and neural retina, and that they extend anteriorly as the double epithelium of the ciliary and iridial parts of the retina. At birth the eye is about three quarters of the adult size. Most growth occurs during the first year. After puberty, growth of the eye is negligible.

portions of the hyaloid vessels eventually degenerate, but their proximal portions persist as the *central artery and vein of the retina.*

The Retina

The retina develops from the walls of the optic cup, an outgrowth of the brain. The outer, thinner layer of the cup becomes the *retinal pigment epithelium,* and the inner, thicker layer differentiates into the complex *neural retina* (Figs. 18–1, 18–3, and 18–4).

During the embryonic and early fetal periods, the two retinal layers are separated by an *intraretinal space,* which represents the cavity of the original optic vesicle (Figs. 18–3 and 18–4). This space gradually disappears as the two layers of the retina fuse, but this fusion is not firm.

The retinal pigment epithelium becomes firmly fixed to the choroid, but its attachment to the neural retina is not so firm; hence, *detachment of the retina* may follow a hard blow to the eye. The detachment consists of separation of the retinal pigment epithelium from the neural retina, i.e., at the site of embryonic adherence of the outer and inner layers of the optic cup.

Because the optic cup is an outgrowth of the forebrain, the layers of the optic cup are continuous with the wall of the brain. Under the influence of the developing lens, the inner layer of the optic cup proliferates and forms a thick neuroepithelium that differentiates into the *neural retina,* the light-sensitive region of the eye. It contains photoreceptors called rods and cones,

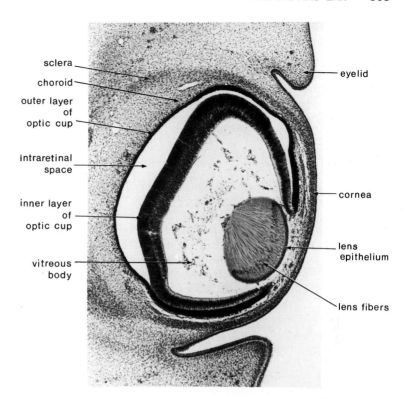

Figure 18–4. Photomicrograph of a sagittal section through the developing eye of a human embryo at about 50 days (×75). The relatively large intraretinal space, derived from the cavity of the optic vesicle, gradually disappears as the inner and outer layers of the optic cup fuse to form the retina. (See Figure 18–3.) (Courtesy of Professor Jean Hay, Department of Anatomy, Faculty of Medicine, University of Manitoba, Winnipeg, Canada.)

bipolar cells, and ganglion cells (Figs. 18–2 and 18–3).

The neural layer of the developing retina is continuous with the inner layer of the optic stalk (Figs. 18–1F and G and 18–2D); consequently, the axons of ganglion cells pass into the inner wall of the optic stalk and gradually convert it into the *optic nerve* (Fig. 18–2B, D, and F). Myelination of the optic nerve fibers is incomplete at birth. After the eyes have been exposed to light for about ten weeks, myelination is complete, but the process normally stops short of the optic disc (Kwitko, 1979). The normal newborn infant can see, but not too well; it is able to fixate points of contrast. Visual acuity has been estimated to be in the range of 20/600.

The Ciliary Body

The pigmented portion of the epithelium of the ciliary body is derived from the outer layer of the optic cup and is continuous with the retinal pigment epithelium (Fig. 18–3). The nonpigmented portion of the ciliary epithelium represents the anterior prolongation of the neural retina in which no neural elements differentiate. The ciliary muscle (the smooth muscle responsi-

ble for focusing the lens) and the connective tissue in the ciliary body develop from mesenchyme or early fibroblasts at the edge of the optic cup between the anterior scleral condensation and the ciliary pigment epithelium (Sellheyer and Spitznas, 1988).

The Iris

The iris develops from the anterior part or rim of the optic cup, which grows inward and partially covers the lens (Fig. 18–3); in this area, the two layers of the optic cup have remained thin. The epithelium of the iris represents both layers of the optic cup. It is continuous with the double-layered epithelium of the ciliary body and with the pigmented and neural layers of the retina (Fig. 18–3D). The dilator and sphincter pupillae muscles of the iris are derived from the neuroectoderm of the optic cup. The vascular connective tissue of the iris is derived from mesenchyme located anterior to the rim of the optic cup.

The iris is bluish in most infants. It acquires its definitive color as pigmentation occurs during the first few months. It is the concentration and distribution of pigment-containing cells *(chromatophores)* in the spongy, vascular, loose connective tissue of the iris that determine eye color. If the melanin pigment is confined to the two-layered pigmented epithelium on the posterior surface of the iris, the eye appears blue. If melanin is also distributed throughout the stroma of the irises, the eyes appear brown.

The Lens

The lens develops from the lens vesicle, a derivative of the surface ectoderm (Figs. 18–1 to 18–4). The anterior wall becomes the *anterior lens epithelium* of the adult lens. The nuclei of the cells of the posterior wall disappear, and the cells lengthen to form *primary lens fibers.* As they grow, they gradually obliterate the cavity of the lens vesicle. New lens fibers are continuously added to the lens from epithelial cells at the *equatorial zone* or region of the lens. As these cells elongate, they lose their nuclei and become *secondary lens fibers.* They are added to the external sides of the primary lens fibers that developed from the posterior wall of the lens vesicle. Although secondary lens fibers continue to form during adulthood and the lens continues to increase in diameter, the primary lens fibers (formed during the embryonic period) must last a lifetime.

The developing lens is supplied by the *hyaloid artery* (Figs. 18–2 and 18–3); however, it becomes avascular in the fetal period. It thereafter depends on diffusion from the aqueous humor in the anterior chamber bathing its anterior surface and from the vitreous humor around the rest of it (Figs. 18–3 and 18–4).

The Vitreous Body

This body forms within the cavity of the optic cup (Figs. 18–3 and 18–4). It is composed of vitreous humor, an avascular mass of transparent, gelled, intercellular substance. The original vitreous humor is derived from the vascular mesenchyme in the optic cup. This primary *vitreous humor* does not increase, but it becomes surrounded by a gelatinous secondary vitreous humor, the origin of which is uncertain. It is generally believed to arise from the inner layer of the optic cup.

The Aqueous Chambers and Cornea

The *anterior chamber* of the eye develops from a cleftlike space, which forms in the mes-

enchyme located between the developing lens and the cornea (Figs. 18–3 and 18–4). The epithelium of the cornea and the conjunctiva are derived from surface ectoderm. The mesenchyme deep to this epithelium forms the substantia propria (dense connective tissue) of the cornea. After the lens is established, it induces the surface ectoderm to develop into the epithelium of the cornea and the conjunctiva.

The **cornea** is formed from two sources: surface ectoderm and mesoderm (Fig. 18–3). The posterior chamber of the eye develops from a space that forms in the mesenchyme posterior to the developing iris and anterior to the developing lens. When the pupillary membrane disappears and the pupil forms (Fig. 18–3), the anterior and posterior chambers of the eye are able to communicate with each other.

The Choroid and Sclera

The mesenchyme surrounding the optic cup differentiates into an inner vascular layer called the choroid and an outer fibrous layer called the sclera (Figs. 18–3 and 18–4). Toward the rim of the optic cup, the choroid becomes modified to form the cores of the *ciliary processes*, consisting chiefly of capillaries supported by delicate connective tissue. The sclera is continuous with the substantia propria of the cornea.

At the attachment of the optic nerve to the eye, the choroid is continuous with the pia-arachnoid of the brain, which forms the internal sheath around the optic nerve (Moore, 1992). The sclera is continuous with the dura mater of the brain, which forms the external sheath around this nerve. The continuity of these layers is understandable when it is recalled that the eyes develop from outgrowth of the brain (Fig. 18–1). The subarachnoid space around the brain also extends around the optic nerves as far as their attachment to the eyes. This relationship of the sheaths of the optic nerve to the meninges of the brain and the subarachnoid space is clinically important (Moore, 1992). An increase in cerebrospinal fluid pressure causes edema of the optic disc and slows venous return from the retina. This occurs because the retinal vessels lie in the extension of the subarachnoid space that surrounds the optic nerve.

The Eyelids

The eyelids develop from two surface ectodermal folds that have cores of mesenchyme

(Figs. 18–3 and 18–4). The eyelids meet and adhere by about the tenth week and remain closed until about the twenty-sixth week (see Chapter 7, p. 85). While the eyelids are adherent, a closed *conjunctival sac* exists anterior to the cornea. When the eyes open, the *conjunctiva* covers the "white" of the eye and lines the eyelids (Moore, 1992).

The eyelashes and lacrimal glands are derived from the surface ectoderm in a manner similar to that described for other parts of the integument (see Chapter 19). The connective tissue and tarsal plates develop from mesenchyme in the cores of the eyelids. The *orbicularis oculi muscle* is derived from mesenchyme in the second branchial or pharyngeal arch (see Chapter 11); as a result, it is supplied by the seventh cranial nerve (CN VII).

Congenital Anomalies of the Eye

Because of the complexity of eye development, many anomalies may occur, but most of them are uncommon. The *critical period of eye development is from 22 to 50 days* after fertilization. Most congenital anomalies of the eye appear to be caused by genetic factors and several environmental teratogens (Stromland et al., 1991) including certain maternal infections (see Chapter 9, p. 137). Most common congenital defects of the eye are related to *defects in closure of the optic fissure* (choroid fissure); it usually closes during the sixth week (Fig. 18–2).

COLOBOMA OF THE EYELID (Fig. 18–5). Defects of the eyelid *(palpebral coloboma)* are uncommon. A coloboma is usually characterized by a small notch in the upper eyelid, but the defect

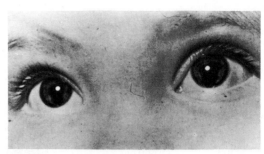

Figure 18–6. Photograph of the eyes of a child showing typical bilateral colobomata of the iris. (From Rahn EK, Scheie HG: The eye. *In* Rubin A (ed): *Handbook of Congenital Malformations.* Philadelphia, WB Saunders, 1967.)

may involve most of the lid. Colobomata in the lower eyelid are also uncommon. Palpebral colobomata appear to result from a local developmental disturbance in the growth of the eyelid.

COLOBOMA OF THE IRIS (Fig. 18–6). In these infants there is a defect in the inferior part of the iris, giving the pupil a "keyhole appearance". The notch may be limited to the iris or it may extend deeper and involve the ciliary body and retina. A typical coloboma of the iris is the result of *failure of closure of the optic fissure* during the sixth week. This may be genetically determined or caused by an environmental factor. Simple colobomata of the iris are frequently hereditary and are transmitted as an autosomal dominant characteristic (Behrman, 1992).

COLOBOMA OF THE RETINA. This defect is characterized by a localized gap in the retina, usually inferior to the optic disc. In most cases the defect is bilateral. A typical coloboma of the retina is the result of *defective closure of the optic fissure.*

CONGENITAL CATARACT (Fig. 18–7). In these infants the lens is opaque and frequently appears grayish-white. Many lens opacities are inherited, but some are caused by infectious agents, e.g., the *rubella virus,* which affects early lens development, (p. 137). The developing lenses are vulnerable to the rubella virus between the fourth and seventh weeks when primary lens fibers are forming (Figs. 18–3 and 18–4). Cataract and other ocular abnormalities caused by the rubella virus could be completely prevented if immunity to rubella were conferred on all women of reproductive age (Warkany, 1981).

CONGENITAL GLAUCOMA (Fig. 18–7). High intraocular pressure and enlargement of the eye in newborn infants is usually due to abnormal development of the drainage mechanism of the aqueous humor during the fetal period (Moore and Persaud, 1993). *Intraocular tension* rises because of an imbalance between production of aqueous humor and its outflow. This imbalance

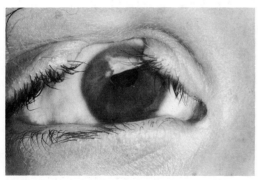

Figure 18–5. Photograph of the eye of a child with a coloboma of the iris and upper eyelid. (From Brown CA: Abnormalities of the eyes and associated structures. *In* Norman AP [ed]: *Congenital Abnormalities in Infancy,* 2nd ed. 1971. Courtesy of Blackwell Scientific Publications).

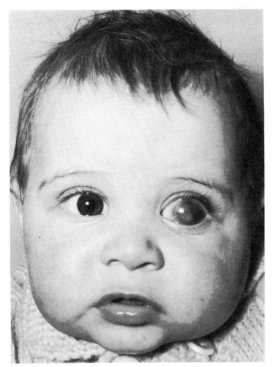

Figure 18–7. Photograph of a child with congenital glaucoma of the left eye. (Courtesy of Dr. C. A. Brown, Consultant Ophthalmologist, Bristol Eye Hospital, England.)

is probably due to the absence of or abnormal development of the *sinus venosus sclerae* or canal of Schlemm (Fig. 18–3D). Congenital glaucoma is usually caused by recessive mutant genes, but the condition may result from a rubella infection during early pregnancy (p. 137). For a description of other eye defects (e.g., *microphthalmos* [very small eye] and *anophthalmos* [absence of the eye]), see Moore and Persaud (1993).

THE EAR

The ear consists of internal, middle, and external parts. The external and middle ears are mainly concerned with the transference of sound waves from the exterior to the internal ear, which contains the *vestibulocochlear organ* concerned with equilibration and hearing.

The Internal (Inner) Ear

This is the first of three anatomical parts of the ear to develop. Early in the fourth week a thickened plate of surface ectoderm, the *otic placode*, appears on each side of the caudal part of the developing hindbrain (Fig. 18–8A and B). Each placode soon invaginates and sinks deep to the surface ectoderm into the underlying mesenchyme. In so doing, it forms an *otic pit* (Fig. 18–8D). The edges of the pit soon come together and fuse to form an *otic vesicle* (otocyst), the primordium of the *membranous labyrinth* (Figs. 18–8D and 18–9E). The otic vesicle soon loses its connection with the surface ectoderm (Fig. 18–8G). A diverticulum protrudes from this vesicle, which elongates to form the *endolymphatic duct and sac* (Fig. 18–9A to E).

Two regions of each otic vesicle soon become recognizable (Fig. 18–9A): a dorsal *utricular portion* from which the endolymphatic duct arises, and a ventral *saccular portion*. Three flat, disklike diverticula grow out from the utricular portion. The central portions of the walls of these diverticula soon fuse and disappear (Fig. 18–9B to E). The peripheral, unfused portions of the diverticula become the *semicircular ducts*. They are attached to the utricle and are later enclosed in the *semicircular canals of the bony labyrinth* (Moore, 1992).

From the ventral saccular portion of the otic vesicle, a tubular diverticulum called the *cochlear duct* grows and coils to form the membranous *cochlea* (Fig. 18–9C to E). The *spiral organ (of Corti)* differentiates from cells in the wall of the cochlear duct (Fig. 18–9F to I). Nerve processes grow from the *spiral ganglion* (cochlear ganglion) to the spiral organ where they terminate on hair cells.

The mesenchyme around the otic vesicle condenses and differentiates into a cartilaginous *otic capsule* (Fig. 18–9F). As the membranous labyrinth enlarges, vacuoles appear in the cartilaginous otic capsule, which coalesce to form the *perilymphatic space*. The membranous labyrinth is soon suspended in a fluid called *perilymph* in the perilymphatic space. The perilymphatic space related to the cochlear duct develops in two divisions, the *scala tympani* and *scala vestibuli* (Fig. 18–9H and I). The cartilaginous otic capsule later ossifies to form the *bony labyrinth of the internal ear* (Moore, 1992).

The Middle Ear

The distal portion of the *tubotympanic recess* of the first pharyngeal pouch, described in Chapter 11, expands and becomes the *tympanic cavity* (Fig. 18–10). The proximal, unexpanded portion becomes the *auditory (eustachian) tube*.

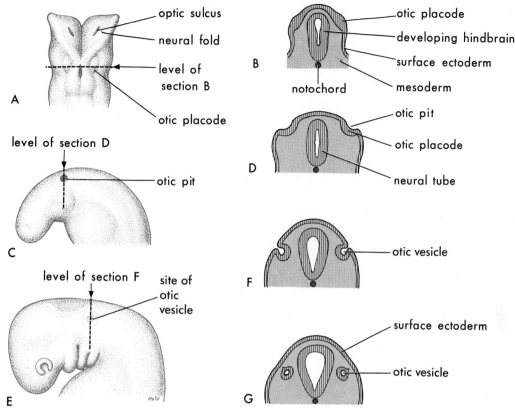

Figure 18–8. Drawings illustrating early development of the internal ear. *A*, Dorsal view of an embryo of 22 days showing the otic placodes. *B, D, F,* and *G,* Schematic sections illustrating successive stages in the development of the otic vesicles. *C* and *E,* Lateral views of the cranial region of embryos of about 24 and 28 days, respectively, showing the external appearance of the developing otic vesicle.

The auditory ossicles (malleus, incus, and stapes) develop by endochondral ossification in the cartilages of the first two pairs of branchial (pharyngeal) arches (see Fig. 11–5). As the tympanic cavity expands, it gradually envelops the *auditory ossicles,* their tendons and ligaments, and the chorda tympani nerve. All these structures receive a more or less complete epithelial investment. Even in adults, the ossicles are covered with an epithelial layer. From a study of early human embryos and fetuses, it has been suggested that an epithelial-type organizer located at the tip of the tubotympanic recess probably plays a role in the early development of the middle ear and tympanic membrane (Michaels, 1988).

During the late fetal period, expansion of the tympanic cavity gives rise to the *mastoid antrum* located in the petromastoid portion of the temporal bone (Moore, 1992). This antrum is well developed at birth; however, no mastoid (air) cells are present. By two years of age the mastoid cells are well developed, and they produce projections of the temporal bones called *mastoid processes.* The middle ear continues to grow through puberty (Behrman, 1992).

The External Ear

The *external acoustic meatus* develops from the dorsal end of the first branchial (pharyngeal) groove (Fig. 18–10). The ectodermal cells at the bottom of this funnel-shaped tube proliferate and form a solid epithelial plate called the *meatal plug.* Late in the fetal period, the central cells of this plug degenerate, forming a cavity which becomes the internal part of the external acoustic meatus (external auditory meatus).

The *tympanic membrane* forms from the first branchial (pharyngeal) membrane (Fig. 18–10A).

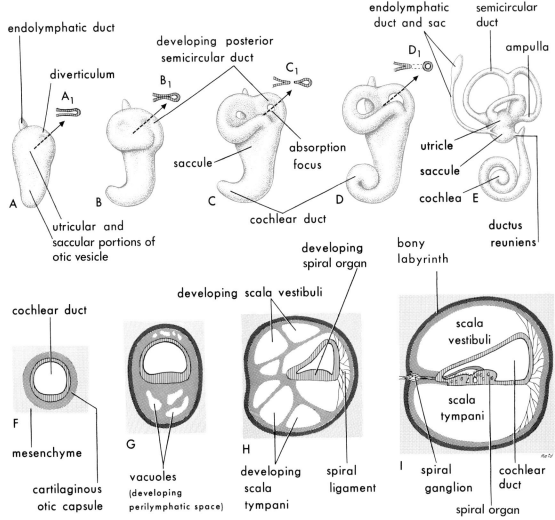

Figure 18–9. Diagrams showing development of the membranous and bony labyrinths of the internal ear. *A* to *E*, Lateral views showing successive stages in the development of the otic vesicle into the membranous labyrinth from the fifth to eighth weeks. *A₁* to *D₁*, Diagrammatic sketches illustrating the development of a semicircular duct. *F* to *I*, Sections through the cochlear duct showing successive stages in the development of the spiral organ (of Corti) and the perilymphatic space from the eighth to the twentieth weeks.

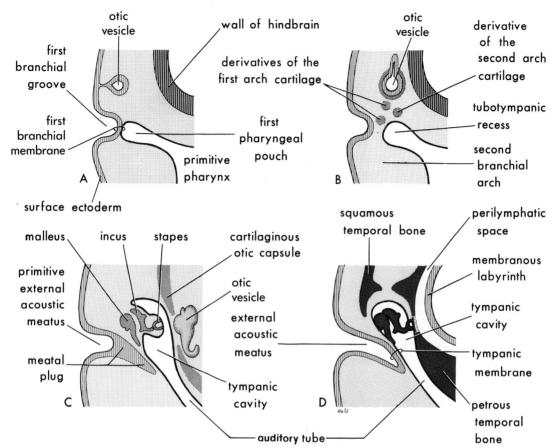

Figure 18–10. Schematic drawings showing development of the external and middle ear. *A*, Four weeks, illustrating the relation of the otic vesicle to the branchial apparatus. *B*, Five weeks, showing the tubotympanic recess and branchial (pharyngeal) arch cartilages. *C*, Later stage, showing the tubotympanic recess (future tympanic cavity and mastoid antrum) beginning to envelop the ossicles. *D*, Final stage of ear development, showing the relationship of the middle ear to the perilymphatic space and the external acoustic meatus.

As development proceeds, mesenchyme grows between the layers of the branchial (pharyngeal) membrane and later differentiates into the collagenic fibers in the tympanic membrane. The external covering of the tympanic membrane (very thin skin) is derived from the surface ectoderm; whereas, its internal lining is derived from the endoderm of the tubotympanic recess.

The *auricle* (pinna) of the external ear forms from six swellings called *auricular hillocks*, which develop around the margins of the first branchial (pharyngeal) groove (Figs. 6–8C and 18–11A). The auricles begin to develop in the cranial part of the future neck region. As the mandible develops the auricles ascend to the level of the eyes.

Congenital Anomalies of the Ear

There are many minor variations in the shape of the auricle of the external ear that are not clinically important. Major anomalies of the auricle are usually associated with numerical chromosomal abnormalities (e.g., trisomy 18 syndrome; see Fig. 9–5) and with the *first arch syndrome* (see Fig. 11–10).

CONGENITAL DEAFNESS. Congenital impairment of hearing may be due to maldevelopment of the sound-conducting apparatus of the middle ear or of the neurosensory or perceptive structures of the internal ear. Most types of congenital deafness are caused by genetic factors. *Rubella infection* during the critical period of development of the internal ear, particularly

auricular hillocks derived from the
first and second branchial arches

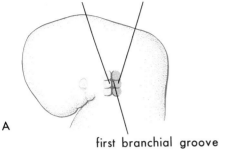

A

first branchial groove

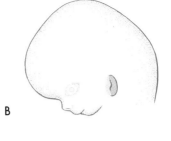

B

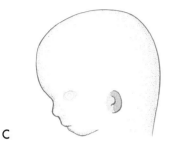

C

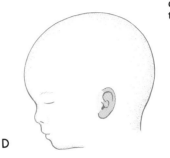

D

Figure 18–11. Drawings illustrating development of the auricle of the external ear. *A*, Five weeks. *B*, Six weeks. *C*, Eight weeks. *D*, 32 weeks. As the mandible and teeth develop, the auricles move from the neck to the side of the head.

during the seventh and eighth weeks (see Fig. 9–12), can cause maldevelopment of the spiral organ (see Chapter 9, p. 137).

Congenital fixation of the stapes, one of the three middle ear bones, results in congenital conductive deafness in an otherwise normal ear. Defects of the other two middle ear bones (malleus and incus) are often associated with the *first arch syndrome* (p. 161).

Auricular appendages or tags anterior to the auricle are common (Fig. 18–12) and result from the development of *accessory auricular hillocks*. They usually consist of skin only, but they may contain some cartilage.

ATRESIA OF THE EXTERNAL ACOUSTIC MEATUS. Congenital blockage of the external ear canal is the result of failure of the meatal plug to canalize (Fig. 18–10*C*). Usually, the deep part of the meatus is open, but the superficial part is blocked by bone or fibrous tissue. Most cases are associated with the *first arch syndrome* (p. 161). Often, abnormal development of both the first and second branchial (pharyngeal) arches is involved. The auricle is also usually severely affected, and anomalies of the middle and/or internal ear are sometimes present (Parrish and Amedee, 1990). For a discussion of other anomalies of the ear (e.g., anotia and microtia), see Moore and Persaud, 1993.

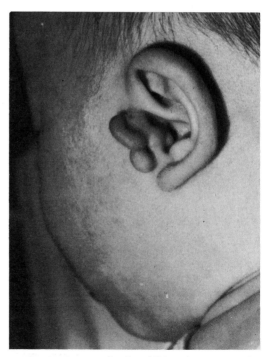

Figure 18–12. Photograph of a child with two auricular appendages or tags, which result from the development of accessory auricular hillocks. (From Swenson O: *Pediatric Surgery.* 1958. Courtesy of Appleton-Century-Crofts).

SUMMARY

The eyes and ears begin to develop during the fourth week. These special sense organs are very sensitive to the teratogenic effects of infectious agents (e.g., cytomegalovirus and rubella virus [p. 137]). The most serious defects result from disturbances of development during the fourth to sixth weeks, but defects of sight and hearing may result from developmental disturbances by certain microorganisms during the fetal period (e.g., rubella virus and *Treponema pallidum,* the microorganism that causes syphilis).

The Eye

The first indication of the eye is the *optic sulcus,* which forms at the beginning of the fourth week. This sulcus soon forms an *optic vesicle* that projects laterally from the side of the forebrain. The optic vesicle contacts the surface ectoderm and induces development of the *lens placode,* the primordium of the lens. As the lens placode invaginates to form a *lens vesicle,* the optic vesicle invaginates to form an *optic cup.* The retina forms from both layers of this cup.

The retina, the optic nerve fibers, the muscles of the iris, and the epithelium of the iris and ciliary body are derived from the *neuroectoderm* of the forebrain. The lens, the epithelium of the lacrimal glands and ducts, the eyelids, the conjunctiva, and the cornea are derived from the *surface ectoderm.* The eye muscles (except those of the iris) and all connective and vascular tissues of the eyelids, cornea, iris, ciliary body, choroid, and sclera are derived from *mesoderm.* The sphincter and dilator muscles of the iris develop from the ectoderm at the rim of the optic cup.

There are many congenital ocular anomalies, but most of them are uncommon. Most anomalies are caused by defective closure of the optic fissure during the sixth week. *Congenital cataract* and glaucoma may result from intrauterine infections (e.g., rubella virus), but most congenital cataracts are inherited.

The Ear

The surface ectoderm gives rise to the *otic vesicle* during the fourth week. It develops into the membranous labyrinth of the internal ear. The bony labyrinth develops from the surrounding mesenchyme.

The epithelium lining the tympanic cavity, mastoid antrum, mastoid cells, and the auditory tube are derived from endoderm of the tubotympanic recess of the first pharyngeal pouch. The *otic vesicle* gives rise to the utricle, saccule, semicircular ducts, and the spiral organ (of Corti).

The auditory ossicles develop from the cartilages of the first two branchial (pharyngeal) arches. The external acoustic meatus develops from ectoderm of the first branchial (pharyngeal) groove and the mesoderm associated with it. The tympanic membrane develops from endoderm of the first pharyngeal pouch, ectoderm of the first branchial (pharyngeal) groove, and mesenchyme between these layers. The auricle of the external ear develops from six *auricular hillocks* that form around the first branchial (pharyngeal) groove.

Congenital deafness may result from abnormal development of the membranous labyrinth and/or the bony labyrinth as well as from abnormalities of the auditory ossicles. Recessive inheritance is the most common cause of congenital deafness, but a prenatal *rubella virus infection* is a major environmental factor known to cause defective hearing. There are many minor anomalies of the auricle, but most of them are clinically unimportant; however, they alert the clinician to the possible presence of associated major anomalies (e.g., of the heart and kidneys). Low-set malformed ears are often associated with numerical chromosomal abnormalities (e.g., trisomy 13; see Chapter 9, p. 122).

Commonly Asked Questions

1. If a woman has rubella (German measles) during the first trimester of her pregnancy, what are the chances that the eyes and ears of the embryo/fetus will be affected? What is the most common manifestation of late fetal rubella infection in babies? If a pregnant

woman is exposed to rubella, can it be determined if she is immune to the infection?

2. My grandmother told me that a good way of preventing the congenital anomalies caused by German measles is by the purposeful exposure of young girls to rubella (German measles). Is this the best way for me to prevent having a blind and deaf baby due to rubella infection during pregnancy? If not, what can be done to provide immunization against rubella infection?

3. A nurse told me that deafness and tooth defects occurring during childhood can result from what she called "fetal syphilis." Is this true? If so, how could this happen? Can these defects be prevented?

4. I recently heard that blindness and deafness can result from herpes virus infections. Is this true? If so, which herpes viruses are involved? What are the infant's chances of normal development?

5. I read in the paper that methyl mercury exposure in utero can cause mental retardation, deafness, and blindness. The mother had apparently been eating contaminated fish. Can you explain how these anomalies could be caused by methylmercury?

The answers to these questions are given on page 336.

REFERENCES

Ars B: Organogenesis of the middle ear structures. *J Laryngol Otol 103:*16, 1989.

Behrman RE: *Nelson Textbook of Pediatrics,* 14th ed. Philadelphia, WB Saunders, 1992.

Brown CA: Abnormalities of the eyes and associated structures. *In* Norman AP (ed): *Congenital Abnormalities in Infancy,* 2nd ed. Oxford, Blackwell Scientific Publications, 1971.

Crowley LV: *An Introduction to Clinical Embryology.* Chicago, Year Book Medical Publishers, 1974.

Jones KL: *Smith's Recognizable Patterns of Human Malformation,* 4th ed. Philadelphia, WB Saunders, 1988.

Kwitko ML (ed): *Surgery of the Infant Eye.* New York, Appleton-Century-Crofts, 1979.

Mann IC: *The Development of the Human Eye,* 3rd ed. London, British Medical Association, 1974.

Martyn LJ: Pediatric ophthalmology. *In* Behrman RE (ed): *Textbook of Pediatrics,* 14th ed. Philadelphia, WB Saunders, 1992.

Michaels L: Evolution of the epidermoid formation and its role in the development of the middle ear and tympanic membrane during the first trimester. *J Otolaryngol 17:*22, 1988.

Moll M: Congenital earpits or auricular sinuses. *Acta Path Microbiol Scand 99:*96, 1991.

Moore KL: *Clinically Oriented Anatomy,* 3rd ed. Baltimore, Williams & Wilkins, 1992.

Moore KL, Persaud TVN: *The Developing Human. Clinically Oriented Embryology,* 5th ed. Philadelphia, WB Saunders 1993.

Nordquist D, McLoon SC: Morphological patterns in the developing vertebrate retina. *Anat Embryol 184:*433, 1991.

O'Rahilly R: The early development of the eye in staged human embryos. *Contr Embryol Carneg Instn 38:*1, 1966.

O'Rahilly R: The early development of the otic vesicle in staged human embryos. *J Embryol Exp Morphol 11:*741, 1963.

O'Rahilly R: The prenatal development of the human eye. *Exp. Eye Res. 21:*93, 1975.

Parrish KL, Amedee RG: Atresia of the external auditory canal. *J La State Med Soc 142:*9, 1990.

Sellheyer K, Spitznas M: Differentiation of the ciliary muscle in the human embryo and fetus. *Graefes Arch Clin Exp Ophthalmol 226:*281, 1988.

Sevel D: A reappraisal of the development of the eyelids. *Eye 2(Pt 2):*123, 1988.

Sevel D, Isaacs R: A re-evaluation of corneal development. *Trans Am Ophthalmol Soc 86:*178, 1989.

Shah CP, Halperin DS: Congenital deafness. *In* Persaud TVN (ed): *Advances in the Study of Birth Defects, Vol 7. Central Nervous System and Craniofacial Malformations.* New York, Alan R Liss, 1982.

Smith B, Guberina C: Congenital ocular anomalies. *In* Kwitko ML (ed): *Surgery of the Infant Eye.* New York, Appleton-Century-Crofts, 1979.

Stromland K, Miller M, Cook C: Ocular teratology. *Surv Ophthalmol 35:*429, 1991.

Tamura T, Smelser JK: Development of the sphincter and dilator muscles of the iris. *Arch Ophthalmol 89:*332, 1973.

Tripathi BJ, Tripathi RC, Livingston AM, Borisuth NSC: The role of growth factors in the embryogenesis and differentiation of the eye. *Am J Anat 192:*442, 1991.

Warkany J: Prevention of congenital malformations. *Teratology 23:*175, 1981.

Wilson RS, Char F: Drug-induced ocular malformations. *In* Persaud TVN (ed): *Advances in the Study of Birth Defects, Vol 7. Central Nervous System and Craniofacial Malformations.* New York, Alan R Liss, 1982.

19

THE SKIN, CUTANEOUS APPENDAGES, AND TEETH

SKIN

The skin consists of two different layers, the *epidermis* and *dermis*. The epidermis is derived from *ectoderm* and the dermis from *mesoderm*.

THE EPIDERMIS (Fig. 19–1). Initially the epidermis consists of a single layer of ectodermal cells. The surface ectodermal cells proliferate and form a protective layer called the *periderm*. Cells from this layer slough off and form part of the *vernix caseosa*, a greasy, cheeselike substance that covers and protects the skin of the fetus from constant exposure to amniotic fluid, which later contains urine produced by the fetus. In addition, the vernix caseosa facilitates birth of the fetus due to its slippery nature.

By about 11 weeks, cells from the basal layer called the *stratum germinativum* have formed an intermediate layer. All layers of the adult epidermis are present at birth. Replacement of peridermal cells continues until about the twenty-first week; thereafter, the periderm gradually disappears as the stratum corneum forms. Proliferation of cells in the stratum germinativum also forms *epidermal ridges*, which extend into the developing dermis (Fig. 19–1C). These ridges begin to appear in embryos of about ten weeks and are permanently established by the seventeenth week.

The epidermal ridges produce ridges and grooves on the surface of the palms of the hands and the soles of the feet, including the digits. The type of pattern that develops is determined genetically and constitutes the basis for using *fingerprints* in criminal investigations and medical genetics. Study of the patterns of the epidermal ridges of the skin is called *dermatoglyphics*. Abnormal chromosome complements affect the development of the ridge patterns, e.g., infants with Down syndrome have distinctive patterns on their hands and feet that are of diagnostic value. For details about the use of dermatoglyphics in medical genetics, see Hirschhorn (1992).

During the early fetal period, cells from the *neural crest* migrate into the dermis and differentiate into *melanoblasts* (see Figs. 17–8 and 19–1C). These cells soon enter the epidermis and differentiate into *melanocytes,* which lie at the dermoepidermal junction (Fig. 19–1D). The *melanocytes produce melanin* and distribute it to the epidermal cells. Very few melanocytes develop in the skin of the palms and soles. Melanin pigment formation mainly occurs after birth when the process is stimulated by ultraviolet radiation. The relative content of melanin in the epidermis accounts for different skin colors.

THE DERMIS (Fig. 19–1). The dermis is derived from the mesoderm underlying the surface ectoderm. By 11 weeks the mesenchymal cells derived from the mesoderm have begun to produce collagenous and elastic connective tissue fibers (Fig. 19–1D). As the epidermal ridges form, the dermis projects superficially into the epidermis and forms *dermal papillae*. Capillary loops develop in some dermal papillae, and

315

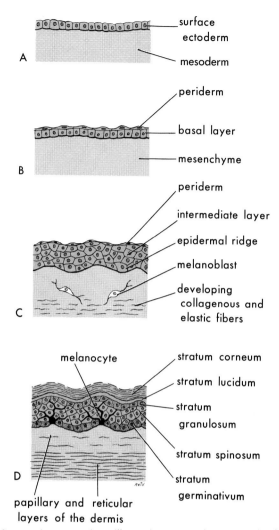

Figure 19–1. Drawings illustrating successive stages in the development of thick skin. *A*, Four weeks. *B*, Seven weeks. *C*, 11 weeks. *D*, Newborn. The epidermis is derived from the surface ectoderm, and the dermis develops from mesenchyme that is derived from the somatic layer of mesoderm. Note the position of the melanocytes in the basal layer of the epidermis and the way their branching dendritic processes extend between the epidermal cells to supply them with melanin.

sensory nerve endings form in others. The major vascular pattern of the fetal dermis is established by the end of the first trimester.

Disorders of Keratinization

Ichthyosis (Gr. *ichthys*, fish) is a general term applied to a group of disorders resulting from excessive keratinization. They are characterized by dryness and *fishskin-like scaling of the skin*, which may involve the entire body surface.

A *harlequin fetus* results from an uncommon keratinizing disorder that is inherited as an autosomal recessive trait (Behrman, 1992). The skin is markedly thickened, ridged, and cracked. Affected infants have a grotesque appearance, and most of them die within the first week of life.

A *collodion baby* is covered at birth by a thick, taut membrane resembling collodion. This membrane cracks with the first respiratory efforts and begins to fall off in large sheets, but complete shedding may take several weeks. For a discussion of other disorders of skin (e.g., albinism, ectodermal dysplasia and angiomas), see Moore and Persaud (1993).

HAIR

Hair begins to develop early in the fetal period (ninth to twelfth week), but it does not become easily recognizable until about the twentieth week (see Fig. 7–1). Hair is first recognizable on the eyebrows, upper lip, and chin. A *hair follicle* begins as a proliferation of the stratum germinativum that extends as a solid downgrowth of the epidermis into the underlying dermis (Fig. 19–2A). The deepest part of the *hair bud* soon becomes club-shaped to form a *hair bulb* (Fig. 19–2B). The epithelial cells of the hair bulb constitute the *germinal matrix*, which later gives rise to the hair.

The hair bulb is soon invaginated by a small mesenchymal *hair papilla* (Fig. 19–2C). The peripheral cells of the developing hair follicle form the *epithelial root sheath*, and the surrounding mesenchymal cells differentiate into the *dermal root sheath* (Fig. 19–2D). As cells in the germinal matrix proliferate, they are pushed toward the surface where they become keratinized (hardened) to form the *hair shaft* (Fig. 19–2C). The hair grows, pierces the epidermis, and protrudes from the surface of the skin. Hairs on the eyebrows and upper lip develop by the end of the twelfth week. These initial hairs, called *lanugo* (L. *lana*, fine) or lanugo hairs, are fine and colorless. They are shed at birth or shortly thereafter.

Anomalies of Hair

CONGENITAL ALOPECIA (ATRICHIA CONGENITA). Absence or loss of hair may occur alone or with other abnormalities of the skin and its deriva-

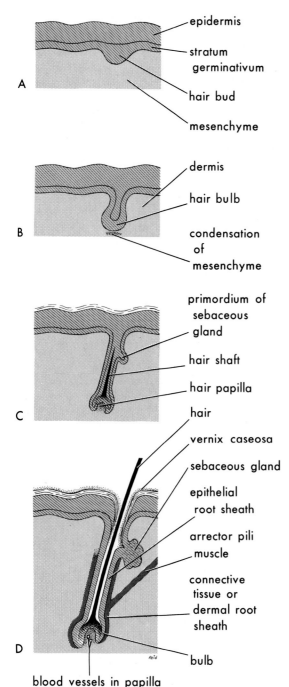

epidermis

stratum germinativum

hair bud

mesenchyme

A

dermis

hair bulb

condensation of mesenchyme

B

primordium of sebaceous gland

hair shaft

hair papilla

hair

C

vernix caseosa

sebaceous gland

epithelial root sheath

arrector pili muscle

connective tissue or dermal root sheath

bulb

D

blood vessels in papilla

Figure 19–2. Drawings showing successive stages in the development of a hair and its associated sebaceous gland. *A*, 12 weeks. *B*, 14 weeks. *C*, 16 weeks. *D*, 18 weeks. Note that the sebaceous gland develops as an outgrowth from the side of the hair follicle. Observe that the hair papillae are rapidly filled with vessels and nerve endings.

tives. The hair loss may be caused by failure of hair follicles to develop, or it may result from follicles producing poor-quality hairs.

HYPERTRICHOSIS. Excessive hairiness (e.g., on the shoulders and back) is the result of the development of excess hair follicles or from the persistence of hairs that normally disappear during the perinatal period. Localized hypertrichosis is often associated with *spina bifida occulta* (see Chapter 17, p. 285).

SEBACEOUS GLANDS

Most of these glands develop as buds from the sides of developing hair follicles (Fig. 19–2C). The glandular buds penetrate the surrounding connective tissue and branch to form the primordia of several alveoli and their associated ducts (Fig. 19–2D). The whitish, creamlike paste called *vernix caseosa* covering the skin of the fetus is formed from the mixture of the oily secretion of the sebaceous glands called *sebum* with degenerated epidermal cells and hairs. Vernix caseosa protects the skin of the fetus against the macerating action of the amniotic fluid.

SWEAT GLANDS

Most of these glands develop as solid epidermal downgrowths into the underlying mesenchyme (future dermis [Fig. 19–3]). As a bud elongates, its end coils to form the primordium of the secretory portion of the gland. The epithelial attachment of the developing gland to the epidermis forms the primordium of the duct (Fig. 19–3C and D). The peripheral cells of the secretory portion of the gland differentiate into secretory and *myoepithelial cells.* The myoepithelial cells, derived from ectoderm, are thought to be specialized smooth muscle cells that aid in expelling sweat from the glands.

The distribution of large sweat glands in humans is very limited. They are mostly confined to the axillae, pubic region, and areolae of the breasts. They develop from the downgrowths of the stratum germinativum of the epidermis that give rise to hair follicles. As a result, the ducts of these glands open, not onto the skin surface as do ordinary sweat glands, but into hair follicles superficial to the openings of the sebaceous glands.

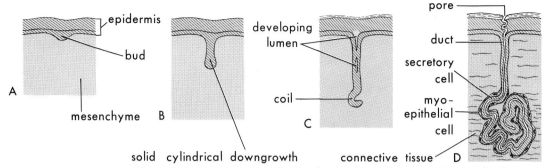

Figure 19–3. Diagrams illustrating successive stages in the development of a sweat gland. It begins to develop at about 20 weeks as a solid downgrowth of epidermal cells into the mesenchyme. The terminal part coils and forms the body of the gland. The central cells degenerate to form the lumen of the gland, and the peripheral cells differentiate into secretory cells and contractile myoepithelial cells.

NAILS

Toenails and fingernails begin to develop at the tips of the digits at about ten weeks (Fig. 19–4). Development of fingernails precedes that of toenails by about four weeks (see Table 7–2). The primordia of the nails first appear as thickened areas or fields of epidermis at the tip of each digit (Fig. 19–4A). Later, these *nail fields* migrate onto the dorsal surface. The nail fields are surrounded laterally and proximally by elevations of the epidermis called *nail folds*. Cells from the proximal nail fold grow over the nail field and become keratinized and consolidated to form the *nail plate*, the primordium of the nail (Fig. 19–4B and C).

The fingernails reach the fingertips by about 32 weeks; the toenails reach the toetips by about 36 weeks (see Fig. 7–9). Nails that have not reached the tips of the digits at birth are an indication of prematurity.

MAMMARY GLANDS

The mammary glands begin to develop during the sixth week as solid growths of the epidermis into the underlying mesenchyme (Fig. 19–5C). These buds occur along two thickened strips of ectoderm called *mammary ridges* (Fig. 19–5A). Each primary mammary bud soon gives rise to several secondary buds, which develop into the *lactiferous ducts* and their branches. The connective tissue and fat of the *mammary gland* develop from surrounding mesenchyme (Fig. 19–5F). No alveoli are present at birth.

At the origin of the mammary gland, the epidermis becomes depressed to form a shallow *mammary pit* (Fig. 19–5E). The nipples are poorly formed and depressed in newborn infants. Soon after birth the nipples usually rise from the mammary pits due to proliferation of the surrounding connective tissues of the *areola*, the circular pigmented area of skin around the

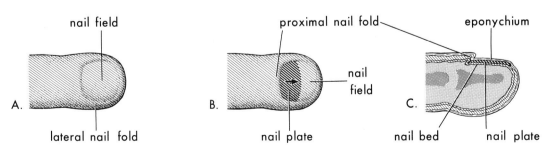

Figure 19–4. Diagrams illustrating successive stages in the development of a fingernail. The fingernails reach the fingertips by 32 weeks and extend beyond them in full-term infants. The first indication of a nail is a thickening of the epidermis, the nail field, at the tip of the digit. The nail field grows dorsally and proximally to occupy the normal position of the nail *(A)*. As the nail develops, it slowly grows toward the tip of the digit *(B)*, which it reaches before birth *(C)*.

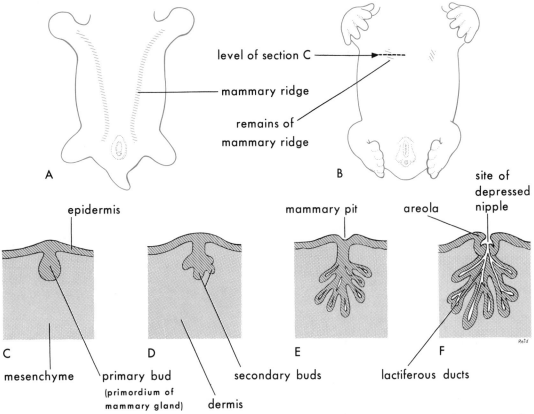

Figure 19–5. Drawings illustrating development of the mammary glands. *A*, Ventral view of an embryo of about 28 days, showing the mammary ridges. *B*, Similar view at six weeks, showing the remains of these ridges. *C*, Transverse section through the mammary ridge at the site of a developing mammary gland. *D*, *E*, and *F*, Similar sections, showing successive stages of development between the twelfth week and birth.

nipple. The smooth muscle fibers of the areola and nipple differentiate from the surrounding mesenchymal cells.

The rudimentary mammary glands of newborn males and females are identical and are often enlarged. They may produce a secretion (often called "witch's milk"). These transitory changes are caused by maternal hormones passing through the placental membrane into the fetal circulation (Chapter 8).

Anomalies of the Mammary Glands

SUPERNUMERARY BREASTS AND NIPPLES (Fig. 19–6). An extra breast *(polymastia)* or nipple *(polythelia)* occurs in about one per cent of the female population and is an inheritable condition. Supernumerary nipples also occur in males. An extra breast or nipple usually develops just inferior to the normal breast. The extra nipples or breasts develop in these positions

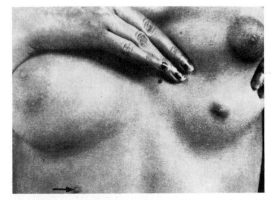

Figure 19–6. Photograph of an adult female with a supernumerary nipple on the right *(arrow)* and a supernumerary breast inferior to the normal left one. (From Haagensen CD: *Diseases of the Breast*, rev. 2nd ed. Philadelphia, WB Saunders, 1974.)

from extra mammary buds along the mammary ridges. Accessory breasts may have normal mammary gland tissue and may become functional during pregnancy, but this is unusual. For other anomalies of the breasts (e.g., absence of nipples), see Moore and Persaud (1993).

TEETH

Two sets of teeth normally develop: the *primary dentition* or deciduous teeth and the *secondary dentition* or permanent teeth (Table 19–1). The teeth develop from ectoderm and mesoderm. The enamel is derived from ectoderm of the oral cavity; all other tissues differentiate from the surrounding mesenchyme, a derivative of mesoderm.

Tooth development appears to be initiated by the inductive influence of the mesenchyme on the overlying ectoderm. This mesenchyme is of neural crest origin. Tooth development is a continuous process, but it is usually divided into stages for descriptive purposes (bud, cap, and bell stages) on the basis of the appearance of the developing tooth. Not all teeth begin to develop at the same time. The first tooth buds appear in the anterior mandibular region; later tooth development occurs in the anterior maxillary region and then progresses posteriorly in both jaws. Tooth development continues for years after birth (Table 19–1).

THE BUD STAGE (Figs. 19–7*B* and 19–8*A* and *B*). Tooth development begins early in the sixth week as linear U-shaped thickenings of the oral epithelium. These bands called **dental laminae** follow the curves of the primitive jaws. Localized proliferations of cells in the dental laminae produce ten round or oval swellings called **tooth**

Table 19–1. ORDER AND TIME OF ERUPTION OF TEETH AND TIME OF SHEDDING OF DECIDUOUS TEETH

Tooth	Eruption Time	Shedding Time
Deciduous		
Medial incisor	6–8 mo	6–7 yr
Lateral incisor	8–10 mo	7–8 yr
Canine	11–20 mo	10–12 yr
First molar	12–16 mo	9–11 yr
Second molar	20–24 mo	10–12 yr
Permanent		
Medial incisor	7–8 yr	
Lateral incisor	8–9 yr	
Canine	10–12 yr	
First premolar	10–11 yr	
Second premolar	11–12 yr	
First molar	6–7 yr	
Second molar	12 yr	
Third molar	13–25 yr	

From Moore, K. L.: *Clinically Oriented Anatomy*, 3rd ed. Baltimore, Williams & Wilkins, 1992.

buds. These buds grow into the underlying mesenchyme and develop into the deciduous ("milk") teeth. The first teeth are called *deciduous teeth* because they are shed during childhood (Table 19–1). There are ten tooth buds in each jaw, one for each deciduous tooth. The tooth buds for the permanent teeth with deciduous predecessors begin to appear at about ten weeks (Fig. 19–8*D*). They develop as outgrowths from the dental lamina. The buds for the second and third permanent molars develop after birth.

THE CAP STAGE (Fig. 19–8*C*). The tooth bud becomes slightly invaginated by mesenchyme that forms the *dental papilla*. This gives the developing tooth a caplike appearance. The dental

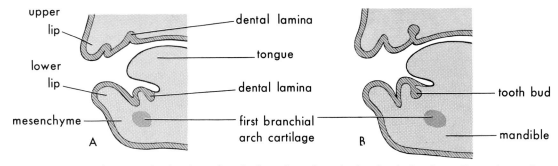

Figure 19–7. Diagrammatic sketches of sagittal sections through the developing jaws, illustrating early development of the teeth. *A*, Early in the sixth week, showing the dental laminae. *B*, Later in the sixth week, showing the tooth buds arising from the dental laminae.

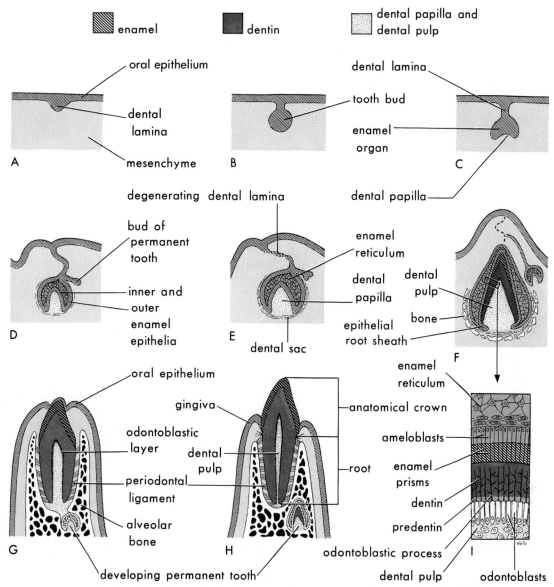

Figure 19–8. Schematic drawings of sagittal sections, showing successive stages in the development and eruption of an incisor tooth. *A*, Six weeks, showing the dental lamina. *B*, Seven weeks, showing the tooth bud developing from the dental lamina. *C*, Eight weeks, showing the cap stage of tooth development. *D*, Ten weeks, showing the early bell stage of the enamel organ of the deciduous tooth and the bud stage of the developing permanent tooth. *E*, 14 weeks, showing the advanced bell stage of the enamel organ. Note that the connection (dental lamina) of the tooth to the oral epithelium is degenerating. *F*, 28 weeks, showing the enamel and dentin layers. *G*, Six months *postnatal,* showing early tooth eruption. *H*, 18 months *postnatal,* showing a fully erupted deciduous incisor tooth. The permanent incisor tooth now has a well-developed crown. *I*, Section through a developing tooth, showing the ameloblasts (enamel producers) and the odontoblasts (dentin producers).

papilla gives rise to the dental pulp. The ectodermal part of the developing tooth is called an **enamel organ** because it produces enamel. As the enamel organ and dental papilla form, the mesenchyme surrounding them condenses to form a capsulelike structure called the *dental sac* (Fig. 19–8E and F). It gives rise to the *cementum* of the tooth and the *periodontal ligament*.

THE BELL STAGE (Fig. 19–8D). As invagination of the enamel organ continues, the developing tooth assumes the shape of a bell. Mesenchymal cells in the dental papilla adjacent to the inner enamel epithelium differentiate into **odontoblasts.** These cells produce *predentin* and deposit it adjacent to the inner enamel epithelium. Later, the predentin calcifies and becomes **dentin.** As the dentin thickens, the odontoblasts regress toward the center of the dental papilla, but their cytoplasmic processes, called *odontoblastic (Tomes') processes*, remain embedded in the dentin (Fig. 19–8F and I).

Cells of the inner enamel epithelium adjacent to the dentin differentiate into *ameloblasts.* These cells produce **enamel** in the form of prisms (rods) over the dentin (Fig. 19–8I). As the enamel increases, the ameloblasts regress toward the outer enamel epithelium. Enamel and dentin formation begins at the tip (cusp) of the tooth and progresses toward the future root.

The *root of the tooth* begins to develop after dentin and enamel formation is well advanced. The inner and outer enamel epithelia come together in the neck region of the tooth; here, they form an epithelial fold called the *epithelial root sheath.* This sheath grows into the mesenchyme and initiates root formation. The odontoblasts adjacent to the root sheath form dentin that is continuous with that of the crown. As the dentin increases, it reduces the pulp cavity to a narrow *root canal* through which the vessels and nerves pass. The inner cells of the dental sac differentiate into *cementoblasts* and produce **cementum,** which is deposited over the dentin of the root. As the teeth develop and the jaws ossify, the outer cells of the dental sac also become active in bone formation. Except over its crown, each tooth becomes surrounded by bone. The tooth is held in its *alveolus* (bony socket) by the strong *periodontal ligament*, a derivative of the dental sac (Fig. 19–8G). Some fibers of this ligament are embedded in the cementum; other parts are fixed to the bony wall of the alveolus.

TOOTH ERUPTION (Fig. 19–8G and H and Table 19–1). As the teeth develop they begin a slow movement toward the exterior. As the root grows, the crown gradually erupts through the oral mucosa. Eruption of the deciduous teeth usually occurs between the sixth and twenty-fourth months after birth. The mandibular teeth usually erupt before the maxillary teeth, and girls' teeth usually erupt earlier than boys' teeth. A child's dentition normally contains 20 deciduous teeth.

The mandibular medial (central) incisors usually erupt six to eight months after birth (Table 19–1), but this process may not begin until 12 to 13 months in some normal children. Despite this, all 20 deciduous teeth are usually present by the end of the second year in healthy children. Delayed eruption of all teeth may indicate systemic or nutritional disturbances such as hypopituitarism or hypothyroidism (Behrman, 1992).

THE PERMANENT TEETH (Figs. 19–8 and 19–9). These teeth develop in a manner similar to that just described for deciduous teeth. As a permanent tooth grows, the root of the corresponding deciduous tooth is gradually resorbed by *osteoclasts*, consequently, when the deciduous tooth is shed, it consists of the crown only and the uppermost portion of the root. The permanent teeth usually begin to erupt during the sixth year and continue appearing until early adulthood (Table 19–1). The permanent teeth are not shed; however, if they are not properly cared for or if disease of the gingiva (gum) develops, they may have to be extracted.

Anomalies of the Teeth

Although most abnormalities of the teeth are genetic disorders, such as *dentinogenesis imperfecta*, environmental factors (e.g., rubella virus, syphilis, radiation, and tetracyclines) can cause tooth defects (pp. 134 and 137–139).

NATAL TEETH. These teeth are erupted at birth. They are observed in about one in 2000 newborn infants (Behrman, 1992). There are usually two in the position of the mandibular incisors. Their presence suggests that early eruption of the other teeth may occur. Obviously, natal teeth may produce maternal discomfort due to biting of the nipple during breast-feeding. In addition, the infant's tongue may be lacerated, or the teeth may detach and be aspirated; for these reasons, natal teeth are sometimes extracted.

DENTINOGENESIS IMPERFECTA. This condition is relatively common in white children. The teeth are brown to gray-blue with an opalescent sheen. The enamel tends to wear down rapidly, exposing the dentin. This anomaly is inherited as an autosomal dominant trait (Thompson et al., 1991).

ENAMEL HYPOPLASIA (Fig. 19–10B). Defective enamel formation results in the presence of grooves, pits, and/or fissures in the enamel of the teeth. These defects are the result of a temporary disturbance in enamel formation. Various factors may injure the ameloblasts (e.g., nutritional deficiency, tetracycline therapy [p. 134], and infectious diseases, such as rubella [p. 137]).

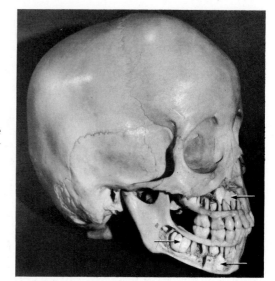

Figure 19–9. Photograph of the skull of a child in the fourth year. The bone of the jaws has been removed to show the relations of the developing permanent teeth *(arrows)* to the deciduous teeth.

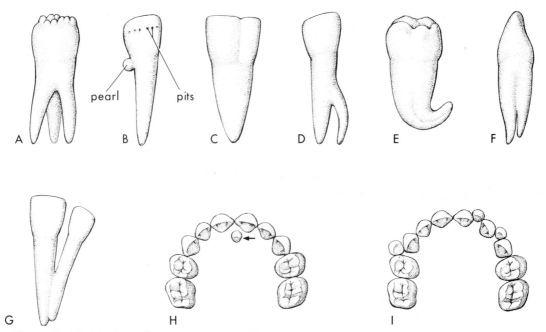

Figure 19–10. Drawings illustrating common abnormalities of teeth. *A*, Irregular raspberrylike crown. *B*, Enamel pearl and pits. *C*, Incisor tooth with a double crown. *D*, Abnormal division of root. *E*, Distorted root. *F*, Branched root. *G*, Fused roots. *H*, Hyperdontia with a supernumerary incisor tooth in the anterior region of the palate *(arrow)*. *I*, Hyperdontia with 13 deciduous teeth in the maxilla (upper jaw) instead of the normal ten.

Tetracyclines are extensively incorporated in the enamel and produce brownish-yellow discoloration and hypoplasia of the enamel. The primary teeth are affected if the tetracyclines are given from 18 weeks (prenatal) to ten months (postnatal), and the permanent teeth are affected from 18 weeks (prenatal) to 12 years. *Tetracyclines should not be administered to pregnant women* or to children if they can be avoided because these drugs adversely affect tooth development.

Rickets, a vitamin D deficiency disease, occurring during the critical period of permanent tooth development, is the most common known cause of enamel hypoplasia. Rickets is characterized by a disturbance of ossification.

ABNORMALITIES OF SHAPE (Fig. 19–10*A* to *G*). Abnormally shaped teeth are relatively common. Occasionally, spherical masses of enamel called *enamel pearls* are attached to the tooth. They are formed by aberrant groups of ameloblasts.

NUMERICAL ABNORMALITIES (Fig. 19–10*H* and *I*). One or more *supernumerary teeth* may develop or teeth may not form. Supernumerary teeth usually appear in the area of the maxillary incisors where they disrupt the position and eruption of normal teeth. The extra teeth commonly erupt posterior to the normal ones.

FUSED TEETH (Fig. 19–10*C* and *G*). Occasionally a tooth bud divides or two buds partially fuse. In some cases the permanent tooth does not form. For other anomalies of teeth, see Moore and Persaud (1993).

SUMMARY

The skin and its appendages develop from ectoderm and mesoderm. The epidermis and its derivatives (hair, nails, and glands) are derived from ectoderm. *Melanocytes* are derived from neural crest cells. The *dermis* is derived from mesoderm. Cast-off cells from the epidermis mix with secretions of the sebaceous glands to form a coating for the skin known as *vernix caseosa.* It protects the epidermis, probably making it more waterproof, and facilitates birth due to its slipperiness.

Hairs develop from downgrowths of the epidermis into the dermis. The sebaceous glands develop as outgrowths from the sides of hair follicles. The sweat and mammary glands develop from epidermal downgrowths. Supernumerary breasts (polymastia) or nipples (polythelia) are relatively common.

The teeth develop from ectoderm and mesoderm. The enamel is produced by cells called *ameloblasts,* which are derived from ectoderm; all other dental tissues develop from mesoderm. The *odontoblasts* produce dentin and the *cementoblasts* form cementum.

The common congenital anomalies of teeth are defective formation of enamel and dentin, abnormalities in shape, and variations in number and position.

Commonly Asked Questions

1. I recently heard someone talking about her baby that she said was born without skin. Is this possible? If so, could such a baby survive?

2. I once saw a dark-skinned person with patches of white skin on his face, chest, and limbs. He even had a white forelock. What is this condition called and what is its developmental basis? Is there any treatment for these skin defects?

3. I was told that some male babies have enlarged breasts at birth. Is this an indication of abnormal sex development? I have also heard that some males develop breasts during puberty. Are they intersexes?

4. A nurse told me about a girl who developed a breast in her axilla during puberty. She also said that this girl had extra nipples on her trunk. What is the embryological basis of these anomalies?

5. I recently read in the newspaper that a baby was born with two teeth. Would these be normal teeth? Is this a common occurrence? Are they usually extracted?

The answers to these questions are given on page 337.

REFERENCES

Avery JK: *Essentials of Oral Histology and Embryology.* St. Louis, Mosby-Year Book, 1992.

Behrman RE (ed): *Nelson Textbook of Pediatrics,* 14th ed. Philadelphia, WB Saunders, 1992.

Beller F: Development and anatomy of the breast. *In* Mitchell Jr, GW, Bassett LW (eds): *The Female Breast and Its Disorders.* Baltimore, Williams & Wilkins, 1990.

Bland KI, Copeland III, EM (eds): *The Breast.* Philadelphia, WB Saunders, 1991.

Booth DH, Persaud TVN: Congenital absence of the breast. *Anat Anz 155:*23, 1984.

Butler PM, Joysey KA (eds): *Development, Function and Evolution of Teeth.* New York, Academic Press, 1978.

Haagensen CD: *Diseases of the Breast,* 3rd ed. Philadelphia, WB Saunders, 1986.

Hirschhorn K: Dermatoglyphics. *In* Behrman RE (ed): *Nelson Textbook of Pediatrics,* 14th ed. Philadelphia, WB Saunders, 1992.

Horn TD: Developmental defects of the skin. *In* Farmer ER, Hood AF (eds): *Pathology of the Skin.* Norwalk, Appleton & Lange, 1990.

Mackie RM: *Clinical Dermatology,* 3rd ed. Oxford, Oxford University Press, 1991.

Moore KL: *Clinically Oriented Anatomy,* 3rd ed. Baltimore, Williams & Wilkins, 1992.

Moore KL, Persaud TVN: *The Developing Human. Clinically Oriented Embryology,* 5th ed. Philadelphia, WB Saunders, 1993.

Moynahan EJ: Abnormalities of the skin. *In* Norman AP (ed): *Congenital Abnormalities in Infancy,* 2nd ed. Oxford, Blackwell Scientific Publications, 1971.

Müller M, Jasmin JR, Monteil RA, Loubiere R: Embryology of the hair follicle. *Early Hum Dev 26:*159, 1991.

Osborne MP: Breast development and anatomy. *In* Harris JR, Hellman S, Henderson IC, Kinne DW (eds): *Breast Diseases,* 2nd ed. Philadelphia, JB Lippincott, 1991.

Persaud TVN: *Environmental Causes of Human Birth Defects.* Springfield, Charles C Thomas, 1990.

Shafer WG, Hine MG, Levy BM: *A Textbook of Oral Pathology,* 4th ed. Philadelphia, WB Saunders, 1983.

Sperber GH: Genetic mechanisms and anomalies in odontogenesis. *J Can Dent Assoc 33:*433, 1967.

Sperber GH: *Craniofacial Embryology,* 4th ed. London, Butterworth, 1989.

Ten Cate AR: Development of the tooth. *In* Ten Cate AR (ed): *Oral Histology. Structure and Function.* St. Louis, CV Mosby, 1989.

Termine JD: Development of dental and paradental structures; Enamel. *In* Provenza DV (ed): *Fundamentals of Oral Histology and Embryology,* 2nd ed. Philadelphia, Lea & Febiger, 1988.

Thompson MW, McInnes RR, Willard HF: *Thompson & Thompson Genetics in Medicine,* 5th ed. Philadelphia, WB Saunders, 1991.

Chapter 1

1. You should not learn how to reproduce the timetables of development. They are presented as an overview of human development before birth. Neither should you try to memorize the criteria for the stages (e.g., that stage 3 begins on day four when there are 12 or more blastomeres present). These stages are used by embryologists when referring to embryos they are describing in detail. You should, however, be able to describe human development to a lay person, and some of the sketches in the timetables would be helpful. You could even use the timetables to explain human development to them.

2. The term *conceptus* is used to refer to the embryo and its membranes (e.g., amnion and chorion); hence, the embryo is only one part of the conceptus. Some people refer to the conceptus as the products of conception, i.e., everything that develops from the zygote.

3. Everyone, especially those in the health sciences, should know about conception, contraception, and how people develop (normally and abnormally). People in the health professions are expected to give intelligent answers to the questions people ask, e.g., When does the baby's heart start to beat? When does it look like a human being? When does it move its limbs?

4. Animal and human embryos look very much alike for the first few weeks, e.g., they both have branchial or pharyngeal arches and tails. After the seventh week, human embryos do not resemble animal embryos, mainly because the head looks human and the tail disappears (see Fig. 6–17).

5. Doctors date pregnancies from the last normal menstrual period (LNMP) because it is a time that is usually remembered by women. It is not possible to detect the precise time of ovulation and fertilization, but there are tests (e.g., ultrasound) that can be done to detect when ovulation is likely to occur and when pregnancy has occurred. These tests are not routinely performed due to the costs involved. When dating pregnancies using LNMP, physicians are aware that the age of the developing human is about two weeks less than the "menstrual age," and they base their decisions on this, e.g., concerning its vulnerability to drugs.

6. *The zygote has the potential to develop into a human being,* just as an acorn has the potential to develop into an oak tree. The zygote is a single cell; whereas, a human being consists of millions of cells. No one knows when an embryo becomes a human being, but many people consider seven- to eight-week-old embryos to be developing human beings. Others consider that it becomes human when it is viable, i.e., after 20 weeks.

Chapter 2

1. The hymen usually ruptures during the perinatal period, forming the vaginal orifice (Fig. 2–3). This opening usually enlarges during childhood as the result of physical activity. Contrary to popular myth, rupture of this fold of mucous membrane surrounding the vaginal orifice, or the absence of bleeding due to tearing of it during the initial intercourse, is not necessarily an indication of the loss of virginity.

2. The term *erection* is rarely used when referring to the sexual excitement of a female, but it is true that the clitoris (homologous to the penis) enlarges ("erects") when it is stimulated and the female is sexually aroused. It is a highly sensitive and important organ related to the sexual excitement of a female.

3. Pregnant women do not menstruate even though there may be some bleeding at the usual time of the menstrual period. This blood leaks from the intervillous space of the placenta (see Chapter 8) due to partial separation of the placenta. As there is no shedding of the endometrium, this is not menstrual fluid. In unusual cases, periodic bleeding may occur every month during pregnancy. Again, this is loss of blood from the placenta and is not menstrual bleeding.

4. It depends on when she forgets to take the pill. If it was around midcycle, ovulation might

occur and pregnancy could result. The taking of two pills the next day would not likely prevent ovulation. Failure to take a pill later in the cycle is not as serious, i.e., if pregnancy is undesirable.

5. *Coitus interruptus* is the term applied to withdrawal of the penis from the vagina before ejaculation occurs. It depends on the self-discipline of the couple to part before the climax of the male (ie., ejaculation). Not only is this difficult to do, it is neither reliable nor psychologically acceptable. Often a few sperms are expelled from the penis with the secretions of one of the auxiliary sex glands (e.g., the seminal vesicles) before ejaculation occurs. One of these sperms could fertilize an ovum.

6. The IUD may inhibit the capacitation of sperms (p. 26) and their transport through the uterus to the fertilization site in the uterine tube; in this case, it would be a *contraceptive device*. More likely, the IUD produces endometrial changes that present a hostile environment for the blastocyst; as a result, it does not implant. In this case it would be a *contraimplantation device* that results in the death and absorption of the embryo when it is a week or so old.

7. The youngest mother on record gave birth at five years and eight months. This was a *highly unusual occurrence* that resulted from precocious ovulation and sexual intercourse. There is a wide variation in the onset of puberty (menarche) in females, but the most common age range in North America is 11 to 13 years.

Chapter 3

1. The ovarian and endometrial (menstrual) cycles cease between 47 and 55 years of age, the average being 48. This results from the gradual cessation of gonadotropin production by the pituitary gland, but it does not mean the ovaries have exhausted their supply of oocytes. This period is called *menopause*. This can be perceived in a positive manner because it is known that there is an increased risk of the Down syndrome or some other trisomy in the children of women who are 35 years of age or older. *Spermatogenesis also decreases after the age of 45*, and the number of nonviable and abnormal sperms increases with age. Nevertheless, sperm production continues until old age, and some very old men have fathered children. The risk of producing abnormal gametes is much less than in women, but old men are more likely to have accumulated mutations that the child might inherit. Mutations may produce congenital anomalies.

2. Considerable research on new contraceptive methods is being conducted, including the development of contraceptive pills for men. This includes experimental work on nonhormonal prevention of spermatogenesis and the stimulation of immune responses to sperms. Arrest of the development of millions of sperms on a continuous basis is much more difficult than arresting the development of a single ovum monthly.

3. It is not known that polar bodies are ever fertilized, but it has been suggested that *dispermic chimeras* result from the fusion of a fertilized ovum with a fertilized polar body. Chimeras are rare individuals who are composed of a mixture of cells from two zygotes. More likely, dispermic chimeras result from the fusion of dizygotic (fraternal) twin zygotes early in development. Dizygotic twins are derived from two zygotes (see Chapter 8). If a polar body was fertilized and remained separate from the normal zygote, it might form a small embryo, but it is doubtful that it would survive.

4. Yes, it is; but this phenomenon is extremely rare. The term *superfecundation* designates the fertilization by separate acts of coitus of two or more ova that were ovulated at approximately the same time. In lower mammals that are characterized by multiple births and promiscuity (e.g., cats and dogs), superfecundity is common. In such cases, litter mates are quite different and have characteristics of the different fathers. The possibility of this process occurring in humans cannot be discounted because evidence exists, from dizygotic (nonidentical) twins belonging to different blood groups, that cannot be accounted for in any other way.

5. Not too many. *Conception* means to become pregnant. *Fertilization* occurs when a sperm fuses with an ovum; and, when this occurs, conception takes place. *Impregnation* means to make pregnant (a male impregnates a female).

6. Essentially, yes. *Mitosis* is the usual process of cell reproduction that results in the formation of daughter cells. *Cleavage* is the series of mitotic cell divisions occurring in the zygote immediately following its formation. This process results in the formation of daughter cells called blastomeres. The expressions "cleavage division" and "mitotic division" mean the same when referring to the dividing zygote; hence, cleavage refers to the repeated mitotic divisions of the zygote.

7. The nutritional requirements of the dividing zygote are not great. The blastomeres are nourished partly by the sparse yolk granules in these cells, but the nutrients mainly come from the secretions of the uterine tubes and later from those of the uterine glands.

8. Yes. One of the blastomeres could be removed, and the Y chromosome could be identified by staining the cell with quinacrine mustard (see Fig. 7–12C). Blastomeres of a female embryo would lack a fluorescent body (Y chromosome). This technique could be available to couples with a family history of sex-linked genetic diseases (e.g., hemophilia or muscular dystrophy) or to women who have already given birth to a child with such a disease and are reluctant to have more children. In these cases, only female embryos developing in vitro would be transferred to the uterus.

Chapter 4

1. "Implantation bleeding" refers to the loss of small amounts of blood from the implantation site of blastocyst that may occur at the expected time of menstruation. Persons unfamiliar with this possible occurrence may interpret the bleeding as light menstrual flow. In such cases, they would give the wrong date for their last menstrual period (LMP). This blood is not menstrual fluid; it is blood from the primitive intervillous space of the developing placenta.

2. Drugs or other agents do not cause congenital anomalies if taken during the first two weeks of development. A teratogenic drug either damages all the embryonic cells, killing the embryo, or it injures only a few cells and the embryo recovers to develop normally. Despite this, it is unwise to give known teratogenic drugs to a female during her reproductive years. If she has a malignant tumor and needs chemotherapy, contraceptive techniques would be used because many chemotherapeutic drugs are teratogenic (see Chapter 9).

3. The term "interception" is sometimes used in reference to *postcoital contraception*. Interceptive pills (e.g., composed of ethinyl estradiol and norgestrel) may be given after a sexual assault to prevent the sperms from fertilizing an ovum (if present). The risk of pregnancy from unprotected midcycle intercourse is up to 30 per cent.

4. The insertion of an *intrauterine device* (e.g., a coil) usually prevents implantation of a blastocyst in the uterus, but it does not prevent sperms from entering the uterine tubes and fertilizing an oocyte if one is present. As the endometrium is hostile to implantation, a blastocyst could develop and implant in the uterine tube (i.e., an ectopic tubal pregnancy; see p. 39).

5. Abdominal pregnancies are very uncommon. Although the pregnancy can result from a primary implantation of a blastocyst in the abdomen, most of them are believed to result from the implantation of a blastocyst that spontaneously aborted from the uterine tube. The risk of severe maternal bleeding and fetal mortality is high in cases of abdominal pregnancy; but, if the diagnosis is made late in pregnancy and the patient (mother) is free of symptoms, the pregnancy may be allowed to continue until the viability of the fetus is ensured (e.g., 32 weeks). It would then be delivered by *cesarean section.*

Chapter 5

1. Yes, if they become pregnant soon after they stop taking the pills. It takes at least three months for normal menstrual cycles to occur. If pregnancy occurs before this time, spontaneous abortions often occur a week or so after the first missed menstrual period. Most of the embryos have been found to have severe chromosomal abnormalities. For this reason, most physicians recommend that other contraceptive techniques be used for two to three months after cessation of birth control pills in order to allow normal menstrual cycles to occur.

2. Yes. Traditionally, the fourth to eighth weeks were considered to constitute the embryonic period, but the third week is now included because important stages of development occur during the third week (e.g., early development of the nervous and cardiovascular systems).

3. "Menstrual extraction" refers to suction or vacuum curettage of the uterus in the first few weeks after a missed menstrual period. It is the most widely used method of early abortion in North America. The conceptus is evacuated utilizing an electrically powered vacuum source.

4. Yes, certain ones can produce congenital anomalies. Antineoplastic agents (antitumor drugs) can produce severe skeletal and neural tube defects in the embryo (e.g., meroanencephaly or partial absence of the brain; see p. 296) if administered during the third week; hence, the brain and skeletal system are most susceptible to disturbance in the third week.

5. Yes, to the mother and her embryo. Increased maternal age is a predisposing factor to

certain medical conditions (e.g., kidney disorders and hypertension). *Toxemia*, for example, occurs more frequently in older pregnant women than in younger ones. Advanced maternal age also produces a significantly increased risk to the embryo/fetus. Most common are birth defects associated with chromosomal abnormalities (e.g., the Down syndrome; see Chapter 9); however, women over 40 often have normal children.

Chapter 6

1. Until the fifth week human embryos resemble the embryos of several other species because of common characteristics (e.g., large head, branchial or pharyngeal arches, and tail); but thereafter, embryos acquire characteristics that are distinctly human (e.g., loss of the tail and the human appearance of the face and limbs, Fig. 6–17). The distinctive feature of early human embryos is the large prominence formed by the heart (Fig. 6–7).

2. Embryos early in the eighth week look different from nine-week-old fetuses because of their webbed toes and stubby tails; but, by the end of the eighth week, embryos and young fetuses appear similar. The name change is made to indicate that a new phase of development (rapid growth and differentiation) has begun.

3. This common question is a difficult one to answer because views are affected by religion and one's peers. The scientific answer is that the embryo has human potential, and no other, from the time of fertilization due to its human chromosome constitution. Three things are definite: (1) human development begins at fertilization, (2) the zygote and early embryo are living organisms, and (3) the embryo acquires distinctive human characteristics during the eighth week.

4. No. During the embryonic period there are more similarities than differences in the external genitalia (see Fig. 14–13). It would be impossible to know whether the primitive sexual organ (genital tubercle at five weeks and phallus at seven weeks) will become a penis or a clitoris. Sexual differences are not clear until the tenth to twelfth weeks. Sex chromatin patterns and chromosome analysis of embryonic cells obtained during amniocentesis can reveal the chromosomal sex of the embryo (see Chapter 7).

5. *Primigravida* is a woman who is pregnant for the first time (L. *primus*, first, + *gravida*, pregnant woman). *Primipara* is a woman who has given birth for the first time to an infant or infants, alive or dead, weighing 500 gm or more, or having a gestation of 20 weeks or more; hence, a mother who had previously had a spontaneous abortion at six weeks would be referred to as a *multigravida* because she has been pregnant more than once. "Primip" is an abbreviation for the term *primipara*, a woman who has given birth to her first child.

Chapter 7

1. It has been reported that mature embryos (eight weeks) and young fetuses (nine weeks) show spontaneous movements, such as twitching of the trunk and limbs. Although the fetus begins to move by the twelfth week, the mother cannot usually feel her baby move until the seventeenth to twentieth weeks. Women who have borne several children usually detect this movement, called *quickening*, sooner than women who are pregnant for the first time because they know what fetal movement feels like.

2. Many pregnant women experience *nausea*, and some of them vomit a little every day ("morning sickness"). Although the urge to vomit usually occurs in the morning, it may occur anytime. Usually eating dry crackers and restricting water intake during meals dispels the nauseated feeling. Some women require medication to relieve the symptoms.

3. No. Although the fetus is competing with the mother for the nutrients and calcium in her blood, the fetus cannot take calcium from the mother's teeth and produce caries (cavities). The fetus needs calcium for its growing skeleton; therefore, the mother's intake of calcium should be sufficient for her and the fetus.

4. At present it is too early to state that periconceptional vitamin supplementation is effective in reducing the incidence of NTDs (e.g., spina bifida), but preliminary studies are encouraging. They have shown that the risk of a mother having a child with a NTD is significantly lowered when vitamin supplementation is received. There is, however, no consensus that vitamins are helpful in preventing these defects in most at-risk pregnancies.

5. There is no risk of damaging the fetus during amniocentesis when ultrasonography is used to locate the position of the fetus; hence, the needle will not injure it. There is a slight risk of inducing an abortion (about 0.5 per cent). Maternal or fetal infection is an unlikely complication when the procedure is performed by a

trained person using modern techniques (e.g., ultrasound).

Chapter 8

1. A stillbirth is the birth of a dead fetus (i.e., stillborn) that weighs at least 500 gm and is at least 20 weeks old. A stillborn (fetus) shows no evidence of life (e.g., breathing or heartbeat). Stillborn infants occur about three times more frequently among mothers over the age of 40 than in women in their 20s. It is true that more male fetuses are stillborn than females. The reason for this is unknown.

2. Sometimes the umbilical cord is abnormally long and wraps around the fetus' neck or a limb. This "cord accident" obstructs blood flow to and from the placenta. As a result, the fetus does not receive sufficient oxygen and nutrients and soon dies. A true knot in the umbilical cord, formed when the fetus passes through a loop in it, also obstructs blood flow through the cord. *Prolapse of the umbilical cord* may also be referred to as a "cord accident." This occurs when the cord prolapses into the cervix at the level of a presenting part (often the head). This creates pressure on the cord and prevents the fetus from receiving adequate oxygen. This may cause fetal death or brain damage. Entanglement of the cord around the fetus can also cause congenital defects (e.g., absence of a forearm).

3. Most "over-the-counter" pregnancy tests are based on the presence of a hormone called hCG (human chorionic gonadotropin). These tests are capable of detecting the relatively large amounts of hCG that are in the woman's blood or urine. Such tests are positive a short time (a week or so) after the first missed period. This hormone is produced by the syncytiotrophoblast of the chorion. These tests usually give an accurate diagnosis of pregnancy, but a doctor should be consulted as soon as possible because some tumors *(choriocarcinomas)* also produce this hormone.

4. The "bag of waters" is a layperson's term for the amniotic sac that is filled with amniotic fluid (largely composed of water). Sometimes this sac ruptures before labor, allowing the fluid to escape. *Premature rupture of the amnion is the most common event leading to premature labor (birth).* The premature rupture of the membranes may complicate the birth process *(wrongly called a dry birth)*. Sometimes sterile saline is infused into the uterus by way of a catheter to alleviate fetal distress, a technique

known as amnioinfusion. Premature rupture of the membranes may also allow a vaginal infection to spread to the fetus. Prolapse of the cord also occurs most commonly following premature rupture of the membranes (amniotic and chorionic sacs).

5. The term "fetal distress" is synonymous with *fetal hypoxia* (a decrease below normal levels of oxygen in the fetal blood). Fetal distress exists when the fetal heart rate falls below 100 beats per minute. *Pressure on the umbilical cord* causes fetal distress in about one in 200 deliveries due to impairment of blood supply to the fetus. In these cases, the fetus compresses the umbilical cord as it passes through the cervix and vagina. Often the reason for fetal distress is unknown.

6. Yes, this statement is true for dizygotic (fraternal) twins but not for monozygotic (identical) twins. Dizygotic (DZ) twinning is an autosomal-recessive trait that is carried by the daughters of mothers of twins; hence, *DZ twinning is hereditary* or, as laypeople say, "it runs in the family." Monozygotic (MZ) twinning, on the other hand, is a random occurrence that is not genetically controlled.

7. Yes. The human immunodeficiency virus (HIV) can cross the placental membrane from the mother's blood and enter the fetus' blood. The HIV-infected fetus may develop AIDS two to ten years after birth.

Chapter 9

1. There is no evidence that the occasional use of aspirin *in the recommended therapeutic dosages* is harmful during pregnancy; however, large doses at subtoxic levels (e.g., for rheumatoid arthritis) have not been proved to be harmless to the embryo and fetus. Hence, women who take a couple of aspirin for an occasional headache need not worry about affecting their embryo/fetus.

2. A woman who is addicted to a habit-forming drug (e.g., heroin) and uses the drug during pregnancy is almost certain to give birth to a child who shows signs of drug addiction. The fetus' chances of survival until birth, however, are not good; the mortality and premature birth rates are high among fetuses of drug-addicted mothers.

3. All drugs prescribed in North America are tested for teratogenicity before they are marketed. The thalidomide tragedy, however, clearly demonstrated the need for improved

methods for detecting potential human teratogens. Thalidomide was not teratogenic in pregnant mice and rats, but it was a potent teratogen in humans during the fourth to sixth weeks of pregnancy. Because it would be unethical to test the effects of drugs on embryos who are to be aborted, there is no way of preventing some human teratogens from being marketed. Human teratological evaluation depends on retrospective epidemiological studies and the reports of astute physicians. This is the way thalidomide teratogenicity was detected. Most new drugs contain a disclaimer in the accompanying package insert, such as, "This drug has not been proven safe for pregnant women." Some drugs may be used if, in the opinion of the physician, the potential benefits outweigh the possible hazards. All teratogenic drugs that are likely to be taken by a pregnant woman are available only through prescription by a physician.

4. Cigarette smoking during pregnancy is clearly harmful to the embryo and fetus; therefore, abstinence from smoking during the embryo's critical period of development (third to eighth weeks) will not prevent its most adverse effect, *intrauterine growth retardation.* Women who stop smoking during the first half of pregnancy have infants with birth weights closer to those of nonsmokers. Decreased placental blood flow, thought to be a nicotine-mediated effect, is believed to cause decreased intrauterine blood flow. There is no conclusive evidence that maternal smoking causes congenital anomalies in infants. The growth of the fetus of a woman who smokes but does not inhale is still endangered because nicotine, carbon monoxide, and other harmful substances are absorbed into the bloodstream through the mucous membranes of the mouth and throat, as well as through the lungs. Hence, refraining from inhalation of the smoke is safer, but smoking in any manner during pregnancy is not advisable.

5. There is ample evidence to indicate that most drugs do not cause congenital anomalies in human embryos; however, a pregnant woman should not take any drugs that are not essential for her health. This should be determined by her physician. A pregnant woman with a severe lower respiratory infection, for example, would be unwise to refuse drugs recommended by her doctor (e.g., antibiotics) to cure her illness; otherwise, her health and that of her embryo or fetus could be endangered. Most drugs, including sulfonamides, meclizine, penicillin, antihistamines, and bendectin, are considered safe. Similarly, local anesthetic agents, dead vaccines, and salicylates (e.g., aspirin) in low doses are not known to cause congenital anomalies.

Chapter 10

1. Yes. When a baby is born with a congenital diaphragmatic hernia (CDH), its liver may be in its chest; however, this is uncommon. Usually, the abnormally placed viscera are hollow ones (e.g., the stomach and intestine). The viscera enter the chest through a developmental defect in the diaphragm, usually on the left side (Figs. 10–8 and 10–9).

2. Yes. A baby born with CDH may survive, but the mortality rate is high (about 75 per cent). Treatment must be given immediately. A feeding tube is inserted into the stomach; and, with continuous suction, the air and gastric contents are aspirated. The displaced viscera are then replaced into the abdominal cavity, and the defect in the diaphragm is surgically repaired. Infants with large diaphragmatic hernias, operated on within 24 hours after birth, have survival rates of 40 to 70 per cent. CDH can be repaired before birth, but this intervention carries considerable risk to the fetus and the mother.

3. It depends upon the degree of herniation of the abdominal viscera. With a moderate degree of herniation, the lungs may be mature but small. With a severe degree of herniation, lung development is reduced, but the lungs often develop following surgery. The mortality rate is high, however (about 76 per cent). Most babies with CDH die, not because there is a defect in the diaphragm or viscera in the chest, but because the lung is hypoplastic due to compression during its development.

4. Yes, it is possible to have a small CDH and not be aware of it. Some small diaphragmatic hernias remain completely asymptomatic into adulthood and are discovered only during a routine radiographic examination of the chest. His lung on the affected side probably developed normally because there would be little or no pressure on his lungs during development.

Chapter 11

1. "Harelip" is the old, incorrect term for cleft lip that many laypersons still use. It was given this name because the hare (a mammal like a large rabbit) has a divided upper lip. It is not an accurate comparison, however, because

the cleft in the hare's lip is a median one. Median cleft of the upper lip is very uncommon in humans.

2. No, both statements are inaccurate. All embryos have grooves in their upper lips where the maxillary prominences meet the merged medial nasal prominences (Fig. 11–18A and B), but normal embryos do not have cleft lips. When lip development is abnormal, the tissue in the floor of the lip groove breaks down, and a cleft lip forms (Fig. 11–18E to H). This anomaly usually results from a combination of genetic and environmental factors.

3. The risk in your case is the same as for the general population; that is, one per 1000.

4. Although environmental factors may be involved, it is reasonable to assume that your son's cleft lip and cleft palate were hereditary and recessive in their expression. This would mean that your husband also carried a concealed gene for cleft lip and that his family was equally responsible for your son's anomalies.

5. Minor anomalies of the auricle of the external ear are common, and usually they are of no serious medical or cosmetic consequence. About 14 per cent of newborn infants have minor morphological abnormalities, and less than one per cent of them have other defects. The child's abnormal ears could be considered branchial anomalies because the external ears develop from six small swellings of the first two pairs of branchial or pharyngeal arches (see Fig. 18–8); however, such minor abnormalities of ear shape would not normally be classified in this way.

Chapter 12

1. The fetus cannot breathe before birth because the airways and primitive alveoli are distended with liquid. The fetal lungs do not function as organs of gas exchange, but breathing movements are practiced by the fetus. Rapid, irregular, respiratory movements occur during the terminal stages of pregnancy. The lungs must develop in such a way that they can assume their breathing role as soon as the baby is born. There is a rapid replacement of the intra-alveolar fluid by air.

2. The stimuli that initiate breathing at birth are multiple. "Slapping the buttocks" used to be a common physical stimulus, but this is usually unnecessary. Under normal circumstances, the infant's breathing begins so promptly which suggests that it is a reflex response to the sensory stimuli of exposure to air and touching. The changes in blood gases after interruption of the placental circulation are important, e.g., the fall in oxygen tension and pH and the rise in pCO_2.

3. *Hyaline membrane disease* (HMD), a common cause of the *respiratory distress syndrome* (RDS), occurs after the onset of breathing in infants with lung immaturity and a *deficiency of pulmonary surfactant*. The incidence of RDS is about one per cent of all live births and is the leading cause of death in newborn infants. It occurs mainly in infants who are born prematurely. HMD is caused by environmental factors (primary surfactant deficiency).

4. A 22-week-old fetus is viable and, if born prematurely and given special care in a neonatal intensive care unit, may survive. Chances of survival, however, are poor for infants who weigh less than 600 gm because the lungs are immature and incapable of adequate alveolar-capillary gas exchange. Furthermore, the fetus' brain is not differentiated sufficiently to allow for regular respiration.

Chapter 13

1. Undoubtedly, the baby had a condition known as *congenital hypertrophic pyloric stenosis.* This is a diffuse hypertrophy (enlargement) and hyperplasia of the smooth muscle in the pyloric part of the stomach. This produces a hard mass, sometimes called a "tumor;" however, it is not a true tumor. It is a benign enlargement and is definitely not a malignant tumor. The muscular enlargement causes the exit canal to be narrow, which allows it to become easily obstructed. In response to the outflow obstruction and vigorous peristalsis, the vomiting is projectile, as in the case of your sister's baby. Surgical relief of the pyloric obstruction is the usual treatment. The cause of pyloric stenosis is not known, but is thought to have a *multifactorial inheritance* (see Chapter 9, p. 139), i.e., genetic and environmental factors are probably involved.

2. It is true that infants with Down syndrome have an increased incidence of *duodenal atresia.* They are also more likely to have an *imperforate anus* and other congenital defects (e.g., of the cardiovascular system, such as *atrial septal defect*; see Chapter 15). These anomalies are likely caused by the abnormal chromosome constitution of the infants (i.e., three instead of two

chromosomes 21). The atresia can be corrected by bypassing the obstruction through an operation that is called a *duodenoduodenostomy.* Often there are other anomalies of the digestive tract, such as *anular pancreas,* in which the pancreas surrounds and usually obstructs the duodenum.

3. In very uncommon cases when the intestines return to the abdomen, they rotate in a clockwise direction rather than in the usual counterclockwise manner. As a result, the cecum and appendix are located on the left side. This is called *situs inversus abdominis.* Left-sided cecum and appendix could also result from a condition known as *mobile cecum.* If the cecum does not become fixed to the posterior abdominal wall, it is freely movable and the cecum and appendix could migrate to the left side.

4. Undoubtedly, the nurse's friend had an *ileal (Meckel) diverticulum,* a fingerlike outpouching of the ileum (see Fig. 13–9). This common anomaly is sometimes referred to as a "second appendix," which is a misnomer. An ileal diverticulum produces symptoms that are similar to those produced by appendicitis. It is also possible that the person had a *duplication of the cecum,* which would result in two appendices.

5. Hirschsprung's disease, also known as *congenital megacolon* (Gr. *megas,* big), is the most common cause of obstruction of the colon in newborn infants. The cause of the condition is thought to be *failure of migration of neural crest cells* into the wall of the intestine (see Fig. 17–8). As these cells form neurons, there is a deficiency of the nerve cells that innervate the muscles in the wall of the bowel. When the wall collapses, obstruction occurs and constipation results. In newborn infants, signs may be noted early, e.g., failure to pass *meconium* (fetal feces).

6. No, she was not. If the baby had an *umbilic-ileal fistula* (Fig. 13–9C), the abnormal canal connecting the ileum and the umbilicus could permit the passage of feces from the umbilicus. This occurrence would be an important diagnostic clue to the presence of such a fistula. Urine could also drip from the umbilicus if the urachus (Fig. 8–16) was patent (i.e., a *urachal fistula was present*).

Chapter 14

1. Most people with a horseshoe kidney have no urinary problems. Most of these abnormal kidneys are discovered at autopsy or in the dissecting room. Nothing needs to be done with this abnormal kidney unless infection of the urinary tract occurs that cannot be controlled. In some of these cases the urologist may divide the kidney into two parts and fix them in positions that do not result in urinary stagnation.

2. His developing kidneys probably fused during the sixth to eighth weeks as they "migrated" from the pelvis (Fig. 14–5). The fused kidneys then ascended toward the normal position on one side or the other. There are usually no problems associated with fused kidneys, but surgeons have to be conscious of the possibility of this condition and recognize it for what it is. Removal of fused kidneys would be a catastrophic error because they represent the only kidneys the person has.

3. Some true hermaphrodites have married, but most of them do not. These people have both ovarian and testicular tissue. Although spermatogenesis is uncommon, ovulation is not. Pregnancy and childbirth have been observed in a few patients with an **XX** sex chromosome complex.

4. By 72 hours after birth a definite gender assignment can be made in most cases. The parents are told that their infant's genital development is incomplete and that tests are needed to determine whether the baby is a boy or a girl. They are usually advised against announcing their infant's birth to their friends until the sex has been assigned. The buccal smear test for the identification of sex chromatin is done as soon as possible. Chromatin-positive cells (those with sex chromatin) almost always indicate a female. Chromatin-negative cells usually indicate a male, but study of the baby's chromosomes may be required before sex can be assigned. Hormone studies may also be required.

5. Virilization or masculinization of the female fetus resulting from congenital adrenal hyperplasia is the most common cause of ambiguous external genitalia resulting in intersexuality. Sometimes the androgens enter the fetal circulation following maternal ingestion of androgenic hormones. In unusual cases the hormones are produced by a tumor on the mother's suprarenal gland. Partial or complete fusion of the urogenital folds or labioscrotal swellings is the result of exposure to androgens prior to the twelfth week of development. Clitoral enlargement will occur after this, but androgens will not cause sexual ambiguity because the other external genitalia are fully formed by this time.

Chapter 15

1. Heart murmurs are sounds transmitted to the thoracic wall that result from turbulence of the blood within the heart or great arteries. Loud murmurs often represent narrowing or *stenosis of one of the semilunar valves* (aortic or pulmonary valves). A ventricular septal defect or a patent foramen ovale may also produce a loud murmur.

2. Congenital heart defects are common. They occur in six to eight of every 1000 newborns and represent about ten per cent of all congenital anomalies. Ventricular septal defects (VSDs) are the most common type of heart anomaly. It occurs more frequently in males than females. The reason for this is unknown.

3. The cause of most congenital anomalies of the cardiovascular system is unknown. In about eight per cent of children with heart disease, there is a clear genetic basis. Most of these are associated with obvious chromosomal abnormalities (e.g., trisomy 21) and deletion of parts of chromosomes. *Down syndrome* is associated with congenital heart disease in 50 per cent of cases. The maternal ingestion of drugs, such as antimetabolites and Coumadin (an anticoagulant), has been shown to be associated with a high incidence of cardiac malformations. There is suggestive evidence that high consumption of alcohol during pregnancy may cause heart defects, but it is impossible to say whether the excessive use of alcohol by your friend caused her baby's heart disease.

4. Several viral infections have been shown to be associated with congenital cardiac defects, but only the *rubella virus* is known to cause cardiovascular disease (e.g., patent ductus arteriosus). *Measles* is a general term that is used for two different viral diseases. Rubeola (common measles) does not cause cardiovascular defects, but *rubella* (German measles) does. *Rubella virus vaccine* is available and is effective in preventing the development of rubella infection in a woman who has not had the disease and is planning to have a baby. It will subsequently prevent the rubella syndrome in her baby as well. Because of potential hazard of the vaccine to the embryo, the vaccine is given only if there is assurance that there is no likelihood of pregnancy for the next two months.

5. This condition is called transposition of the great arteries (TGA) because the position of the great vessels (aorta and pulmonary arteries) is reversed. Survival after birth depends on mixing between the pulmonary and systemic circulations (e.g., via an ASD or patent foramen ovale). TGA occurs in slightly more than one per 5000 live births and is more common in male infants (almost 2:1). Most infants with this severe cardiac anomaly die during the first months of life, but corrective surgery can be done in those who survive for several months. Initially, an ASD may be created to increase mixing between the systemic and pulmonary circulations. Later an arterial switch operation (reversing the aorta and pulmonary artery) can be performed; but, more commonly, a baffle is inserted in the atrium to divert systemic venous blood through the mitral valve, left ventricle, and pulmonary artery to the lungs, and pulmonary venous blood through the tricuspid valve and right ventricle to the aorta. This physiologically corrects the circulation.

6. Very likely the one twin has a condition known as *dextrocardia.* Usually this is of no clinical significance. In some cases the heart is simply displaced to the right; and in others, there is a complete transposition of the right and left chambers. In the condition represented by your friend, the heart presents a mirror picture of the normal cardiac structure. This results during the fourth week of development when the heart tube rotates to the left rather than to the right. Similar evidence of asymmetry often occurs in the direction of the hair whorl at the back of the head. It is usually clockwise, but it may be counterclockwise in one of the twins. The cause of these types of asymmetry is unknown, but the differences probably arise very early in development.

Chapter 16

1. The ingestion of drugs did not cause the child's short limbs. The infant appears to have a skeletal disorder known as *achondroplasia* (Fig. 9–11). This type of short-limbed dwarfism has an incidence of 1:10,000 and shows an autosomal dominant inheritance. About 80 per cent of these infants are born of normal parents, and presumably the condition results from fresh mutations (changes of genetic material) in the parents' germ cells. Most achondroplastic people have normal intelligence and lead normal lives within their physical capabilities. If the parents of an achondroplastic child have more children, the risk of having another child with this condition is slightly higher than the population risk;

however, the risk for the achondroplastic person's own children is 50:50.

2. Brachydactyly is also an autosomal dominant trait, i.e., it is determined by a dominant gene. If your sister (likely bb) marries the brachydactylous man (likely Bb), the risk is 50 per cent for a brachydactylous child and 50 per cent for a normal child. It would be best for her to discuss her obvious concern with a medical geneticist.

3. Bendectin, an antinauseant, does not produce limb defects in human embryos. Several epidemiological studies have failed to show an increased risk of birth defects after exposure to Bendectin or its separate ingredients during early pregnancy. In the case you describe, the mother took the drug over three weeks after the end of the critical period of limb development (24 to 36 days after fertilization). Consequently, even a known limb teratogen such as *thalidomide* could not have caused failure of the child's hand to develop if ingested during such a late period of embryonic development. Most limb reduction defects have a genetic basis.

4. Congenital absence of a muscle (e.g., the palmaris longus in the forearm or part of a pectoral muscle as in this case) is common. When unilateral absence of the sternal head of the pectoralis major muscle is associated with cutaneous syndactyly of the hand, the condition is referred to as the *Poland syndrome* or anomaly. It has an incidence of one in 20,000; there may be other associated upper limb defects (e.g., brachydactyly). It has been estimated that ten per cent of people with syndactyly also have absence of part of the pectoralis major muscle. It has also been suggested that the Poland syndrome may result from defective development of the subclavian artery, which results in an early deficit of blood flow to the pectoral region and the upper limb. The cutaneous syndactyly of the hand can be easily corrected surgically, and plastic surgery can be done on the thorax to improve the appearance of the chest; hence, the defects are not serious and they usually do not cause physical disabilities.

5. In the thoracic region the costal processes of developing vertebrae give rise to ribs; whereas, in the cervical region, they usually form part of the transverse processes of the vertebrae. In about 0.5 per cent of people, a cervical costal process develops into a *cervical rib* (rib in the neck), which is usually several inches long. The cervical rib may compress your sister's subclavian artery and brachial plexus of nerves

on the affected side (Moore, 1992). This usually causes tingling and/or pain, which begins around puberty when the neck grows. Some people never suffer neurovascular symptoms; others feel numbness and pain when they carry something heavy (e.g., a suitcase). If the symptoms are severe, the rib is usually surgically removed to relieve the pressure on the nerves and vessels of the upper limb.

6. The person has a skull anomaly known as *scaphocephaly*, which resulted from premature closure of the sagittal suture of his skull during early childhood. Normally, this suture begins to close on the internal aspect of the cranial vault or calvaria during the early twenties and fusion progresses throughout life. Scaphocephaly is not a birth injury. Although the calvaria undergoes changes of shape during birth called *molding*, the calvaria usually returns to its normal shape within a day or so. Scaphocephaly does not cause compression of the brain or cranial nerves, and it is usually not associated with complications requiring therapy.

Chapter 17

1. Neural tube defects such as meroanencephaly (anencephaly) and spina bifida cystica have a multifactorial inheritance, i.e., both genetic and environmental factors are involved. It is believed that nutritional factors may be implicated. After the birth of one child with NTD, whether meroanencephaly or spina bifida cystica, the risk of a subsequent child having a neural tube defect is divided about equally between the two defects. The recurrence risk in the United Kingdom, where NTDs are common (e.g., 7.6 per 1000 in South Wales and 8.6 per 1000 in Northern Ireland), is about one in 25. It is probably about one in 50 in North America. NTDs can be detected prenatally by a combination of ultrasound scanning (see Fig. 17–12) and measurement of alpha-fetoprotein amniotic fluid (p. 90).

2. The condition you described is called *hydranencephaly*, an extremely rare anomaly. Most of both cerebral hemispheres are reduced to membranous sacs that contain CSF (Behrman, 1992; Moore and Persaud, 1993 [pp. 299 and 300]). If you hold a light against the infant's head in a dark room, it will light up like a lantern. Absence of cerebral hemispheres can result from different developmental disturbances. The condition most likely resulted from vascular occlusion of both internal carotid arteries due to a

severe intrauterine infection. In some cases hydranencephaly appears to be a severe type of intrauterine hydrocephalus (hence, the prefix *hydra-* in the designation). These infants usually do not survive longer than two or three months.

3. Mental retardation and growth retardation are the most serious aspects of the *fetal alcohol syndrome.* Average IQ scores are 60 to 70. It has been estimated that the incidence of mental retardation resulting from heavy drinking during pregnancy may be as high as one per every 400 live births. Heavy drinkers are those who consume five or more drinks on occasion, with a consistent daily average of 45 ml absolute alcohol. At present, there is no safe threshold for alcohol consumption during pregnancy. Most obstetricians recommend complete abstinence from alcohol during pregnancy.

4. There is no conclusive evidence to indicate that maternal smoking affects the mental development of a fetus (Chapter 9, p. 132); however, maternal cigarette smoking compromises oxygen supply to the fetus because blood flow to the placenta is decreased during smoking. As it is well established that heavy maternal smoking seriously affects physical growth of the fetus and is a major cause of intrauterine growth retardation, it is not wise for mothers to smoke heavily during pregnancy. The reduced oxygen supply to the brain could affect intellectual development, even though it would probably be undetectable. Abstinence gives the fetus the best chance for normal development. Mental retardation has many causes (p. 298).

5. Most laypeople use the designation "spina bifida" in a general way. Many of them are unaware that the common type, spina bifida occulta, is usually clinically insignificant. It is an isolated finding in up to 20 per cent of radiographically examined vertebral columns. Most people are unaware that they have this vertebral defect, and most doctors would not tell them about it because it produces no symptoms unless it is associated with an NTD or an abnormality of the spinal nerve roots. The various types of *spina bifida cystica* are of clinical significance. Meningomyelocele is a more severe defect than meningocele because neural tissue is included in the lesion. Because of this, the function of abdominal and limb muscles may be affected. Meningoceles are usually covered with skin, and motor function in the limbs is usually normal unless there are associated developmental defects in the spinal cord or brain. Management of infants with spina bifida cystica is complex and involves several medical and surgical specialties. Spinal meningocele is obviously easier to correct surgically than spinal meningomyelocele, and the prognosis is also better.

Chapter 18

1. The chance of significant damage to the embryo/fetus depends primarily on the timing of the infection with the rubella virus. In cases of primary maternal infection during the first trimester of pregnancy, the overall risk of embryonic/fetal infection is about 20 per cent (Moore and Persaud, 1993). It is estimated that about 50 per cent of the pregnancies will end in spontaneous abortion, stillbirth, or congenital anomalies (deafness, cataract, glaucoma, and mental retardation). When infection occurs at the end of the first trimester, the probability of congenital anomalies is only slightly higher than for an uncomplicated pregnancy. Certain infections occurring late in the first trimester, however, may result in severe eye infections (e.g., chorioretinitis), which may affect visual development. Deafness is the most common manifestation of late fetal rubella infection (i.e., during the second and third trimesters).

If a pregnant woman is exposed to rubella, an antibody test can be performed. If determined to be immune, she can be reassured that her embryo/fetus will not be affected by the virus. Preventative measures are essential for the protection of the embryo. It is especially important that girls have immunity to rubella before they reach child-bearing age, either by contracting the disease or by active immunization (e.g., with live-virus vaccine).

2. The purposeful exposure of young girls to rubella (German measles) is not recommended by physicians. Although complications resulting from such infections are relatively uncommon, neuritis and arthritis occasionally occur (inflammation of nerves and joints, respectively). *Encephalitis* (inflammation of the brain) occurs in about one out of 6000 cases; furthermore, the rubella infection is often subclinical (difficult to detect) and yet represents a risk to pregnant women. The chance of injury to embryos is possible because the danger period is greatest when the eyes and ears are developing. This occurs early enough in pregnancy that some women would be unaware that they are pregnant. A much better way of providing immunization against rubella is use of live-virus vaccine (Behrman, 1992). This is given to children over 15

months of age and to nonpregnant postpubertal females who can be reasonably relied upon not to become pregnant within three months of immunization.

3. Congenital syphilis (fetal syphilis) results from the transplacental transmission of a microorganism called *Treponema pallidum.* The transmission from untreated pregnant women may occur throughout pregnancy but is most likely during the last trimester. Deafness and tooth deformities commonly develop in these children. These anomalies can be prevented by treating the mother during pregnancy. The microorganism that causes syphilis is very sensitive to penicillin, an antibiotic that does not harm the fetus.

4. There are several viruses in the herpes virus family that can cause blindness and deafness during infancy. *Cytomegalovirus* can cross the placenta and be transmitted to the infant during birth, or it can be passed to the baby in the breast milk. Herpes simplex viruses (usually type 2 or genital herpes) are usually transmitted just before or during birth. The chances for normal development of these infants is not good. Some of them develop microcephaly, seizures, deafness, and blindness.

5. Methylmercury has been shown to be teratogenic in human embryos, especially to the developing brain (p. 137). Because the eyes and internal ears develop as outgrowths from the brain, it is understandable how their development could also be affected. Besides the methylmercury that passes from the mother to the embryo/fetus via the placenta, the newborn infant may receive more methylmercury from the breast milk. Sources of methyl mercury have included fish from contaminated water, flour made from methylmercury-treated seed grain, and meat eaten from animals raised on such seed grain.

Chapter 19

1. Congenital absence of skin is a very uncommon anomaly. Only patches of skin (several centimeters in diameter) are absent, most often from the scalp, but there may be patches of skin missing from the trunk and limbs. The skin defects are usually in the median plane of the scalp in the parietal and occipital areas. These infants usually survive because healing of the lesions is uneventful and takes one or two months. A hairless scar persists. The cause of congenital absence of hair, called *aplasia cutis congenita,* is usually unknown. Most cases are sporadic, but there are several well-documented pedigrees demonstrating autosomal dominant transmission of the defect.

2. The white patches of skin on a dark-skinned person result from a condition called *partial albinism* (piebaldism). This defect, which also affects light-skinned persons, is a heritable disorder transmitted by an autosomal dominant gene. Ultrastructural studies show that there is an absence of melanocytes in the depigmented areas of skin. Presumably there is a genetic defect in the differentiation of melanoblasts (see Fig. 19–1). These skin and hair defects are not amenable to treatment, but they can be covered with cosmetics and hair dyes.

3. The breasts, including the mammary glands within them, of males and females are similar at birth. Breast enlargement in newborn male and female infants is a common occurrence due to stimulation by maternal hormones; hence, this is a normal occurrence in male infants and does not indicate abnormal sex development. Similar physiological pubertal gynecomastia occurs in some males during their early teens due to decreased levels of testosterone. The breast enlargement is usually transitory. *Familial gynecomastia* is an X-linked or autosomal dominant, sex-limited trait. Gynecomastia also occurs in some males with the *Klinefelter syndrome* (XXY syndrome), as described in Chapter 9 and illustrated in Figure 9–7. These men are not intersexes because their external and internal genitalia are normal, except that their testes are small due to degeneration of the seminiferous tubules.

4. An extra breast (polymastia) or nipple (polythelia) is common, as described in the text. The axillary breast may enlarge during puberty or it may not be noticed until pregnancy occurs. The embryological basis of these extra breasts and nipples is the presence of mammary ridges that extend from the axillary to the inguinal regions (see Fig. 19–5A). Usually, only one pair of breasts and nipples develop, but they can develop anywhere along the mammary ridges. The extra breast or nipple is usually just superior or inferior to the normal breast (see Fig. 19–6).

5. Teeth that are present at birth are called **natal teeth** (L. *natalis,* to be born). A more appropriate designation would be *congenital teeth* (L. *congenitus,* born with). Natal teeth are erupted at birth and are observed in about one in 2000 newborn infants. There are usually two in the position of the mandibular medial (central)

incisors. This usually suggests that early eruption of other teeth will occur. Obviously natal teeth may produce maternal discomfort due to biting of the nipples during feeding. In addition, the infant's tongue may be lacerated or the teeth may detach and be aspirated into the lungs. For these reasons, natal teeth are sometimes extracted, but often they fall out on their own. Such teeth should not be considered supernumerary until they have been identified as such by x-ray examination. A natal tooth may be a prematurely erupted deciduous tooth, in which case early eruption of the other deciduous teeth may be expected.

INDEX

Note: Page numbers in *italics* refer to illustrations; page numbers followed by t refer to tables. Emphasis is given to boldface terms and page numbers.

A

Abdominal pregnancy, 39, 41
Abortion, definition of, **6**, 78
  elective, 6
  missed, 6
  spontaneous, 6, 32, 39, *43*
    of early embryos, 43
  threatened, 6
Abortus, definition of, 6
Accessory ribs, 259–260, *260*
Acetabulum, development of, abnormal, congenital hip dislocation from, 268
Achondroplasia, 128, *128*, **268**
Acoustic meatus, external, at 6 weeks, 67, *70*
  atresia of, 312
  development of, 309, *311*
  origin of, 159, *160*
Acrania, 263, *263*
  meroanencephaly associated with, 296
Acrosin, in acrosome reaction, 26
Acrosome, 17
Acrosome reaction, 26, *27*
Adenocarcinoma, of vagina from *in utero* DES (diethylstilbestrol) exposure, 134
Adenohypophysis, development of, 290, *292*, 292t, *293*
Adrenal glands, congenital hyperplasia of, 213, *222*
  development of, 212–213, *214*
Adrenal medulla. See also *Suprarenal medulla.*
  origin of, 61, *62*
Afterbirth, 94
  expulsion of, 106
Age, estimation of, in embryonic period, 69, 73
  in fetal period, 78–80
  fertilization, establishing, 69, 78
  gestational, establishing, 78
    size of chorionic sac and, 97
  maternal, autosomal trisomies and, 122, 124t

Alar plates, in spinal cord development, 275, *279*, *281*, **282**
Alcohol, as teratogen, 129t, 133
  maternal use of, fetal growth and, 88
  mental retardation from, **133**, 298
Allantois, *50*, 51
  derivatives of, 94
  fate of, 111, *111*
  importance of, 111
Alopecia, congenital, 316–317
Alpha-fetoprotein (AFP), assay of, in fetal status assessment, 90
  high levels of, in spina bifida cystica, 286
Alveolar ducts, formation of, 185
Alveolar period, in lung development, *184*, 185
Alveolus (alveoli), dental, 322
  pulmonary, formation of, *184*, 185
Amelia, 267, *267*
  causes of, 136, **268**
Ameloblasts, *321*, 322
Aminopterin, as teratogen, 129t, 135, *135*
Amnioblasts, 37
Amniocentesis, diagnostic, 89, *89*
  in spina bifida detection, 286
Amnion, *106*, 108, *110*
  formation of, 37
Amniotic band disruption complex (ABDC), 108
Amniotic band syndrome, 108
Amniotic cavity, formation of, 35, *36*, 37
Amniotic fluid, composition of, 109
  exchange of, 109
  origin of, 108–109
  significance of, 109–110
Amniotic sac, *106*, 108, *109*, *110*
  rupture of, 108
Ampulla, of uterine tube, 23
  fertilization in, 26
Anal canal, *199*, 200
Anal membrane, *199*, 200
Anaphase lagging, mosaicism from, 124
Anatomical position, 9, *10*

Androgen insensitivity syndrome, 220–221, *221*
Androgens, as teratogens, 129t, 133–134
Anencephaly, 296, *296*. See also *Meroanencephaly.*
  acrania with, 263
Aneuploidy, **120**, *121*, 122, *123*, 124, *125*
Angelman syndrome, 127
Angioblastic cords, 227
Angioblasts, 54–55
Angiogenesis, *54*, 54–55, *55*
Angiotensin-converting enzyme (ACE) inhibitors, as teratogens, 135
Ankyloglossia, 167
Anlage, definition of, 6
Annulus. See *Anulus.*
Anomaly, congenital. See *Birth defects; Congenital anomalies.*
Anorectal agenesis, 200, 201
Antibiotics, as teratogens, 129t, 134
Antibodies, placental transport of, 102
Anticoagulants, as teratogens, 134–135
Anticonvulsants, as teratogens, 135
Antineoplastic agents, as teratogens, 135
Antithyroid substances, as teratogens, 136
Antituberculosis agents, as teratogens, 134
Antrum, 20
  mastoid, development of, 309
Anular epiphyses, in ossification of vertebrae, 258, *258*
Anulus fibrosus, 256, *257*
Anus, agenesis of, 200, 201
  imperforate, *200*, 201
  membranous atresia of, *200*, 201
  stenosis of, *200*, 201
Aorta(e), arch of. See *Aortic arch(es).*
  ascending, formation of, 237, *238*
  coarctation of, 243, *245*
  in primitive circulation, *230*, 231
Aortic arch(es), 152, *153*, 154, 155, 229, *230*, **242–243**, *243*, *244*, *245*, *246*, *246*

Aortic arch(es) *(Continued)*
  anomalies of, 243, *245*, 246, *246*
  derivatives of, *242–243, 243, 244, 245*
  in branchial arches, 152, *153*, 154, *155*
  in primitive circulation, *230*, 231
  origin of, 242
Aortic sac, 229, *230*
Aortic vestibule, 237
Aorticopulmonary septum, formation of, 237, *238, 239*
Apertures, median and lateral, 288
Apical ectodermal ridge, in limb development, 264, *264*
Appendicular skeleton, 263
Appendix, subhepatic, 197
  vermiform, 193, *195*
Aqueductal stenosis, congenital, hydrocephalus from, 297
Aqueous chambers, development of, *304, 305*, 306
Arachnoid villi, in CSF absorption, 288
Areola, development of, 318–319, *319*
Arrector pili muscle, 317
Arteriocapillary-venous system, 100, *100*
Arteriocapillary-venous system, formation of, 56
Artery (**arteries**), carotid, common, origin of, 242
  internal, origin of, 242
  central, of retina, origin of, *303*, 304
  great, transposition of, 242
  hyaloid, 301, *302, 303, 304*
    in developing lens, *303, 304*, 306
  intercostal, in vertebral column development, 256
  intersegmental, in vertebral column development, 256, *257*
  pulmonary, left, origin of, 243
    right, origin of, 243
  renal, supernumerary, 208
  spiral, 37, 98, *99*, 101
  subclavian, right, origin of, 243
  superior mesenteric, 193, *195*
  umbilical, 99, 100, *101, 108*
    fate of, 249
Arthrogryposis multiplex congenita, 273
Articulation, 255. See also *Joint(s)*.
Aspirin, as possible teratogen, 136
Atresia, biliary, 193
  duodenal, 190, *192*
  esophageal, 181, *182*, 188–189
  intestinal, 197–198
  membranous, of anus, *200*, 201
  of external acoustic meatus, 312
  rectal, *200*, 201
  vaginal, 224
Atrial septal defects (**ASDs**), 237, *240*
Atrichia congenita, 316–317
Atrioventricular (AV) canal, partitioning of, 231, *232*
Atrioventricular (AV) node, development of, 237

Atrioventricular (AV) septal defects, with primum atrial septal defects, endocardial cushion and, 237, *240*
Atrium, left, adult, formation of, 232
  primitive, partitioning of, 231–232, *233–236*
  right, adult, formation of, 232, *236*
Auditory meatus, external. See *Acoustic meatus, external*.
Auditory ossicles, development of, 309, *311*
Auditory tube, development of, 308, *311*
  origin of, 159, *160*
Auricle, appendages of, 312, *312*
  development of, 232, *236*
  formation of, 311, *312*
Auricular cysts, congenital, 161, *162*
Auricular hillocks, 311, *312*
  accessory, 312
Auricular sinuses, congenital, 161, *162*
Autonomic ganglia, origin of, 298
Autosomes, trisomy of, 122, *123*, 124t
Axial skeleton, origin of, 49, 53

B

"Bag of waters." See *Amniotic sac*.
Balanced translocation carriers, 125, *126*
Basal plates, in spinal cord development, 275, *279, 281, 282–283*
Benzodiazepines, as teratogens, 137
Bifid nose, 177, *177*
Bile, formation of, in fetus, 191
Bile duct, extrahepatic, atresia of, 193
  formation of, 191, *191*
Biliary apparatus, development of, 190, 191
Biliary atresia, extrahepatic, 193
Binge drinking, fetal alcohol effects from, 133
Birth(s), premature, 6
  process of, **104**, *104, 105*, 106
  time of, 85
Birth control pills, 20
  teratogenicity of, 133–134
Birth defects, 118–140. See also *Congenital anomalies*.
Bladder. See *Gallbladder; Urinary bladder*.
Blastocyst(s), abnormal, 32
  definition of, 1
  formation of, *30*, **31**
  implantation of, 32, *35*, 39, *41*, 41–43, *42*. See also *Implantation, of blastocyst*.
Blastomeres, 1, *30*, 31
Bleeding, implantation, 45
Blood, flow of, impaired uteroplacental, fetal growth and, 88
  formation of, *54*, 54–55
  transfusion of, fetal, intrauterine, 90
  umbilical cord, sampling of, percutaneous, in fetal assessment, 91
Blood cells, primitive, formation of, 55

Blood islands, formation of, 55
Blood vessels. See also *Artery (arteries); Vein(s)*.
  formation of, *54*, 54–55, *55*
  renal, multiple, 208
Body cavities, 142–148. See also *Cavity (cavities); Intraembryonic coelom*.
Body wall(s), in vertebral column development, 256
  lateral, in development of diaphragm, *146, 147*, 148
Bone, development of, 252, *254*, 255
  formation of, endochondral, **252**, 253, *254*, 255
  intramembranous, 252, 253
  histogenesis of, 252–253
Bony labyrinth, of internal ear, formation of, 308, *310*
Bowman capsule, formation of, 206, *207*
Brachial plexus, cervical rib pressure on, 260
Brachydactyly, 268, *270*
  causes of, 271
Brain, congenital anomalies of, *295*, 295–298, *296, 297*
  damage to, from *in utero* exposure to organic mercury, 137
    from maternal alcohol abuse, **133**, *133*, 298
  development of, **286**, *287*, 288–290, *289, 290*, 291–292, *293*, 293–298, *294, 295, 296, 297*
  development of, critical period in, *130*, 131
  flexures of, 286, *287*, 288
  ventricles of, fourth, 288, *289*
    lateral, formation of, 294
    third, 289, *291*
      formation of, 293–294
  vesicles of, 286, *287*
Brain stem, development of, 288, *289*
Branch villi. See also *Chorionic villi*.
  development of, 57
Branchial apparatus, 152–178
  anomalies of, 161, *162, 163*
  remnants of, 161
Branchial arch(es), 152–159
  at four weeks, 63, *65, 68*
  cartilage component of, derivatives of, 154, *157*, 157t, 158
  cartilaginous viscerocranium from, 260
  contents of, 152, *153*, 154, *155*
  fate of, 154, *156*
  first, *153*, 154
  in skeletal muscle development, 271
  muscular component of, derivatives of, 157t, 158, *158*
  nerves of, derivatives of, 157t, 158–159
  second, *153*, 154
Branchial arch arteries, 155, 158–159. See also *Aortic arch(es)*.
Branchial cysts, 161, *162*
Branchial fistula, 161, *162*

Branchial grooves, *153, 156*, 159, *160*
Branchial membranes, *153, 155*, 159, 161
Branchial sinuses, 161, *162, 163*
Branchial vestiges, 161, *162*
Breasts, accessory, 320
　anomalies of, *319*, 319–320
　development of, 318–320, *319*
　supernumerary, *319*, 319–320
Bronchi, development of, **182**, *183*, 184–185
Bronchioles, respiratory, formation of, *184*, 185
Bronchopulmonary segments, formation of, 184
Brown fat, 84
Bulbar ridges, formation of, 232, 237, *238*
Bulbourethral glands, development of, 217, *218*
Bulboventricular loop, formation of, 231
Bulbus cordis, partitioning of, **232**, 237, *238*
Busulfan, as teratogen, 129t, 135

C

C cells. See also *Parafollicular cells*.
　origin of, 159
Caffeine, as possible teratogen, 133
Calices (calyces), renal, development of, 206, *206*
Calvaria, 260
　defective formation of, *295*, 295–296
　growth of, postnatal, 261
　molding of, 260
Canal(s), of Schlemm, abnormality in, congenital glaucoma from, 307–308
　pericardioperitoneal, 142, 143, *145, 146*
Canalicular period, in lung development, *184*, 185
Capacitation, of sperms, 26, *27*
Carbon dioxide, placental transport of, 102
Cardiac jelly, 231
Cardiac muscles, development of, 272
Cardiac skeleton, formation of, 237
Cardinal veins, common, 143, *146*, 229, *229*
　in primitive circulation, *230*, 231
Cardiogenic area, 227, *227*
Cardiogenic mesoderm, formation of, 53
Cardiovascular system. See also specific structures, e.g., *Heart; Vein(s).*
　development of, **227–250**
　primitive, development of, *54*, 54–55, *55*
Carotid arteries, common, origin of, 242
　internal, origin of, 242
Cartilage(s), branchial arch, derivatives of, 154, *157*

Cartilage(s) *(Continued)*
　development of, 252, *254*, 255
　histogenesis of, 252
　laryngeal, origin of, *157*, 157t, 158, 181
　Meckel's, derivatives of, 154, *157*, 157t, 158, **260**
　Reichert's, derivatives of, *157*, 157t, 158, **260**
Cartilaginous joints, 255, *256*
Cartilaginous neurocranium, 260, *261*
Cartilaginous rod, in branchial arch, *153*, 154, *155*
Cartilaginous viscerocranium, 260, *261*
Cataract, congenital, 307
　in congenital rubella syndrome, 137
Cauda equina, 283, *283*
Caudate nuclei, 294
Cavity (cavities), embryonic body, 142–148
　division of, 143, *145, 146, 147*, 148
　pericardial, 142, *144, 146*
　peritoneal, 142–143, *144, 145*
　pleural, 142
Cecal diverticulum, 193, *195*
Cecum, 193, *195*
　mobile, 197
　subhepatic, 197, *197*
Cell(s), chromaffin, origin of, 298
　cultures of, in fetal status assessment, 90
　hemopoietic (hematopoietic), in intracartilaginous ossification, 255
　Kupffer, of liver, 190
　microglial, in spinal cord development, 275, *280*
　Schwann, 284
　Sertoli, *215*, 216
Cell theory, 8
Cell(s). See also specific cell, e.g. *Osteoblasts.*
Cementoblasts, 322
Cementum, production of, 322
Central canal, origin of, *287*, 288
Central nervous system (CNS). See also *Brain; Spinal cord.*
　origin of, 49, 51, **275**
Centrum, in vertebral column development, 256, *258*
Cerebellum, development of, 288, *289*
　origin of, *287*, 288
Cerebral aqueduct, formation of, 288, *289, 290*
Cerebral cortex, abnormal histogenesis of, mental retardation from, 295
　development of, 294–295
Cerebral hemispheres, origin of, 289, *290, 291*, 293
Cerebral peduncles, formation of, 289, *290*
Cerebral vesicles, formation of, 289, *290*
Cerebrospinal fluid (CSF), 288
　excess, in hydrocephalus, *297*, 297–298
Cervical flexure, 286, *287*, 288

Cervical ribs, 260, *260*
Cervical sinus, formation of, 64, *70*, 154
Cervix, implantation of blastocyst in, 39, *41*
Chemicals, as teratogens, 129t, 137
Chickenpox virus, as teratogen, 138
Childbirth, **104**, *104, 105*, 106
Choanae, primitive, 169
Chondrification, of vertebrae, 256, *258*
Chondroblasts, in cartilage formation, 252
Chondrocranium, 260, *261*
Chondroid tissue, in intracartilaginous ossification, 255
Chordee, 222, *223*
Chordoma, origin of, 256
Chorion, 39, *41*, 94
　smooth, 95, *96, 97*
　villous, 95, 96, 97, *97*
Chorion frondosum, 96
Chorion laeve, 96
Chorionic cavity, 39, *41*
Chorionic plate, 97, *98, 99*, 101
Chorionic sac, development of, 39, *40, 41*
　size of, in gestational age determination, 97
Chorionic villi, degeneration of, 96
　development of, 55–57, *56*
　primary, formation of, 39
　sampling of, in fetal assessment, *89*, 89–90
　secondary, development of, 55–56, *56*
　stem, 97–98, *99*
　　fibrinoid material on surfaces of, 100, *100*
Chorionic villus sampling (CVS), in fetal assessment, *89*, 89–90
Choroid, development of, *304, 305*, 306
Choroid plexuses, 288, *289*
　development of, 288
Chromaffin cells, origin of, 298
Chromatophores, eye color and, 306
Chromosome(s), abnormalities of, in spontaneous abortions, 43
　numerical, 18, **119–125**, *121, 122, 123*, 124t, *125*
　structural, **125**, *126, 127*, 127–128, *128*
　crossing over of, 29
　deletion of, 125, *126*, 127
　diploid number of, restoration of, 29
　duplication of, *126*, 127
　early research on, 8
　inversion of, *126*, 127
　microdeletions of, 125, 127
　nondisjunction of. See also *Nondisjunction of chromosomes.*
　sex. See *Sex chromosomes.*
　translocation of, 125, *126*
　Y, in sex determination, 213
Cigarette smoking, fetal growth and, 88
　teratogenicity of, 132–133
Ciliary body, development of, *304*, 305

Ciliary processes, formation of, 306
Circulation, fetal, 246, *247*, 249
  placental, 98–99, *100*, *101*
    fetal, *99*, 100, *100*, *107*, *108*
    maternal, *99*, 100–101
    postnatal, *248*, 249
    primitive, *230*, 231
  uteroplacental, impaired, fetal growth
    and, 88
    primitive, 37
Cleavage, definition of, 1
Cleft(s), facial, 176–177, *177*
Cleft foot, 268, *269*
Cleft hand, 268, *269*
Cleft lip, 173, *173*, *174*, *175*, 176, *176*,
    177
  bilateral, 173, *173*, 176
  causes of, *173*, *174*, 176
  median, 176, *177*
  unilateral, *173*, *174*
Cleft palate, *175*, 176, *176*
  causes of, *175*, 176
Clitoris, development of, *219*, 220
Cloaca, 199, *199*
  partitioning of, *199*, 200–201
Cloacal membrane, *48*, 49, *50*, *60*, 61,
    199, *199*
Cloacal sphincter, 200–201
Clubfoot, 139
  congenital, 268, *271*
Coarctation of aorta, 243, *245*
Cocaine, as teratogen, 129t, 137
Cochlea, formation of, 308, *310*
Cochlear duct, development of, 308,
    310
Coelom, extraembryonic, formation of,
    36, 37, *37*, *39*, *40*
  intraembryonic, development of, *52*,
    53, 142
Colliculi, formation of, 288, *290*
Collodion baby, 316
Coloboma, of eyelid, 307, *307*
  of iris, 307, *307*
  of retina, 307
Compaction, of blastomeres, *30*, 31
Conal growth hypothesis, 242
Conceptus, definition of, 6
Conchae, nasal, 169, *172*
Conducting system, of heart, abnormali-
    ties of, 237
  development of, 237
Cones, in neural retina, 304
Congenital adrenal hyperplasia (CAH),
    213, *222*
  female pseudohermaphroditism from,
    221, *222*
Congenital anomalies, causes of, **118**,
    118t, 129t
  chromosome abnormalities as, nu-
    merical, 119–125, *121*, *122*,
    123, 124t, *125*
    structural, 125, *126*, *127*, 127–
    128, *128*
  environmental factors as, 128,
    129t, *130*, **131–139**. See also
    Teratogen(s).
  genetic factors as, 119–128

Congenital anomalies *(Continued)*
  mutant genes as, 128, *128*
  from abnormal neurulation, 51
  from multifactorial inheritance, 139–
    140
  incidence of, 118t, 118–119
  of anus, 200, *201*
  of aortic arches, 243, *245*, 246, *246*
  of brain, 295, **295–298**, *296*, *297*
  of branchial apparatus, 161, *162*, *163*
  of ear, 311–312, *312*
  of eye, 307, 307–308, *308*
  of heart, 237, 239, *240–241*, 242,
    242
  of kidney, 208, *209*, 210, *210*
  of limbs, 267, **267–268**, *269–271*, 271
  of liver, 191, 193
  of mammary glands, *319*, 319–320
  of midgut, *196*, 196–198, *197*, *198*
  of muscles, 272–273
  of ribs, 259–260, *260*
  of skull, 263, *263*, *264*
  of spinal cord, *284*, **284–286**, *285*,
    286
  of teeth, 322, *323*, 324
  of thyroid gland, 165, *165*
  of tongue, *165*, 167
  of ureters, 208, *209*, 210, *210*
  of uterus, 224, *224*
  of vagina, 224, *224*
  of vertebrae, 258–259, *260*, *263*
Congenital aqueductal stenosis, hydro-
    cephalus from, 297
Congenital diaphragmatic hernia
    (CDH), *149*, 149–150, *150*
Congenital hypertrophic pyloric steno-
    sis, 190
Congenital rubella syndrome (CRS),
    137
Conjoined twins, *114*, 115
Conjunctiva, 307
Conjunctival sac, 307
Connecting stalk, 39, *40*, *60*, 61
Contiguous gene syndromes, 127
Contraceptives, oral, 20
  teratogenicity of, 133–134
Contractions, uterine, in labor, 104
Conus arteriosus, 237
Conus medullaris, 283, *283*
Copula, *166*, 167
Cordocentesis, in fetal status assess-
    ment, 91
Cornea, development of, *304*, *305*, 306
Cornu, greater, origin of, *157*, 157t,
    158
  lesser, origin of, *157*, 157t, 158
Corona radiata, *15*, 18, 20, *21*
Coronary sinus, formation of, 232, *236*
Corpus luteum, *19*, 20, *21*
Corpus striatum, development of, 294
Cortex, of cerebrum, 294–295
  of indifferent gonad, 213, *214*
  suprarenal, congenital hyperplasia of,
    213, *222*
  development of, 212–213
Cortical cords, *215*, 216
Corticosteroids, as teratogens, 135

Costal processes, in rib development,
    258, 259
Costodiaphragmatic recesses, 148, *148*
Costovertebral joints, in rib develop-
    ment, *258*, 259
Cotyledons, of placenta, 97, 98, *107*
Craniofacial dysmorphism, from *in utero*
    exposure to isotretinoin, 136
Craniosynostosis, 263, *264*
Cranium bifidum, 295, 295–296
Cri du chat syndrome, 125, *127*
Critical periods of development, *130*,
    131–132
Crown-heel length (CHL), in embry-
    onic measurement, 73, 75
Crown-rump length (CRL), in embry-
    onic measurement, 73, 75
  in fetal age estimation, 79–80
Cultures, cell, in fetal assessment, 90
Cumulus oophorus, 20
Cuneate nucleus, origin of, *287*, 288
Cutaneous nerve area, 266
Cyst(s), auricular, congenital, 161, *162*
  branchial, 161, *162*
  lingual, congenital, *165*, 167
  thyroglossal duct, 165, *165*
Cystic duct, formation of, 191, *191*
Cytogenetics, molecular, 127
Cytomegalovirus (CMV), as teratogen,
    129t, 137–138
Cytotrophoblast, 35
  formation of, 32
Cytotrophoblastic shell, 97, *99*
  formation of, *56*, 57

D

Deafness, congenital, 311–312
  from antituberculosis agents, 134
  in congenital rubella syndrome, 137
Decidua, 94, *95*
Decidua basalis, 94, *95*, 97, *98*
Decidua capsularis, 94, *95*
Decidua parietalis, 94, *95*, *98*
Deletion, chromosomal, 125, *126*, 127
Dental laminae, 320, *320*
Dental papilla, formation of, 320–321
Dental sac, formation of, 321
Dentin, formation of, *321*, 322
Dentinogenesis imperfecta, 322
Dentition. See also *Teeth*.
  primary and secondary, 320
Dermal papillae, formation of, 315
Dermal root sheath, 316, *317*
Dermatoglyphics, 315
Dermatomes, cutaneous innervation of
    limbs and, 266–267
  definition of, 266
Dermis, development of, 315–316
Dermomyotome, in musculoskeletal sys-
    tem development, 252
Development, critical periods in, 59,
    130, **131–132**
  periods of, postnatal, ossification of
    vertebrae in, 258, *258*
  prenatal, 1, *2–5*, 6
    1st week, *2*, 26–33

Development *(Continued)*
    2nd week, *2,* 35–44
    3rd week, *3,* 45–58
    4th week, *3,* 59–63, 64t, *65–67,*
        68–69
    5th week, *3,* 59–63, 64, 64t, *70*
    6th week, *3,* 59–63, 64, 64t, 67,
        70–71
    7th week, *4,* 59–63, 64t, 67, *71–*
        72
    8th week, *4,* 59–63, 64t, 67, *72–*
        73
    9th week, *4*
    10th week, *4*
    fetal, *5,* 78–92. See also *Fetal pe-*
        riod.
    ossification of vertebrae in, 256,
        258
    stages of, 1, *2–5,* 6
Diabetes mellitus, maternal, teratoge-
    nicity of, 139
Diaphragm, congenital defects in, 149–
    150
    descent of, 149
    development of, 148–150
    innervation of, 148–149
    positional changes in, 148–149, *149*
    primitive, 148
Diaphragmatic atresia, 198
Diaphyseal-epiphyseal junction, in in-
    tracartilaginous ossification, *254,*
    255
Diaphysis, in intracartilaginous ossifica-
    tion, 253, *254*
Diazepam, as teratogen, 137
Diencephalon, development of, 286,
    287, **289–290,** *291*
    in pituitary gland development, 290
Diethylstilbestrol (**DES**), as teratogen,
    129t, 134
    in inhibition of implantation, 41–43
Differentiation, in embryonic period,
    59
Diffusion, placental transport by, 101–
    102
Digestive system, development of, 188–
    202. See also specific organs, e.g.,
    Stomach.
Digit(s), absence of, 268, *269*
    development of, at 8 weeks, 67, 72,
        73
Digital rays, *264,* 264–265, *265*
    at 6 weeks, 67, *70*
    formation of, 64, *70, 72*
Dilantin, as teratogen, 129t, 135
Dislocation, of hip, congenital, 139,
    268
Diverticulum (diverticula), cecal, 193,
    195
    hepatic, 190
    ileal, 110, 198, *198*
    laryngotracheal, formation of, 180
    Meckel's, 110, 198, *198*
    metanephric, 206, *206*
Dizygotic (**DZ**) twins, *112,* 113
Dorsal gray horns, in spinal cord devel-
    opment, *279, 281, 282*

Dorsal gray matter, in spinal cord de-
    velopment, *279,* 282
Dorsal mesentery, *60,* 61, 143, *144*
    of esophagus in development of dia-
        phragm, *146, 147,* 148
Dorsal mesogastrium, *189,* 189–190
Dorsal root ganglia. See Spinal ganglia.
Dorsal roots, of spinal nerves, *281, 282,*
    283
Dorsal septum, in spinal cord develop-
    ment, *279, 281,* 282
Down syndrome, 18, **122,** *122,* 124t
    incidence of, 124t
    tongue anomalies in, 167
Drug(s), as teratogens, 129t, **132–137**
    maternal use of, fetal growth and, 88
    ovulation-inducing, multiple births
        from, 111
    placental transport of, 102–103
Duct(s), alveolar, formation of, 185
    bile, extrahepatic, atresia of, 193
        formation of, 191, *191*
    cochlear, development of, 308, *310*
    cystic, formation of, 191, *191*
    ejaculatory formation of, 217, *218*
    endolymphatic, formation of, 308,
        309
    genital. See *Genital duct(s).*
    hepatic, accessory, 191, 193
    lactiferous, development of, 318, *319*
    mesonephric, *216,* 217
    müllerian, 217
    paramesonephric, *216,* 217
    semicircular, development of, 308,
        310
    submandibular, formation of, 168
    wolffian, 217. See also *Mesonephric*
        duct.
Ductus arteriosus, fate of, 249
    origin of, 243, *244, 245*
    patent, *243,* 246, *246*
Ductus deferens, *12,* 14
    formation of, 217, *218*
Ductus epididymis, formation of, 217,
    218
Ductus venosus, fate of, 249
    in fetal circulation, 246, *247*
Duodenum, atresia of, 190, *192*
    development of, 190
    obstruction of, from mixed rotation
        and volvulus, 196
    stenosis of, 190, *192*
Dural venous sinuses, in CSF absorp-
    tion, 288

E

Ear, congenital anomalies of, 311–312,
    312
    development of, 308–313
    external, development of, 309, 311
    internal (inner), development of, 308,
        309, 310
    middle, development of, 308–309,
        311
Early pregnancy factor (**EPF**), 29, **45**
    in pregnancy tests, 45

Ectoderm, 61, *62*
    embryonic, formation and derivatives
        of, *46,* 49
    in epidermal development, 315, *316*
Ectodermal ridge, apical, in limb devel-
    opment, 264, *264*
Ectopic pregnancies, 39, 41, *41, 42*
Edwards, *in vitro* fertilization and, 8
Edwards syndrome. See *Trisomy 18.*
Efferent ductules, formation of, 217,
    218
Ejaculation, 23
Ejaculatory duct(s), *12,* 14
    formation of, 217, *218*
Electrolytes, placental transport of, 102
Embryo(s), age of, estimation of, 69, 73
    "blighted," 125
    definition of, 1, 6
    development of, control of, 61, 63
    early, spontaneous abortion of, 43
    folding of, 59, *60,* 61
    measuring, methods of, 73, *73–75*
    tetraploid, 125
    transfer of, 29
    trilaminar, formation of, 45, *46–47*
    triploid, 125
Embryoblast, 1, 31
Embryology, descriptive terms in, *9,* 10
    Greek contributions to, 7
    historical highlights in, 7–8, 10
    importance of, 6
    in Koran, 7
    in Middle Ages, 7
    in Renaissance, 7
    in Sanskrit treatise, 7
    in 17th century, 7–8
    in 18th century, 8
    in 19th century, 8
    recent advances in, 8, 10
Embryonic body cavity(ies), 142–148
    division of, **143,** *145, 146, 147,* 148
Embryonic development, early, 35–39
Embryonic disc (disk), bilaminar, forma-
    tion of, 35, 37
    layers of, 37
Embryonic ectoderm, formation and de-
    rivatives of, *46,* 49
Embryonic endoderm, formation and
    derivatives of, *46,* 49
Embryonic mesoderm, derivatives of,
    49
Embryonic period, *3–4,* 59
    control of development during, 61,
        63
    definition of, 1, 6, 59
    3rd week in, *3,* 45–58
    4th week in, 59–63, 64t, *65–67, 68–*
        69, 144, 145
    5th week in, 59–63, **64,** 64t, *70, 146,*
        147
    6th week in, 59–63, **64,** 64t, *70–71,*
        146, 147
    7th week in, 59–63, 64t, *67, 71–72,*
        146
    8th week in, 59–63, 64t, *67, 72–73,*
        146
Embryonic pole, *31,* 32

Embryotroph, 35
Enamel, hypoplasia of, 322, *323*, 324
  production of, *321*, 322
Enamel pearls, 324
Endocardial cushion(s), **AV** septal defects and, with primum type ASD, 237, *240*
  development of, 231, *232*, *233*, *234*
Endocardium, *228*, 231
Endochondral bone formation, 252, 253, *254*, *255*
Endoderm, 61
  embryonic, formation and derivatives of, *46*, 49
Endolymphatic duct and sac, formation of, 308, *310*
Endometrium, 13, *13*
  in menstrual cycle, *19*, 20, 22
Endothelial heart tubes, formation of, *54*, 55, 227, *228*
Entoderm. See *Endoderm.*
Environmental factors, congenital anomalies from, **128**, 129t, *130*, 131–139. See also *Teratogen(s).*
Epiblast, *36*, 37
  formation of, 45, *47*
Epicardium, *228*, 231
Epidermal ridges, formation of, 315, *316*
Epidermis, development of, 315, *316*
Epididymis, *12*, 14
Epiphyseal cartilage plate, in intracartilaginous ossification, *254*, 255
Epiphyses, anular, in ossification of vertebrae, 258, *258*
  in intracartilaginous ossification, *254*, 255
Epiploic foramen, 190
Epispadias, 223, 224
  exstrophy of bladder and, 210
Epithelial root sheath, 316, *317*
  formation of, *321*, 322
Epithelium, pigmented, of retina, origin of, 304
Erectile tissue, of penis, *12*, 14
Erythropoiesis, in fetus, at 9 to 12 weeks, 83
  at 26 to 29 weeks, 85
Esophagus, atresia of, *182*, 188–189
  tracheoesophageal fistula associated with, 181, *182*, 188
  development of, 188–189, *189*
  stenosis of, 189
Estrogen(s), in inhibition of implantation, 41–43
  placental secretion of, 103
  production of, 20
Eustachian tube. See also *Auditory tube.*
Eustachian tube, development of, 308
Exencephaly, 296
Exocoelomic membrane, formation of, *36*, 37
Expected date of confinement (EDC), 85
Extraembryonic coelom, formation of, *36*, 37, *37*, 39, *40*
Extraembryonic mesoderm, formation of, *36*, 37, *37*

Extraembryonic mesoderm *(Continued)*
  somatic, 39, *40*
  splanchnic, formation of, 39, *40*
Eye(s), at 6 weeks, 67, *70*
  at 8 weeks, 67
  congenital anomalies of, *307*, 307–308, *308*
  development of, **301–308**
    critical period of, 307
  in fetus, at 26 to 29 weeks, 85
    at 30 to 34 weeks, 85
  movements of, at 14 weeks, 83
Eyelid(s), coloboma of, 307, *307*
  development of, *304*, *305*, 306–307
Eye(s). See also specific parts, e.g., *Retina.*

F

Face, clefts of, 176–177, *177*
  development of, *168*, **168–169**, *170–171*
Facial expression, muscles of, development of, 271
Facial nerve, origin of, 157t, 158
Fallopian tubes. See *Uterine tube(s).*
Fat, brown, 84
Female pronucleus, 27, *28*
Female pseudohermaphroditism, 221–222, *222*
Feminization, testicular, 220–221, *221*
Fertilization, 11, 14, **26–31**
  assisted in vivo, 31
  in vitro, 8, 29
  phases of, 26–27, *28*, *29*
  probable time of, in estimation of embryonic age, 69
  results of, 29
Fertilization age, establishing, 69, 78
Fetal alcohol effects (**FAE**), 133
Fetal alcohol syndrome (**FAS**), 88, 129t, **133**, *133*
Fetal hydantoin syndrome, 135
Fetal hypoxia, causes of, 101
Fetal period, 5, 6, 78–92. See also *Development, periods of, prenatal.*
  assessing health of fetus during, 88–92
  9th to 12th week in, 80, *81–82*, 83, *147*
  13 to 16 weeks, *81*, *82*, 83, *83*
  17 to 20 weeks, *81*, *82*, 83–84, *84*
  21 to 25 weeks, *81*, *82*, 85, *86*
  26 to 29 weeks, *81*, *82*, 85
  30 to 34 weeks, *81*, *82*, 85
  35 to 38 weeks, *81*, *82*, 85, *87*
Fetomaternal junction, 97–98, *99*
Fetoscopy, in fetal assessment, 90–91
Fetus(es), age of, estimating, 78–80
  at 9 to 12 weeks, 80, *81*, *82*, 83, *147*
  at 13 to 16 weeks, *81*, *82*, 83, *83*
  at 17 to 20 weeks, *81*, *82*, 83–84, *84*
  at 21 to 25 weeks, *81*, *82*, 85, *86*
  at 26 to 29 weeks, *81*, *82*, 85
  at 30 to 34 weeks, *81*, *82*, 85
  at 35 to 38 weeks, *81*, *82*, 85, *87*
  circulation in, 246, *247*, 249
  definition of, 6

Fetus(es) *(Continued)*
  drug addiction in, 102–103
  external characteristics of, 79–80, 80t
  growth of, at 13 to 16 weeks, 83
    at 35 to 38 weeks, 85
    factors influencing, 85, 88
  harlequin, 316
  infections in, 103
    mental retardation from, 298
  movements of, at 17 to 20 weeks, 83–84
  skull of, 260–261
  starvation of, 88
  status of, assessing, procedures for, 89–92
    alpha-fetoprotein assay as, 90
    cell cultures as, 90
    chorionic villus sampling as, 89–90
    cordocentesis as, 91
    diagnostic amniocentesis as, 89, *89*
    fetoscopy as, 90–91
    intrauterine fetal transfusion as, 90
    percutaneous umbilical cord blood sampling as, 91
    sex chromatin patterns as, 90, *90*
    ultrasonography as, *91*, 91–92
  triploid, 125
  weight of, in fetal age estimation, 79
Fibrinoid material, of surfaces of villi, 100, *100*
Fibrous joints, 255, *256*
Filum terminale, 283, *283*
Fingernails, development of, 318, *318*
Fingerprints, 315
Fingers. See *Digit(s).*
First arch syndrome, 161, *163*
  atresia of external acoustic meatus in, 312
  auricular anomalies with, 311
  congenital fixation of stapes in, 312
Fistula(s), anal agenesis with, *200*, 201
  anorectal agenesis with, *200*, 201
  branchial, 161, *162*
  lingual, congenital, *165*, 167
  piriform sinus, 161
  tracheoesophageal, 181–182, *182*, 188
Fleming, embryological studies of, 8
Flexures, brain, 286, *287*, 288
Fluids, intravenous, placental transport of, 102
Fluorescent in situ hybridization (**FISH**), in chromosome identification, 127
Follicle, hair, development of, 316, *317*
  ovarian, development of, *16*, *19*, 20
  primordial, in fetus, *215*, 216
Follicle stimulating hormone (**FSH**), in ovarian cycle, *19*, 20
  in ovulation, 20
Fontanelles, 260, *262*
Foot, cleft, 268, *269*
  length of, in fetal age estimation, 79
Foot plates, 264, *265*
Foramen, interventricular, 232, *233*, *239*
  of Luschka, 288
  of Magendie, 288

Foramen *(Continued)*
  omental, 190
Foramen ovale, after birth, 232, *248*
  before birth, 232, *235*, *236*, *247*
  closure of, postnatal, 249
  formation of, 232, *235*, *236*
  in fetal circulation, 246, *247*
  patent, 237, *240*, *241*
Foramen primum, formation of, 231,
  233, *234*
  patent, 237, *240*
Forebrain, development of, 286, *287*,
  289–290, *291*
Foregut, 61
  derivatives of, 188–193. See also spe-
    cific structure, e.g., *Esophagus.*
Forked ribs, 260, *260*
Fragile X syndrome, 128
Fraternal twins, *112*, 113
Frontonasal prominence (FNP), 168,
  169
Fructose, as energy source for sperm,
  24
Fused ribs, 260
Fused teeth, *323*, *324*

G

Galen, embryological studies of, 7
Gallbladder, formation of, 191, *191*
Gametes. See also *Oocyte(s); Sperm(s).*
  abnormal, 18–19
  formation of, 14–19
  intrafallopian transfer of (GIFT), 31
  male and female, comparison of, 18
  transportation of, 23–24
  viability of, 24
Gametogenesis, 14–19. See also *Gametes; Germ cells.*
  meiosis in, 15
Ganglion (ganglia), autonomic, origin
  of, 298
  sensory, formation of, 51
  spinal, development of, *281*, *282*,
    282–283
  spiral, 308, *310*
Gases, placental transport of, 102
Gastrulation, **45**, *46–48*, 49, *50*
  germ layers formed during, 61
Gene(s), inactivation of, on X chromosome, 119–120
  mutation of, anomalies caused by,
    128, *128*
Genetic factors, congenital anomalies
  from, 119–128. See also *Congenital
  anomalies.*
  fetal growth and, 88
Genital duct(s), development of, *214*,
  216, 216–217, *218*, 220
  embryonic, vestigial structures de-
    rived from, 217, *218*
  female, development of, 217, *218*
  indifferent (undifferentiated) stage of,
    214, 216–217
  male, development of, 217, *218*
Genital glands, female, auxiliary, 217
Genital system, congenital anomalies of,
  220–222, *221*, *222*, *223*, *224*, *224*

Genital system *(Continued)*
  development of, 213, *214–215*, *216*,
    216–217, *218–219*, 220–222,
    221, *222*, *223*, 224, *224*. See also
    specific structures, e.g.,
    Gonad(s).
Genital tubercle, development of, *219*,
  220
Genitalia, external, *12*, 14, *14*
  ambiguous, 220
  development of, *219*, 220
  indifferent/undifferentiated stage of,
    219, 220
Germ cells. See also *Oocyte(s); Sperm(s).*
  formation of, 14–19
  haploid, 15
  primordial, in gonadal development,
    213, *214*, *215*, 216
  in yolk sac wall, 110
Germ layers, derivatives of, 61, *62*
  formation of, 45, *46–48*, 49, *50*
Germinal matrix, 316
Gestational age, establishing, 78
  size of chorionic sac and, 97
  time units for, comparison of, 79t
Glands. See specific gland(s).
Glandular hypospadias, 222, *223*
Glandular plate, 212, *219*
Glans penis, development of, *219*, 220
Glaucoma, congenital, 307–308, *308*
Glomerular capsule, formation of, 206,
  207
Glomerulus, 206, *207*
Glossopharyngeal nerve, origin of,
  157t, 158
Glucose, fetal growth and, 88
  placental transport of, 102
Gonad(s), development of, 213, *214–
  215*, 216
  indifferent or undifferentiated, 213,
    214–215
Gonadal ridge, 213, *214*
Gonadotropin-releasing hormones
  (GnRH), 20
Graaf, Reinier de, embryological studies
  of, 7
Graafian follicle, 20. See also *Follicle,
  ovarian.*
Greater peritoneal sac, 190
Greatest length (GL), in embryonic
  measurement, 73, *75*
Greeks, embryological studies of, 7
Growth, in embryonic period, 59
  of fetus, at 13 to 16 weeks, 83
    at 35 to 38 weeks, 85
    factors influencing, 85, 88
Gut, primitive, yolk sac in, 110

H

Hair, abnormalities of, 316–317
  development of, 316, *317*
  loss of, 316–317
Hair bud, 316, *317*
Hair bulb, 316, *317*
Hair follicle, development of, 316, *317*
Hair papilla, mesenchymal, 316, *317*
Hair shaft, 316, *317*

Hamm, embryological studies of, 8
Hand(s), absence of, 268, *269*
  cleft, 268, *269*
Hand plates, 264, *265*
  formation of, 64, *70*
Harlequin fetus, 316
Harvey, William, embryological studies
  of, 7
Haversian systems, in intramembranous
  ossification, 253
Head fold, 59, *60*, 61, 142, 286
  in early heart development, 229, *229*
Head growth, in 5th week, 64, *70*
Heart, conducting system of, abnormalities of, 237
  development of, 237
  congenital anomalies of, **237**, 239,
    240–241, 242, *242*
  defects of, in congenital rubella syn-
    drome, 137
  development of, completion of, **231–
    232**, *232*, 233–236, 237, *238*, *239*
    early, **227**, *228*, *229*, 229, *230*, 231
  muscles of, development of, 272
  primitive, formation of, *54*, 55
Heart prominence, at 6 weeks, 64, *67*,
  70, *71*
Heart tube, endothelial, formation of,
  54, 55, **227**, *228*
Hematoma, placental separation and,
  106
Hematopoietic cells, in intracartilagin-
  ous ossification, 255
Hematopoietic tissue, of liver, 190
Hemispheres, cerebral, origin of, 289,
  290, *291*
Hemivertebra, 259, *260*
Hemolytic disease of newborn (HDN),
  102
Hemopoiesis, in embryonic liver, 190
Hemopoietic cells, in intracartilaginous
  ossification, 255
Hepatic diverticulum, 190
Hepatic ducts, accessory, 191, 193
Hermaphrodites, true, 220
Hermaphroditism, 220
Hernia, congenital diaphragmatic
  (CDH), *149*, 149–150, *150*
Hernia, midgut, reduction of, 193
  umbilical, 196
Herniation, umbilical, at 7 weeks, 67,
  72
Heroin, maternal use of, fetal growth
  and, 88
Herpes simplex virus, as teratogen,
  129t, 138
Hindbrain, development of, 286, *287*,
  288, *289*
Hindgut, 61
  derivatives of, 198–201
Hip, congenital dislocation of, 139, 268
Hippocrates, embryological studies of, 7
His, Wilhelm, embryological studies
  of, 8
Homologs, 119
Hormone(s), human chorionic gonado-
  tropin (hCG), in pregnancy tests,
  45

Hormone(s) *(Continued)*
placental secretion of, 103
production of, by syncytiotrophoblast, 35
human chorionic somatomammotropin (hCS), placental secretion of,
103
placental transport of, 102
steroid, placental secretion of, 103
Horseshoe kidney, 208, *210*
Human immunodeficiency virus (**HIV**),
as teratogen, 129t, 138
Human parvovirus, as teratogen, 129t
Hutchinson's teeth, in congenital syphi-
lis, 139
Hyaline membrane disease (HMD), 185
Hyaloid artery, 301, *302, 303, 304*
in developing lens, *303, 304,* 306
Hyaluronidase, in acrosome reaction, 26
Hydramnios. See *Polyhydramnios.*
Hydrocephalus, *297,* 297–298
in spina bifida cystica, 285
Hymen, formation of, 217, *218, 219*
imperforate, 224
Hyoid arch, 63, *65, 68,* 153, 154, *155*
Hyoid bone, origin of, 157, 157t, 158
Hypertrichosis, 317
Hypoblast, *36,* 37
formation of, *31, 32, 45, 47*
Hypobranchial eminence, *166, 167,*
181
Hypoglycemic drugs, as possible terato-
gens, 136
Hypophyseal pouch, 293, *294,* See also
Rathke's pouch.
Hypophysis cerebri, development of,
290, *292,* 292t, 293
Hypospadias, 222, *223,* 224
Hypoxia, fetal, causes of, 101

I

Ichthyosis, 316
Identical twins, *112,* 113, *114,* 115
Ileal diverticulum, 110, 198, *198*
Immature infants, definition of, 78
Imperforate anus, 200, *201*
Imperforate hymen, 224
Implantation of blastocyst, 32, **35,** 39,
41, 41–43, *42*
bleeding at time of, 45
cervical, 39, *41*
completion of, 35–39
ectopic, 39
inhibition of, 41–43
sites of, extrauterine, 39, 41, *41, 42*
intrauterine, 39, *41*
In vitro fertilization (**IVF**), 8, *29*
Incisive fossa, 173
Incus, development of, 309, *311*
origin of, 154, 157, 157t
Induction, of embryonic development,
63
Infants, full term, characteristics of, 85
immature, definition of, 78
premature, definition of, 78
Infection(s), as teratogens, 129t, **137–**
139

Infection(s) *(Continued)*
fetal, 103
mental retardation from, 298
Infectious agents, placental transport of,
101, 103
Inferior vena cava, in fetal circulation,
246, *247*
Infundibular stem, 292t, 293, *294*
Infundibulum, 293, *294*
Inheritance, multifactorial, 118
anomalies caused by, 139–140
cleft palate from, 176
Inner cell mass, 1, 31. See also *Em-
bryoblast.*
Insula, 295
Insulin, fetal growth and, 88
in pregnancy, 135–136
secretion of, by fetal pancreas, 193
Intercalated discs (disks), in cardiac
muscle development, 272
Intercostal arteries, in vertebral column
development, 256
Intermediate zone, in spinal cord devel-
opment, 275, *279, 281*
Internal capsule, 294
Intersegmental arteries, in vertebral
column development, 256, *257*
Intersexuality, 220
Interstitial cells of Leydig, 216
Interventricular foramen, 232, *233,*
239
Interventricular septum, 232, *232, 233,*
238, *239*
Intervertebral disc (disk), in vertebral
column development, 256
Intervillous space, *95,* 98, *98, 99*
Interzonal mesenchyme, in synovial
joints, 255, *256*
Intestines, atresia of, 197–198
fixation of, 193, *195*
in fetus at 9 to 12 weeks, *81,* 83
obstruction of, congenital, *192*
stenosis of, 197–198
Intracartilaginous ossification, 253, *254,*
255
Intraembryonic coelom, development
of, *52, 53,* 142
Intraembryonic ectoderm. See *Embryonic ectoderm.*
Intraembryonic endoderm. See *Embryonic endoderm.*
Intraembryonic mesoderm, formation
of, *46,* 49
in musculoskeletal system development, 252
Intramembranous bone formation, 252,
253
Intramembranous ossification, 253
Intraretinal space, 304, *304, 305*
Intrauterine device (IUD), 43
Intrauterine fetal transfusion, 90
Intrauterine growth retardation (**IUGR**),
from polychlorinated biphenyls,
137
nicotine and, 132
Intravenous fluids, placental transport
of, 102
Iodine, radioactive, as teratogen, 136

Ionizing radiation, as teratogen, 129t,
139
mutagenicity of, 18
Iris, coloboma of, 307, *307*
development of, *304,* 305–306
muscles of, origin of, 272
Isochromosome, *126,* 127–128
Isotretinoin, as teratogen, 129t, 136

J

Jaundice, from biliary atresia, 193
Jaws, development of, 154, *156,* 157,
168, *170–171*
Joint(s), cartilaginous, 255, *256*
costovertebral, in rib development,
258, 259
development of, 255, *256*
fibrous, 255, *256*
laxity of, generalized, congenital hip
dislocation from, 268
neurocentral, in ossification of vertebrae, 258, *258*
synovial, 255, *256*

K

Keratinization, disorders of, 316
Kidney(s), agenesis of, 208, *209*
oligohydramnios and, 109
blood vessels of, multiple, 208
congenital anomalies of, **208,** *209,*
210, *210*
development of, **204,** 206, *206, 207,*
208
double, 208, *209,* 210
ectopic, 208, *209*
fetal, 206
horseshoe, 208, *210*
pancake, 208, *209*
pelvic, 208
permanent, development of, 206,
206, 207
positional changes of, *207,* 208
supernumerary, 208
unilateral fused, 208, *209*
Koran, in history of embryology, 7
Kupffer cells, of liver, 190

L

Labia majora, development of, *219,* 220
Labia minora, development of, *219,* 220
Labioscrotal swellings, development of,
219, 220
Labor, definition of, 104
stages of, **104,** *104, 105,* 106
Labyrinth, bony, of internal ear, forma-
tion of, 308, *310*
membranous, origin of, 308
Lactiferous ducts, development of, 318,
319
Lacunae, in syncytiotrophoblast, 35
derivative of, 98
Lacunar networks, formation of, 37, *37,*
38
Lanugo, 84
Laryngeal aditus, primitive, 180, *181*

Laryngeal cartilages, origin of, *157*, 157t, 158, 181
Laryngeal muscles, development of, 181
Laryngotracheal diverticulum, formation of, 180
Laryngotracheal tube, formation of, 181, *181*
Larynx, development of, 181
Last normal menstrual period (**LNMP**), in estimation of embryonic age, 69
Lateral gray horns, in spinal cord development, 282
Lead, as teratogen, 137
Leeuwenhoek, Antony van, embryological studies of, 8
Length, measurements of, in embryonic measurement, 73, 75
Lens, development of, 301, *302*, *303*, *304*, *305*, 306
Lens pit, formation of, 301, *302*
Lens placodes, formation of, 301, *302*
Lens vesicle, formation of, 301, *302*
Lentiform nuclei, 294
Leonardo da Vinci, embryological studies of, 7
Lesser sac of peritoneum. See *Omental bursa.*
Levan, embryological studies of, 8
Ligament(s), anterior, of malleus, formation of, 154, 157t
 periodontal, 321, *321*, 322
 sphenomandibular, formation of, 154, 157t
 stylohyoid, origin of, *157*, 157t, 158
 umbilical, medial, origin of, 249
 median, origin of, 94, 111
Ligamentum arteriosum, origin of, 249
Ligamentum teres, origin of, 249
Ligamentum venosum, origin of, 249
Limb(s), cutaneous innervation of, dermatomes and, 266–267
 defects in, *267*, **267–268**, *269–271*, 271
 causes of, **268**, 271
 development of, 263–267, *264*, *265*, *266*
 critical period of, 268
 lower, in embryo, at 5 weeks, 64
 at 7 weeks, 67, 72
 at 8 weeks, 67, *73*
 in fetus, at 9 to 12 weeks, 80, *81–82*, 83
 at 30 to 34 weeks, 85
 muscles of, development of, 271
 upper, in embryo, at 5 weeks, 64, *70*
 at 6 weeks, 67
 at 7 weeks, 67, 72
 at 8 weeks, 67, *73*
 in fetus, at 30 to 34 weeks, 85
 at 12 weeks, 80
Limb buds, **63**, 263–264, *264*, *265*, 265–266
 at four weeks, 63, *65*, *69*
Lingual cysts and fistulas, congenital, *165*, 167
Lip, cleft, 173, *173*, *174*, *175*, 176, *176*, 177

Lip *(Continued)*
 bilateral, 173, *173*, 176
 median, 176, *177*
 unilateral, 173, *174*
Lithium carbonate, as teratogen, 129t, 136–137
Liver, anomalies of, 191, 193
 development of, 190–191, 193
Lobster-claw deformities, 268, *269*
Lumbar puncture, 283–284
Lumbar rib, 259
Lung(s), aeration of, postnatal, 249
 development of, **182**, *183*, 184–185
 alveolar period of, *184*, 185
 canalicular period of, *184*, 185
 pseudoglandular period of, *184*, 184–185
 terminal sac period of, *184*, 185
 in congenital diaphragmatic hernia, 150
 in fetus, at 26 to 29 weeks, 85
 maturation of, *184*, 184–185
Lung bud, 182, *183*
 formation of, 180
Luteinizing hormone (**LH**), in ovarian cycle, *19*, 20
 in ovulation, 20
Lymphatic nodules, origin of, 159
Lysergic acid diethylamide (**LSD**), in pregnancy, 137

M

Macroglossia, 167
Macrostomia, 177, *177*
Male pronucleus, *28*, 29
Male pseudohermaphroditism, 220
Malformation. See *Congenital anomalies.*
Malleus, development of, 309, *311*
 origin of, 154, *157*, 157t
Malnutrition, maternal, fetal growth and, 88
Malpighi, Marcello, embryological studies of, 7–8
Mammary glands. See *Breasts.*
Mammary pit, 318, *319*
Mammary ridges, 318, *319*
Mandible, development of, 169
 origin of, 154
Mandibular arch, 63, 65, *68*
 fate of, 154
Mandibular prominences, 168, 169
 fate of, 154
Marijuana, as possible teratogen, 137
 maternal use of, fetal growth and, 88
Mastoid antrum, development of, 309
 origin of, 159
Mastoid process, development of, 309
Maxilla, development of, 168–169, *170*
 intermaxillary segment of, 169
 premaxillary part of, 169
Maxillary prominences, 168
 fate of, 154
Meatal plug, formation of, 309, *311*
Meckel's cartilage, derivatives of, 154, *157*, 157t, 158, 260

Meckel's diverticulum, 110, 198, *198*. See also *Ileal diverticulum.*
Medial umbilical ligament, origin of, 249
Median eminence, origin of, 292t, 293, *294*
Median sac diameter (**MSD**), in gestational age determination, 97
Medulla, of indifferent gonad, 213, *214*
 suprarenal, development of, 213
 origin of, 61, *62*
Medulla oblongata, origin of, 287, 288
Medullary center, formation of, 295
Meiosis, in gametogenesis, 15
 species variation and, 29
Meiotic cell divisions, in oogenesis, 17–18
Melanin, production of, 315
Melanoblasts, 315, *316*
Melanocytes, 315, *316*
Membrane(s), amniochorionic, 95, 108
 anal, *199*, 200
 branchial, *153*, *155*, 159, 161
 cloacal, *48*, 49, *50*, *60*, 61, 199, *199*
 fetal, 94
 oronasal, 169
 oropharyngeal, *48*, 49, *50*, *60*, 61, **152**, *153*
 placental, 98–100, *100*, *101*
 placental, in amniotic fluid exchange, 109
 pleuropericardial, 143, *146*
 pleuroperitoneal, 143, *147*
 in development of diaphragm, *147*, 148
 synovial, 255
 tympanic, formation of, 309, 311, *311*
 origin of, *160*, 161
 urogenital, *199*, 200
Membranous labyrinth, origin of, 308
Membranous neurocranium, 260, *261*, *262*
Membranous ventricular septal defect, 239
Membranous viscerocranium, 260, *261*
Menarche, 11
Mendel, Gregor Johann, principles of heredity and, 8
Meninges, 288
Meningocele, cranium bifidum with, *295*, 296
 spina bifida cystica with, *284*, 285
Meningoencephalocele, *295*, 296
Meningohydroencephalocele, *295*, 296
Meningomyelocele, spina bifida cystica with, *284*, 285, *286*
Menopause, 22
Menstrual cycle, *19*, *20*, 22–23
 menstrual phase of, *19*, 22
 pregnancy phase of, 20
 proliferative phase of, *19*, 22
 secretory phase of, *19*, 22
Mental retardation, 298
 causes of, 131, 295
 from alcohol, 129t, *133*, 133
 from chromosomal aberration, 118t, 119

Mental retardation *(Continued)*
    from fragile X syndrome, 128
    from *in utero* exposure to organic
        mercury, 137
    in microcephaly, 297
6-Mercaptopurine, as teratogen, 135
Mercury, organic, as teratogen, 137
Meroanencephaly, 51, **296**, *296.* See
    also *Anencephaly.*
    acrania with, 263, *263*
Meromelia, 136, *136*, **267**, *267*
    causes of, **268**, 271
    from thalidomide, 136, *136*
Mesencephalon, development of, 288–
    289, *289, 290*
Mesenchymal hair papilla, 316, *317*
Mesenchyme, formation of, 49
    in gonadal development, 213
    in muscle development, 271
    in musculoskeletal system develop-
        ment, 252
    interzonal, in synovial joints, 255,
        256
Mesenteric artery, superior, 193, *195*
Mesentery (mesenteries), dorsal, *60*, 61,
    143, *144*
    of esophagus in development of dia-
        phragm, *146, 147*, 148
Mesoderm, **61**
    cardiogenic, formation of, 53
    embryonic, derivatives of, 49
    extraembryonic, formation of, *36*, 37,
        37
        somatic, formation of, 39, *40*
        splanchnic, formation of, 39, *40*
    in dermal development, 315, *316*
    intraembryonic, formation of, *46*, 49
        in musculoskeletal system develop-
            ment, 252
    metanephric, 206, *206*
    paraxial, formation of, 51, 52
        in musculoskeletal system develop-
            ment, 252, *253*
    somatic, in skeletal muscle develop-
        ment, 271
    splanchnic, in visceral muscle devel-
        opment, 272
Mesogastrium, dorsal, *189*, 189–190
    ventral, 190
Mesonephric ducts, *216*, 217
Mesonephroi, 204, *205*
Mesothelium, in gonadal development,
    213
Metabolism, placental, 101
Metanephric diverticulum, 206, *206*
Metanephric mesoderm, 206, *206*
Metanephric tubules, 206, *206*
Metanephroi, 204
Metencephalon, development of, 286,
    287, 288, *289*
Methadone, as teratogen, 137
Methotrexate, as teratogen, 129t
Methyl mercury, as teratogen, 129t,
    137
Microcephaly, 297, *297*
Microencephaly, 297
Microglial cells, in spinal cord develop-
    ment, 275, *280*

Microglossia, 167
Microscopes, early, *8*
Microstomia, congenital, 177, *177*
Midbrain, development of, 286, *287,*
    288–289, *289, 290*
Midbrain flexure, 286, *287*
Middle Ages, in history of embryology,
    7
Midgut, *60*, 61
    anomalies of, *196*, 196–198, *197, 198*
    derivatives of, 193, 196–198
    fixation of, 193, *195*
    nonrotation of, 196, *197*
    rotation of, 193, *195*
        mixed, volvulus and, 196–197, *197*
Midgut loop, 193
Midgut volvulus, 197, *197*
Minamata disease, from *in utero* expo-
    sure to organic mercury, 137
Miscarriage, definition of, 6
Molding, of skull, 260
Molecular biology, recent advances in,
    8, 10
Molecular cytogenetics, 127
Monosomy, 18, 120, *121*, 122
Monozygotic (MZ) twins, *112*, 113, *114,*
    115
"Morning-after" pill, in inhibition of
    implantation, 41–43
Morphogenesis, in embryonic period,
    59
Morula, 30, *31*
    definition of, 1
Mosaicism, 124
Mother(s), malnutrition in, fetal growth
    and, 88
Mouth. See *Stomodeum.*
Müllerian ducts, 217
Müllerian-inhibiting factor (**MIF**), 216
Multifactorial inheritance. See *Inheri-
    tance, multifactorial.*
Muscle(s), anomalies of, 272–273
    branchial arch, derivatives of, 157t,
        158, *158*
    cardiac, development of, 272
    development of, 271–273, *272*
    laryngeal, development of, 181
    orbicularis oculi, origin of, 307
    pectoralis major, absence of, 273
    skeletal, development of, 271–272,
        272
    smooth, development of, 272
    variations in, 273
    visceral, development of, 272
Muscular component, of branchial arch,
    154, *155*
Muscular system. See also *Muscle(s).*
    development of, 271–273, *272*
Musculoskeletal system, development
    of, 252–274. See also Muscle(s);
    specific structures, e.g., *Joint(s).*
Myelencephalon, development of, 286,
    287, 288
Myelination, of nerves, 284
Myelocele, spina bifida with, *284*, 285,
    285
Myeloschisis, spina bifida with, *284,*
    285, 285–286

Myoblasts, in limb development, 265
    in muscle development, 271
Myocardium, in embryo, *228*, 231
    primitive, 231
Myoepithelial cells, in sweat gland de-
    velopment, 317
Myofibrils, in skeletal muscle develop-
    ment, 271
Myometrium, 13, *13*
Myotomes, occipital, in tongue muscle
    development, 271, *272*

N

Nail fields, 318, *318*
Nail folds, 318, *318*
Nail plate, 318, *318*
Nails, development of, 318, *318*
Narcotics, maternal use of, fetal growth
    and, 88
Nasal cavities, development of, 169,
    172
Nasal pits, 168, 169, *170*
Nasal placodes, in facial development,
    168, 169, *170*
Nasal prominences, in facial develop-
    ment, 168, 169, *170*
Nasal sacs, development of, 169, *172*
Nasal septum, 169, *172*
Nasopalatine canal, 173
Natal teeth, 322
Neonate, circulation in, *248*, 249
    skull of, 260–261
Nephron, formation of, 206
Nerve(s), branchial arch, derivatives of,
    157t, 158–159
    facial, origin of, 157t, 158
    glossopharyngeal, origin of, 157t, 158
    in branchial arch, *153*, 154, *155*
    myelination of, 284
    of limbs, dermatomes and, 266–267
    olfactory, 169, *172*
    optic, development of, *303*, 305
        origin of, 289, *291*
    phrenic, formation of, 148
    spinal, dorsal roots of, *281, 282*, 283
    supplying diaphragm, 148–149
    trigeminal, origin of, 157t, 158
    vagus, origin of, 157t, 158–159
Nervous system. See also *Nerve(s).*
    central. See also *Brain; Spinal cord.*
    development of, 275–299
    peripheral, development of, 298
    origin of, 275
Neural canal, in nervous system devel-
    opment, 275, *277, 279, 281*
Neural crest, derivatives of, 51
    formation of, 51, *53*
    in peripheral nervous system devel-
        opment, 275
Neural crest cells, derivatives of, 61, *62*
    formation of, 51
    in branchial arch development, 152
    in development of peripheral nervous
        system, 298
    in epidermal development, 315
    in musculoskeletal system develop-
        ment, 252

Neural crest cells *(Continued)*
  in salivary gland development, 167
  in spinal ganglia development, 282, *282*
  laryngeal cartilages derived from, 181
Neural groove, formation of, 51, *52, 53*
Neural plate, formation of, *48, 49, 50, 51, 53*
Neural retina, development of, 304–305
  origin of, 304
Neural tube, defects in **(NTDs)**, 51, *284*, **284–286**, *285, 286*
  of brain, 295
  derivatives of, 275
  formation of, **51**, *52, 53, 63, 65, 66*
  in vertebral column development, 256, *258*
Neuroblasts, in spinal cord development, 275, *279, 280*
Neurocentral joints, in ossification of vertebrae, 258, *258*
Neurocranium, 260
  cartilaginous, 260, *261*
  membranous, 260, *261, 262*
Neurohypophysis, development of, *292*, 293
  origin of, 290, 292t
Neurons, in spinal cord development, 275, *279*
Neuropores, 63, *65–67*
  in nervous system development, 275, *276, 277*
Neurulation, *48, 49, 50*, 51, *52–53*
  abnormal, congenital anomalies resulting from, 51
Nipples, supernumerary, *319*, 319–320
Nondisjunction of chromosomes, 18
  congenital anomalies from, 119–125, *120*
  early abortions and, 43
Nose, bifid, 177, *177*
Nostril, single, 177, *177*
Notochord, formation of, *48, 49, 50*
  in vertebral column development, 256, *257, 258*
Notochordal process, 46, *48, 49*
Nucleus pulposus, in vertebral column development, 256, *257*
  origin of, 49
Nutritional substances, placental transport of, 102

O

Occipital myotomes, in tongue muscle development, 271, *272*
Odontoblastic processes, *321*, 322
Odontoblasts, *321*, 322
Oesophagus. See *Esophagus.*
Olfactory bulbs, 169
Olfactory nerves, 169, *172*
Olfactory receptor cells, 169
Oligodendrocytes, 284
Oligohydramnios, 109
  renal agenesis associated with, 208
  teratogenicity of, 139
Omental bursa, 190

Omental foramen, 190
Omphalocele, congenital, 196, *196*
Oocyte(s), parts of, *15*
  primary, in fetus, 216
  production of, 11
  release of, 12
  sperm compared with, *15*, 18
  transport of, *21, 22, 23*
  viability of, 24
Oogenesis, 17–18
  spermatogenesis compared to, *16*
Oogonia, 17
  in fetus, *215*, 216
Optic cups, formation of, 301, *302, 305*
Optic fissures, development of, 301, *302*
Optic nerve, development of, *303*, 305
  origin of, 289, *291*
Optic stalks, in eye development, 301, *302*
Optic sulci, in eye development, 301, *302*
Optic vesicles, development of, 301, *302*
  formation of, 289
Oral contraceptives, 20
  teratogenicity of, 133–134
Orbicularis oculi muscle, origin of, 307
Organ of Corti. See *Spiral organ of Corti.*
Organogenesis, definition of, 61
  teratogens during, 131
Oronasal membrane, 169
Oropharyngeal membrane, *48, 49, 50, 60, 61*, **152**, *153*
Osseous syndactyly, 268
Ossicles, auditory, development of, 309, *311*
Ossification, intracartilaginous, 253, *254*, 255
  intramembranous, 253
  of vertebrae, 256, 258, *258, 259*
Ossification centers, primary, 253, *254, 255, 258*
  between 9 to 12 weeks, 80
  for centrum in ossification of vertebrae, 256, *258*
  secondary, 255, *258*
  in ossification of vertebrae, 258, *258*
Osteoblasts, in intramembranous ossification, 253
Osteoclasts, in intramembranous ossification, 253
Osteocytes, in intramembranous ossification, 253
Osteoid tissue, in intramembranous ossification, 253
Otic capsule, development of, 308, *310*
Otic pits, at 4 weeks, 63, *65*
  formation of, 308, *309*
Otic placode, 308, *309*
Otic vesicle, formation of, 308, *309*
Ovarian cycle, 17, *19*, **20**, *21*
Ovary (ovaries), 11–12, *12, 13*. See also *Gonad(s).*
  development of, 213, *214–215*, 216
Ovogenesis. See *Oogenesis.*

Ovotestes, in true hermaphrodites, 220
Ovulation, 12, 20, *21*
  failure of, drugs for, multiple births from, 111
Ovum (ova). See *Oocyte(s).*
Oxazepam, as teratogen, 137
Oxycephaly, 263, *264*
Oxytocin, uterine contractions and, 104

P

Painter, chromosome studies of, 8
Palatal shelves, 169, *172*
Palate, cleft, *175*, 176, *176*
  development of, *169*, 172, 173, *174–175, 176*, 176–177, *177*
  hard, formation of, 169, *172*
  primary, formation of, 168, **169**, *172*
  secondary, 169, *172*
    formation of, 168, **169**, *172*, 173
  soft, formation of, *172*, 173
Palatine processes, 169, *172*
Palatine raphe, 169, *172*
Palatine tonsil, origin of, 159, *160*
Palpebral coloboma, 307
Pancreas, development of, 193, *194*
Pancreatic buds, 193
Parafollicular cells, origin of, 159
Paralysis, sphincter, in spina bifida, 286
Paramesonephric ducts, *216*, 217
Paranasal sinuses, development of, 169
Parathyroid glands, origin of, 159, *160*
Paraurethral glands, formation of, 217
Paraxial mesoderm, formation of, 51, *52*
  in musculoskeletal system development, 252, *253*
Parotid glands, 167
Pars distalis, origin of, 292t, 293, *294*
Pars intermedia, origin of, 292t, 293, *294*
Pars nervosa, origin of, 292t, 293, *294*
Pars tuberalis, origin of, 292t, 293, *294*
Parturition, 104, *104, 105*, 106
Patent ductus arteriosus **(PDA)**, **243**, *246*, 246
Patent foramen ovale, 237, *240, 241*
Patent foramen primum, 237, *240*
Pectoralis major muscle, absence of, 273
Penicillin, in pregnancy, 134
Penile hypospadias, 222, *223*
Penis, *12, 14*
  development of, *219*, 220
Penoscrotal hypospadias, 222, *223*
Pentasomy, of sex chromosomes, 124
Percutaneous umbilical cord blood sampling **(PUBS)**, in fetal status assessment, 91
Pericardial cavity, 142, *144, 146*
  formation of, 53
Pericardioperitoneal canals, **142**, 143, *145, 146*
Perichondrium, in intracartilaginous ossification, 253
Periderm, 315, *316*
Perilymph, 308
Perilymphatic space, formation of, 308, *310*

Perimetrium, 13, *13*
Perinatal medicine, 88
Perinatology, 88–92
Perineal body, *199*, 200
Perineal hypospadias, 222
Periodontal ligament, 321, *321*, 322
Periosteum, in intracartilaginous ossification, 253, 255
Peripheral nervous system, development of, 298
origin of, 275
Peritoneal cavity, 142–143, *144*, *145*
formation of, 53
Peritoneal sac, greater, 190
Phalanges. See *Digit(s)*.
Phallus, development of, *219*, 220
Pharyngeal apparatus, 152–178. See also *Branchial apparatus*.
Pharyngeal arches. See *Branchial arch(es)*.
Pharyngeal pouches, *153*, *155*, *156*, 159
1st, *153*, *155*, *156*, 159
derivatives of, 159, *160*
2nd, *155*, 159
derivatives of, 159, *160*
3rd, *155*, 159, *160*
4th, 159
derivatives of, 159, *160*
5th, 159
Pharynx, primitive, 159
Phencyclidine (PCP, "Angel Dust"), as possible teratogen, 137
Phenobarbital, in pregnancy, 135
Phenotypes, 119
Phenylketonuria (PKU), maternal, as teratogen, 139
Phenytoin, as teratogen, 129t, 135
Philtrum, of lip, formation of, 168, *171*
Photoreceptors, in neural retina, 304
Phrenic nerves, formation of, 148
Pia mater, *283*, 288, *289*
Pierre Robin syndrome, 161
Pigmented epithelium, of retina, origin of, 304
Pinna. See also *Auricle*.
Pinna, formation of, 311
Pinocytosis, placental transport by, 102
Piriform sinus fistulas, 161
Pituitary gland, development of, 290, *292*, 292t, 293
Placenta, 94–103
after birth, 106, *107*
circulation in, 98–99, *100*, *101*
fetal, *99*, 100, *100*, *107*, *108*
maternal, *99*, 100–101
development of, **55–57**, *56*, *57*, 96–98
endocrine secretion by, 103
fetal portion of, origin of, 94, **97**
fetal surface of, after birth, 106, *107*
functions and activities of, 94, 101–103
intervillous space of, primordium of, 37
maternal portion of, origin of, 94, **97**
maternal surface of, after birth, 106, *107*

Placenta *(Continued)*
metabolic function of, 101
shape of, determination of, 98
transport function of, 101–103
Placenta previa, 39
Placental barrier. See *Placental membrane*.
Placental insufficiency, fetal growth and, 88
Placental membrane, 98–100, *100*, *101*
in amniotic fluid exchange, 109
Placental septa, 98, *99*
Plagiocephaly, 263, *264*
Planes, of body, *9*, 10
Plasma, primitive, formation of, 55
Pleura, development of, *183*, 184
Pleural cavity(ies), 142
formation of, 53
Pleuropericardial membranes, 143, *146*
Pleuropericardial opening, 143
Pleuroperitoneal membranes, 143, *147*
in development of diaphragm, *147*, 148
Pleuroperitoneal opening, 143
Poland syndrome, 273
Polychlorinated biphenyls (**PCBs**), as teratogens, 129t, 137
Polydactyly, 128, 268, *270*
Polyhydramnios, 109
esophageal atresia associated with, 182, 188–189
tracheoesophageal fistula associated with, 182
Polymastia, 319
Polyploidy, 124–125
Polythelia, 19
Pons, development of, 288, *289*
origin of, *287*, 288
Pontine flexure, 286, *287*, 288
Porta hepatis, biliary atresia at, 193
Posterior root ganglia. See *Spinal ganglia*.
Potassium iodide, as teratogen, 136
Prader-Willi syndrome, 127
Prechordal plate. See *Prochordal plate*.
Predentin, production of, *321*, 322
Pregnancy, abdominal, 39, 41
corpus luteum of, 20
ectopic, 39, 41, *41*, *42*
multiple, 111, *112*, 113–115. See also *Twins*.
fetal growth and, 88
tests for, 45
tubal, 39, *41*, *42*
uterine growth during, 103, *103*
Pregnancy phase, of menstrual cycle, 20
Pregnancy tests, 35
Pregnancy wastage, 32
Premature birth, 6
Premature infants, definition of, 78
Prenatal period, stages of, 1, *2–5*, 6. See also *Development, periods of, prenatal*; specific stage.
Primary sex cords, 213, *214*, *215*
Primitive knot. See *Primitive node*.
Primitive node, formation of, 48, 49

Primitive streak, fate of, *48*, 49
formation of, **45**, *46*, *48*, 49
Primordial follicles, in fetus, *215*, 216
Primordial germ cells, in gonadal development, 213, *214*, *215*, 216
Primordium, definition of, 6
Primum atrial septal defects, AV septal defects with, endocardial cushion and, 237, *240*
Prochordal plate, 49
Proctodeum, 199, *199*
in development of stomach, 188, *189*
Progesterone, secretion of, by corpus luteum, 20
placental, 103
Progestins, as teratogens, 133
Progestogens, as teratogens, 129t, 133–134
Proliferative phase, of menstrual cycle, *19*, 22
Pronephroi, 204, *205*, *206*
Pronucleus, female, 27, *28*
male, *28*, 29
Propylthiouracil, as teratogen, 136
Prostaglandins, in sperm transport, 23
uterine contractions and, 104
Prostate, development of, 217, *218*
Pseudoglandular period, in lung development, *184*, 184–185
Pseudohermaphroditism, female, 221–222, *222*
male, 220
Psychoactive drugs, as teratogens, 137
Puberty, 11
Pulmonary alveoli, formation of, 185
Pulmonary artery, left, origin of, 243
right, origin of, 243
Pulmonary surfactant, production of, 185
by 24 weeks, 85
Pulmonary trunk, formation of, 237, *238*
Pulmonary vein, primitive, 232
Pupillary light reflex, in fetus, 85
Purkinje fibers, 272
Pyloric stenosis, congenital hypertrophic, 190
Pyramids, origin of, *287*, 288

Q

Quickening, 83–84

R

Rachischisis, 259, *263*
meroanencephaly associated with, 296
myloschisis associated with, 285
Radiation, ionizing, as teratogen, 129t, 139
mutagenicity of, 18
teratogenic effects of, period of greatest sensitivity to, 131
Rathke's pouch, in pituitary gland development, 293, *294*
Reciprocal translocation, 125, *126*

Recombinant DNA technology, 8, 10
Rectum, atresia of, *200*, 201
    formation of, *199*, 200
Reflex, pupillary light, in fetus, 85
Reichert's cartilage, derivatives of, *157*, 157t, 158, 260
Renal agenesis, oligohydramnios and, 109
Renal pelvis, formation of, 206, *206*
Renal vessels, multiple, 208
Reproduction, 11–24
    organs of, female, 11–14, *12, 13, 14*
        male, *12, 14*
Reproductive cycles, female, **19–23**
    menstrual, *19, 20,* 22–23
    ovarian, *19, 20, 21*
Respiratory bronchioles, formation of, *184,* 185
Respiratory distress, esophageal atresia and, 188–189
    in tracheoesophageal fistula, 182
    neonatal, patent ductus arteriosus and, 243, 246
Respiratory distress syndrome (**RDS**), 185
Respiratory system, 180–185. See also specific parts, e.g., *Lung(s).*
    development of, 180–185
Rete ovarii, *215,* 216
Rete testis, formation of, *215,* 216
Retina, central artery of, origin of, *303,* 304
    central vein of, origin of, *303,* 304
    coloboma of, 307
    detachment of, 304
    development of, *302–303, 304,* 304–305, *305*
    neural, development of, 304–305
        origin of, 304
    origin of, 289
Retinal pigment epithelium, origin of, 304
Retinoic acid, as teratogen, 136
    limb development and, 264
Ribs, accessory, 259–260, *260*
    anomalies of, 259–260, *260*
    cervical, 260, *260*
    development of, *258,* 259
    forked, 260, *260*
    fused, 260
    lumbar, 259
Rickets, enamel hypoplasia from, 324
Rods, in neural retina, 304
Root canal, formation of, *321,* 322
Root of tooth, development of, *321,* 322
Rubella virus, as teratogen, 129t, 131, **137**
    congenital cataract from, 307
    congenital deafness from, 311–312

S

Sac. See specific structure, e.g., *Yolk sac.*
Saccular portion, of otic vesicle, 308, *310*

Sacrococcygeal teratoma, 49
Salicylates, as possible teratogens, 136
Salivary glands, development of, 167–168
Sanskrit treatise in history of embryology, 7
Scala tympani, development of, 308, *310*
Scala vestibuli, development of, 308, *310*
Scaphocephaly, 263
Schleiden, Matthias Jakob, embryological studies of, 8
Schwann, Theodor, embryological studies of, 8
Schwann cells, 284
Sclera, development of, *304, 305,* 306
Sclerotome, in musculoskeletal system development, 252
    in vertebral column development, 256, *257*
Scoliosis, 259
Scrotum, development of, *219,* 220
Sebaceous glands, development of, 317
Sebum, 317
Secretory phase, of menstrual cycle, *19,* 22
Secundum atrial septal defects, 237, *240*
Semen, ejaculation of, 14
Semicircular canals, of bony labyrinth, 308
Semicircular ducts, development of, 308, *310*
Seminal vesicle, formation of, 217, *218*
Seminiferous cords, *215,* 216
Sensory ganglia, formation of, 51
Septum (septa), aorticopulmonary, formation of, 237, *238, 239*
    dorsal, in spinal cord development, *279, 281,* 282
    interventricular, 232, *232, 233, 238, 239*
    placental, 98, *99*
    tracheoesophageal, 181, *181,* 188
    urorectal, *199,* 200, 210, *211*
    ventral median, in spinal cord development, *281,* 282
Septum primum, development of, 231, *233, 234*
Septum secundum, development of, 231–232, *233, 234, 235, 236*
Septum transversum, *60,* 61, 142–143, *144, 145, 147,* 148
    in development of diaphragm, 148
Sertoli cells, *215,* 216
Sex, determination of, 213, *215*
    error in, 220
    primary, determination of, 29
Sex chromatin, mass of, 119
    patterns of, in fetal status assessment, 90, *90*
    studies of, in detecting trisomies of sex chromosomes, 124
Sex chromosomes, pentasomy of, 124
    tetrasomy of, 124
    trisomy of, 122, 124, 124t, *125*

Sex cords, primary, 213, *214, 215*
Sex organs, female, 11–14, *12, 13, 14*
    male, *12, 14*
Sinoatrial node (SA node), development of, 237
Sinuatrial node. See *Sinoatrial node (SA node).*
Sinus(es), auricular, congenital, 161, *162*
    branchial, 161, *162, 163*
    cervical, formation of, 64, *70,* 154
    coronary, formation of, 232, *236*
    dural venous, in CSF absorption, 288
    paranasal, development of, 169
    thyroglossal duct, 165, *165*
    urogenital, *199,* 200, 210
Sinus tubercle, *216,* 217
Sinus venosus, 143
    fate of, 232, *236*
    formation of, *230,* 231
    in primitive circulation, *230,* 231
    right atrium and, 232, *236*
Sinus venosus sclerae, abnormality in, congenital glaucoma from, 307–308
Sinusoids, formation of, 37
Skeletal muscles, development of, 271–272, *272*
Skeletal system, development of, critical period for, 131
Skeleton, appendicular, 263
    axial, origin of, 49, 53
    cardiac, formation of, 237
    in fetus, at 16 weeks, 83
Skin, development of, 315–316, *316*
    in fetus, at 17 to 20 weeks, 84
        at 21 to 25 weeks, 85
Skull, anomalies of, 263, *263, 264*
    development of, **260–261,** *261, 262,* 263
    fetal, 260–261
    growth of, postnatal, 261, 263
    molding of, 260
    newborn, 260–261
Smoking, maternal, fetal growth and, 88
    possible teratogenicity of, 132–133
Smooth muscles, development of, 272
Somatic mesoderm, in skeletal muscle development, 271
Somatopleure, formation of, *52, 53*
Somites, 63, *65, 67, 68, 69*
    development of, 51, *52, 53*
    in musculoskeletal system development, 252, *253*
    in skeletal muscle development, 271
Sonograms. See *Ultrasonography.*
Spallanzani, embryological studies of, 8
Species variation, from fertilization, 29
Spemann, Hans, embryological studies of, 8
Sperm, abnormalities of, morphological, 18–19
    capacitation of, 26, *27*
    maturation of, 14
    mature, 15, *17*
    ovum compared with, *15, 18*
    parts of, *15*

Sperm (Continued)
production of, 14
transport of, 23–24
viability of, 24
Spermatids, 16, 17
Spermatocytes, 16, 17
Spermatogenesis, oogenesis compared to, 16
Spermatogonia, 15, 17, 215, 216
Spermatozoon. See Sperm.
Spermiogenesis, 17, 17
Sphenomandibular ligament, formation of, 154, 157t
Sphincter, cloacal, 200–201
paralysis of, in spina bifida, 286
Spina bifida cystica, 284, 284, 285, 285–286
Spina bifida occulta, 258–259, 284, 285
hypertrichosis in, 317
Spinal cord, congenital anomalies of, 284, 284–286, 285, 286
development of, 275, 276–281, 282, 282–286, 283, 284, 285, 286
positional changes of, 283, 283–284
Spinal ganglia, development of, 281, 282, 282–283
Spinal nerves, dorsal roots of, 281, 282, 283
Spine. See Vertebral column.
Spiral arteries, 37, 98, 99, 101
Spiral ganglion, 308, 310
Spiral organ of Corti, development of, 308, 310
Splanchnic, definition of, 39
Splanchnic mesoderm, in visceral muscle development, 272
Splanchnopleure, formation of, 52, 53
Spleen, development of, 193, 194
Spontaneous abortion, 32
of early embryos, 43
Stapes, congenital fixation of, 312
development of, 309, 311
Starvation, fetal, 88
Stem villi, 97–98, 99. See also Chorionic villi.
development of, 56, 56, 57
fibrinoid material on surfaces of, 100, 100
Steptoe, in vitro fertilization and, 8
Steroid hormones, placental secretion of, 103
Stigma, 20, 21
Stomach, development of, 189, 189–190
origin of, 189
Stomodeum, 61, 152, 153, 154, 168, 168, 170, 293, 294
in development of stomach, 188, 189
in pituitary gland development, 290
Stratum germinativum, formation of, 315
Stylohyoid ligament, origin of, 157, 157t, 158
Styloid process, 157, 158
Subarachnoid space, 283, 288
Subclavian artery, right, origin of, 243
Sublingual glands, development of, 168

Submandibular duct, formation of, 168
Submandibular glands, development of, 168
Substantia nigra, 289, 290
Sudden infant death syndrome (**SIDS**), 237
Sulcus, terminal, 166, 167
Sulcus limitans, in spinal cord development, 275, 279, 281
Superior mesenteric artery, 193, 195
Supernumerary arteries, 208
Supernumerary breasts and nipples, 319, 319–320
Supernumerary kidneys, 208
Supernumerary teeth, 323, 324
Suprarenal glands, congenital hyperplasia of, 213, 222
development of, 212–213, 214
Suprarenal medulla, origin of, 61, 62
Surfactant, pulmonary, production of, 85, 185
Sutures, cranial, 260, 262
Sweat glands, development of, 317, 318
Syncytial knots, 99–100, 100
Syncytiotrophoblast, formation of, 32
in implantation, 35
of placenta, hormone secretion by, 103
Syndactyly, 265, 268, 269, 271
Synovial joints, 255, 256
Synovial membrane, 255
Syphilis, congenital, 138–139

T

Tail, in embryo at 4 weeks, 63, 64t, 65, 68, 69
Tail fold, 60, 61
Talipes equinovarus, 268
Taste buds, development of, 167
Tectum, origin of, 288
Teeth, anomalies of, 322, 323, 324
deciduous, 320
development of, 320–322
bud stage of, 320, 320, 321
cap stage of, 320–321, 321
tetracyclines and, 131, 134
eruption of, 321, 322
fused, 323, 324
Hutchinson's, in congenital syphilis, 139
natal, 322
numerical abnormalities of, 323, 324
permanent, 321, 322, 323
shape of, abnormalities of, 323, 324
supernumerary, 323, 324
Tegmentum, 289
Tela choroidea, 288, 289
Telencephalic vesicles, formation of, 289, 290
Telencephalon, 289
development of, 286, 287, 293, 293–294, 294
Teratogen(s), 129, 129t, 130, 131–139
alcohol as, 129t, 133, 133

Teratogen(s) (Continued)
aminopterin as, 129t, 135, 135
androgens as, 129t, 133–134
antibiotics as, 129t, 134
busulfan as, 129t, 135
chemical, 129t, 137
cocaine as, 129t, 137
cytomegalovirus as, 129t, 137–138
definition of, 119
diethylstilbestrol as, 129t, 134
drugs as, 129t, 132–137
herpes simplex virus as, 129t, 138
human immunodeficiency virus as, 129t, 138
human parvovirus as, 129t
ionizing radiation as, 129t, 139
isotretinoin as, 129t, 136
lithium as, 129t, 136–137
maternal factors as, 139
mechanical factors as, 139
methotrexate as, 129t
methyl mercury as, 129t, 137
phenytoin as, 129t, 135
polychlorinated biphenyls (PCBs) as, 129t, 137
progestogens as, 129t, 133–134
rubella virus as, 129t, 137
testing of, 132
tetracycline as, 129t, 134
thalidomide as, 129t, 132, 136
Toxoplasma gondii as, 129t, 138
Treponema pallidum as, 129t, 138–139
trimethadione as, 129t, 135
valproic acid as, 129t, 135
varicella virus as, 129t, 138
Venezuelan equine encephalitis virus as, 129t
warfarin as, 129t, 134
Teratology, definition of, 118
Teratoma, sacrococcygeal, 49
Terminal sac period, in lung development, 184, 185
Terminal sulcus, 166, 167
"Test tube babies," 29. See also In vitro fertilization.
Testicular feminization, 220–221, 221
Testis-determining factor (**TDF**), 213, 215
Testis (testes), 12, 14. See also Gonad(s).
descent of, 217
development of, 213, 214–215, 216
undescended, 220
Testosterone, as teratogen, 133
Tetracyclines, as teratogens, 129t, 134
enamel hypoplasia from, 324
Tetralogy of Fallot, 242, 242
Tetraploidy, 125
Tetrasomy, of sex chromosomes, 124
Thalidomide, as teratogen, 129t, 132, 136, 136
limb defects from, 136, 267, 267
Theca folliculi, 19, 20
Thymus, origin of, 159, 160
Thyroglossal duct cysts and sinuses, 165, 165

Thyroid drugs, as teratogens, 136
Thyroid gland, congenital anomalies of, 165, *165*
  development of, *160*, 161, *165*, 166
  ectopic, 165
Thyroid tissue, accessory, 165
Tjio, embryological studies of, 8
Toenails, development of, 318
Tongue, bifid, 167
  cleft, 167
  congenital anomalies of, *165*, 167
  development of, 165, *166*, 167
  muscles of, development of, 271, *272*
Tongue buds, 165, *166*, 167
Tongue-tie, 167
Tonsil, palatine, origin of, 159, *160*
Tonsillar crypts, origin of, 159
Tooth. See *Teeth.*
Toxoplasma gondii, as teratogen, 129t, 138
Trachea, development of, 181–182, *182*
Tracheoesophageal fistula, 181–182, *182*, 188
Tracheoesophageal folds, development of, 180, *181*
Tracheoesophageal septum, 181, *181*, 188
Tranquilizers, as teratogens, 136
Transfusions, fetal, intrauterine, 90
Translocation, chromosomal, 125, *126*
Transport, placental, 101–103
Transposition of great arteries (TGA), 242
Transvaginal sonography, in crown-rump length measurements of embryo, 73, *74*
Treacher Collins syndrome, 161
Treponema pallidum, as teratogen, 129t, 138–139
Trigeminal nerve, origin of, 157t, 158
Trimester, definition of, 6, 79
Trimethadione, as teratogen, 129t, 135
Triplets, 115, *115*
Triploidy, 124–125
Trisomy, 18, 122, *123*, 124
  of autosomes, 122, *123*, 124t
  of sex chromosomes, 122, 124, 124t, *125*
Trisomy 13, 122, *123*, 124t
Trisomy 18, 122, *123*, 124t
Trisomy 21, 122, *122*, 124t
Trophoblast, *30*, 31
Truncal ridges, formation of, 237, *238*
Truncus arteriosus, 229, *229*
  abnormal division of, 239, *241*, 242
  partitioning of, 232, 237, *238*
  persistent, 239, *241*
Tubal pregnancy, 39, *41*, 42
Tubotympanic recess, 308, *311*
  origin of, 159, *160*
Tubules, metanephric, 206, *206*
Tunica albuginea, *215*, 216
Turner syndrome, 18, *121*, 122
Turricephaly, 263, *264*
Twins, conjoined, *114*, 115
  dizygotic (DZ), *112*, 113
  fraternal, *112*, 113

Twins *(Continued)*
  identical, *112*, 113, *114*, 115
  monozygotic (MZ), *112*, 113, *114*, 115
Tympanic cavity, development of, 308–309, *311*
Tympanic membrane, formation of, 309, 311, *311*
  origin of, *160*, 161

U

Ultimobranchial body, origin of, 159, *160*
Ultrasonography, in detecting spina bifida, *286*
  in diagnosing polyhydramnios, 109
  in estimation of age, in embryonic period, 69
    in fetal period, 78, 79–80
  in fetal status assessment, *91*, 91–92
  in pregnancy confirmation, 45
  transvaginal, in crown-rump length measurements of embryo, 73, *74*
Umbilical arteries, 99, 100, *101*, 108
  fate of, 249
Umbilical cord, *60*, 61
  after birth, 106, *107*, 108, 109
  knots in, 106, *108*
Umbilical hernia, 196
Umbilical herniation, at 7 weeks, 67, 72
Umbilical ligament, medial, origin of, 249
  median, origin of, 94, 111
Umbilical vein(s), 99, 100, *101*, 108
  fate of, 249
  in fetal circulation, 246, *247*
  in primitive circulation, *230*, 231
Urachus, origin of, 94, 111
Ureter(s), congenital anomalies of, **208**, *209*, 210, *210*
  development of, 204
  orifices of, ectopic, 210, *211*
Urethra, *12*
  development of, *211*, 212, *219*
  in transport of semen, 14
  spongy, development of, *219*, 220
Urethral glands, formation of, 217
Urethral groove, development of, *219*, 220
Urinary bladder, development of, 210, *211*
  exstrophy of, 210, 212, *212*
Urinary system, development of, 204–212. See also specific structure, e.g., *Kidney(s).*
  duplications of, 208, *209*, 210
Urine, formation of, in fetus, 204
  at 9 to 12 weeks, 83
Urogenital folds, development of, *219*, 220
Urogenital membrane, *199*, 200
Urogenital sinus, *199*, 200, 210
Urogenital system, development of, 204–225. See also *Genital system; Urinary system.*
Urorectal septum, *199*, 200, 210, *211*

Uterine cycle, *19*, 20, 22–23
Uterine tube(s), 12, *12*, 13
  development of, 217, *218*
  implantation in, 39, *41*, 42
  rupture of, from tubal pregnancy, 39
Uteroplacental circulation, impaired, fetal growth and, 88
  primitive, 37
Uterovaginal primordium, *216*, 217
Uterus, anomalies of, 224, *224*
  bicornuate, 224, *224*
  contractions of, during labor, 104
  double, 224, *224*
  growth of, during pregnancy, 103, *103*
  septate, 224, *224*
  structure of, *12*, 12–13, *13*
  unicornuate, 224, *224*
Utricular portion, of otic vesicle, 308, *310*
Uvula, 169, *172*
  formation of, 173

V

Vagina, *12*, *13*, 13–14
  absence of, 224
  adenocarcinoma of, from *in utero* DES exposure, 134
  anomalies of, 224, *224*
  atresia of, 224
  development of, 217, *218*
Vaginal plate, formation of, 217
Vagus nerve, origin of, 157t, 158–159
Valproic acid, as teratogen, 129t, 135
Varicella virus, as teratogen, 129t, 138
Vas deferens, *12*, 14. See also *Ductus deferens.*
  formation of, 217
Vein(s), cardinal, common, 143, *146*, 229, *229*
  in primitive circulation, *230*, 231
  central, of retina, origin of, *303*, 304
  pulmonary, primitive, 232
  umbilical, fate of, 249
    in fetal circulation, 246, *247*
    in primitive circulation, *230*, 231
  vitelline, 229, *229*, *230*, 231
Vena cava, inferior, in fetal circulation, 246, *247*
Venezuelan equine encephalitis virus, as teratogen, 129t
Ventral gray horns, in spinal cord development, 279, *281*, 282
Ventral median fissure, in spinal cord development, 279, *281*, 282
Ventral median septum, in spinal cord development, *281*, 282
Ventral mesogastrium, 190
Ventral roots, in spinal cord development, *281*, 282
Ventricle(s), lateral, origin of, 289
  of brain, fourth, 288, *289*
  lateral, formation of, 294
  third, 289, *291*
    formation of, 293–294

Ventricle(s) *(Continued)*
  primitive, partitioning of, 232, *232,*
    233
Ventricular septal defects (**VSDs**), 239,
  241
Vermiform appendix, 193, *195*
Vernix caseosa, 84
  formation of, 315, *317*
Vertebrae, anomalies of, 258–259, *260,*
  263
  number of, variation in, 258
  typical, chondrification of, 256, *258*
    ossification of, 256, 258, *258, 259*
Vertebral column, cleft, 259, *263*
  development of, 255–256, *257, 258,*
    258–259, 259
    chondrification of vertebrae in,
      256, *258*
    ossification of vertebrae in, 256,
      258, *258, 259*
    precartilaginous mesenchymal stage
      in, 255–256, *257*
Vesicle(s), brain, 286, *287*
  lens, formation of, 301, *302*
  optic, development of, 301, *302*
  otic, formation of, 308, *309*
Vestibular glands, greater, formation of,
  217
Vestibulocochlear organ, 308
Villi, branch, 98
  branch, development of, 57
  chorionic. See *Chorionic villi.*

Villi *(Continued)*
  stem. See *Stem villi.*
Villous chorion, *95, 96, 97, 97*
Virus(es), as teratogens, 129t, 137–138
  rubella, as teratogen, 129t, 131, 137
    congenital cataract from, 307
    congenital deafness from, 311–312
Visceral muscles, development of, 272
Viscerocranium, 260
  cartilaginous, 260, *261*
  membranous, 260, *261*
Vitamins, placental transport of, 102
Vitelline veins, *229, 229, 230,* 231
Vitreous body, development of, *304,*
  305, 306
Vocal cords, development of, 181
Volvulus, malfixation of gut and, 198
  midgut, 197, *197*
  mixed rotation and, 196–197, *197*
  nonrotation of midgut and, 196
Vomiting, projectile, in pyloric obstruc-
  tion, 190

W

Warfarin, as teratogen, 129t, 134
Waste products, placental transport of,
  102
Weight, fetal, gain of, at 21 to 25
  weeks, 85
  in fetal age estimation, 79
Wharton's jelly, 106, *108*

Winiwarter, von, embryologic studies
  of, 8
Wolffian ducts, 217

X

XO chromosome abnormality, 122

Y

Y chromosome, *16,* 18, *90,* 119, **213,**
  215
Yolk sac, derivatives of, 94
  fate of, 110, *110*
  in midgut development, 193
  primary, formation of, *36,* 37
  role of, 110
  secondary, formation of, 39, *40*
Yolk stalk, 110, *110*
  at 4 weeks, *60,* 61
  at 7 weeks, 67, *71, 72*

Z

Zona pellucida, *15,* 18, **20**
  degeneration of, *30,* 31
Zona reaction, 27, 29
Zygote, abnormal, 32
  cleavage of, *30,* **31–32**
    initiation of, 29
  definition of, 1
  formation of, 26, *28*